What People Are Saying About This Book

"This book is absolutely outstanding – one of the best pieces of work on celiac disease, I have ever read for completeness of information!"
Dr. Carlo Catassi, Co-Medical Director, Center for Celiac Research, Baltimore, MD

"Shelley Case is one of the foremost experts on the gluten-free diet. There is a lot of 'bad' information out there about the diet, but Shelley's book can be trusted to be current, accurate, and thoroughly researched."
Danna Korn, Founder of R.O.C.K. (Raising Our Celiac Kids) and Author of *Kids with Celiac Disease: A Family Guide to Raising Happy, Healthy, Gluten-Free Children* and *Wheat-Free, Worry-Free: The Art of Happy, Healthy Gluten-Free Living*

"Each edition of Shelley Case's *Gluten-Free Diet: A Comprehensive Resource Guide* gets better and better with more practical information for all people with wheat and gluten sensitivities. A 'must have' resource for the newly diagnosed person with celiac disease."
Janet Y. Rinehart, Former President, Celiac Sprue Association/USA, Inc.

"Having been diagnosed with celiac disease and practicing as a Registered Dietitian for over 20 years, I know the importance of professional-looking, detailed, and accurate information. Shelley's book accomplishes this and much more! I highly recommend this book to people with celiac disease, as well as dietitians, physicians and other health professionals."
Mark A. Dinga, MEd, RD, LD, Pittsburgh, Pennsylvania

"This book is a wonderful guide to navigating the sometimes frustrating, often overwhelming, journey to a healthy gluten-free lifestyle."
Peggy Wagener, Publisher, *Living Without* magazine, Illinois

"This is a phenomenal book. Shelley has managed to research, compile and organize volumes of valuable information and present it in a logical manner that is easy to understand. It is the most thorough gluten-free reference book on the market today."
Connie Sarros, Author of *Wheat-Free, Gluten-Free Cookbooks*

"Shelley has produced a thoughtful, well-researched book. As a leading nutrition expert in celiac disease, she has given the celiac community the foundation for a long, healthy gluten-free lifestyle."
Elaine Monarch, Founder/Executive Director, Celiac Disease Foundation, California

"This comprehensive book provides a wealth of critically important information for anyone who lives gluten-free. Get your copy right away!"
Carol Fenster, PhD, Author of *Gluten-Free 101, Cooking Free* and *1000 Gluten-Free Recipes*

"This guide is full of information on what's safe and healthy for people with celiac disease, and is presented in a practical, clearly organized, 'no-nonsense' format. It is a must for the celiac bookshelf."
Bev Ruffo, Honorary Life Member, Canadian Celiac Association

"Shelley Case's book is a must for everyone's library. I use it in my cooking classes and for grocery shopping. It is an excellent gift for the newly diagnosed, as well as family and friends who are looking for gluten-free sources."
LynnRae Ries, Author of *What? No Wheat? A Lighthearted Primer to Living the Gluten-Free, Wheat-Free Life* and *Waiter, Is there Wheat in My Soup?*

"Shelley's book is stuffed with practical information and helpful hints. I consult it frequently and have learned more about the gluten-free diet from it than from any other single resource."
Lani K. Thompson, Publisher, *Clan Thompson Gluten-Free Databases*, Bridgton, Maine

"I highly recommend this book as a true 'resource' for those who are gluten-sensitive."
Ann Whelan, Editor and Publisher, *Gluten-Free Living Magazine*, New York

"I've recommended Shelley Case's book to my patients with celiac disease since its very first edition. I trust the research and respect the dedication that she put into writing this educational book. The material is equally useful for those newly diagnosed learning about hidden gluten to those seeking ways to increase variety in their diets with new products, grains, recipes and meal plans."
Melinda Dennis, MS, RD, LDN, Nutrition Coordinator, Celiac Center at Beth Israel Deaconess Medical Center

"Shelley Case should be congratulated for her efforts in contributing such a valuable reference tool to the field of celiac disease."
Mavis Molloy, RDN, Dietitian, Member of the Professional Advisory Board, Canadian Celiac Association

"I needed this book before I accumulated the mountain of computer printouts and handouts that adorn my office. Buy it or spend the next 20 years of your life unnecessarily duplicating this research."
Jacqueline Maxwell, Jackson, Tennessee and Area Celiac Support Group

"I am so impressed by this book. This is exactly the concise compilation of facts and sources of information that I have been looking for. I will be enthusiastically sharing information about this book with our members and local stores."
Sallie Smith, Gluten-Free Support Group of Northwestern Pennsylvania

"Shelley's book is a wonderful well-researched resource and an indispensable tool for people with celiac disease and for any health professional who is working with the celiac community."
Mary K. Sharrett, MS, RD, LD, CNSD, Nutrition Support Dietitian, Children's Hospital and Founder/Dietitian Advisor of the Gluten-Free Gang, Columbus, Ohio

"I heard about this book at a Celiac Support Group meeting, immediately ordered it and read it cover to cover. Even though my son was diagnosed 2 years ago with celiac disease, and I read everything I can find, I learned a great deal from this book. Thank you for writing such an excellent reference book for people with celiac disease."
Susan Garramone, Hopedale, Massachusetts

"A concise resource with all the key information clinicians AND patients frequently need to get started. We recommend this book to all patients referred to us in our GI nutrition clinic with celiac disease."
Carol Rees Parrish, RD, MS, Nutrition Support Specialist, University of Virginia Health System, Digestive Health Center of Excellence, Charlottesville, Virginia

"Shelley certainly does her research! She goes beyond merely listing ingredients as safe or unsafe. Her book describes the background as to why ingredients are categorized as such. I recommend this comprehensive resource to everyone requiring a gluten-free diet."
Trisha B. Lyons, RD, LD, Dietitian, MetroHealth Medical Center, Cleveland, Ohio

"I've really enjoyed this reference book. It's a good 'common sense' approach to gluten-free living."
Becky Warlick, RN, MSN, Duke University Medical Center, Durham, North Carolina

"This is a must-have book for dietitians, doctors and patients. It is a critical component to the nutrition education sessions I provide and is an excellent resource for products and recipes."
Jacquelyn Stern, RD, LD, Digestive Disorders Associates, Annapolis, Maryland

"People who purchase our cookbooks often ask us where to purchase gluten-free ingredients. We feel comfortable recommending Shelley's book as we know it is complete and accurate."
Donna Washburn, P.HEc. *and* **Heather Butt, P.HEc.**, Authors of *125 Best Gluten-Free Recipes*, *The Best Gluten-Free Family Cookbook* and *Complete Gluten-Free Cookbook*

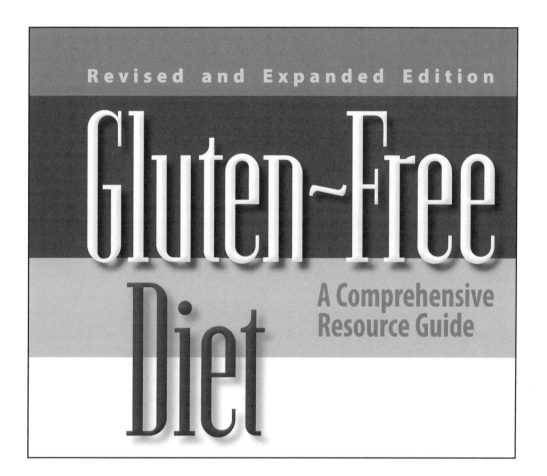

Revised and Expanded Edition

Gluten~Free Diet

A Comprehensive Resource Guide

Shelley Case

BSc (Nutrition & Dietetics), RD

Registered Dietitian

Gluten-Free Diet – A Comprehensive Resource Guide

by
Shelley Case, BSc (Nutrition & Dietetics), RD (Registered Dietitian)

First Edition – May 2001
Revised Edition – April 2002
Third Printing – July 2003
Fourth Printing – May 2004
Fifth Printing – January 2005
Expanded Edition – April 2006
Revised-Expanded Edition – October 2008
Eighth Printing (Revised) – January 2010
Ninth Printing – December 2010

Published by:
Case Nutrition Consulting Inc.

1940 Angley Court
Regina, Saskatchewan
Canada S4V 2V2

www.glutenfreediet.ca
Email: info@glutenfreediet.ca
Phone/FAX: 306-751-1000

Library and Archives Canada Cataloguing in Publication

Case, Shelley

Gluten-free diet : a comprehensive resource guide / Shelley Case. – Rev. and expanded ed.

Includes index.
ISBN 978-1-897010-54-9

1. Gluten-free diet – Handbooks, manuals, etc.   2. Gluten-free diet – Recipes.   I. Title.

RM237.86.C38 2008   613.2'6   C2008-906051-2

Cover Design by:
Brian Danchuk, Brian Danchuk Design, Regina, Saskatchewan

Printed and Produced in Canada by:
Friesens Book Division
One Printers Way, Altona, MB, Canada R0G 0B0
(204) 324-6401   Fax: (204) 324-1333
                 www.friesens.com

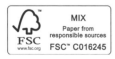

DEDICATION

To GOD
✦ who gives meaning and purpose to my life
✦ for His amazing love, wisdom, strength and answers to prayer
✦ for His countless blessings, especially my family

To my husband, Blair
✦ the love of my life for over 30 years
✦ for your incredible devotion, patience and support

To my daughters, Erin and Jennifer
✦ for your encouragement and unconditional love

To my mother, Helen
✦ for your wonderful support, generosity and encouragement

To my late father, Gord
✦ whose entrepreneurial spirit taught me that anything was possible

ACKNOWLEDGMENTS

When I contemplate the African proverb, "It takes a whole village to raise a child," I think of the amazing group of people involved in creating this book. I would like to acknowledge all of them and also the spirit of their contributions. From family and friends, to dietitians, physicians, authors, government departments in Canada and the USA, the food industry and others in the gluten-free community, their generosity in providing information and help was truly amazing. I am very blessed to have received such assistance and kindness. I would especially like to thank all those who purchased my first books because, frankly, without you this expanded edition would not have been possible. The writing of this acknowledgment is a daunting task because there are so many to whom I owe so much over the past nine years.

First and foremost, a huge debt of gratitude goes to my mom for all of her incredible support in the production and distribution of every edition of the *Gluten-Free Diet* over the past nine years. The countless hours of editing and proofing, often into the wee hours of the night, and all the other "behind the scenes" work is deeply appreciated. Her dedication is amazing. Thanks, mom, for everything!

To my husband, Blair, words cannot express my sincere appreciation for his wonderful encouragement, patience, understanding, continued support and love. Throughout my career, especially during the last nine years of researching and writing each edition and frequently being away from home on speaking engagements, he kept the home-front running smoothly while successfully managing his thriving business. His selfless devotion to our family and to others is one of the many character qualities I have always admired.

To my precious daughters Erin and Jennifer a big thanks for their awesome support and encouragement; you're the best!

To Wolf Rinke for inspiring me to "dream big" and change career paths.

I'm forever grateful to Enid Young, past president of the Regina chapter of the Canadian Celiac Association, who believed in my idea for this book from the very beginning and encouraged and supported me in so many ways, including reviewing the numerous manuscripts.

To my dear friends, mentors and dietitian colleagues, Marion Zarkadas and Beth Armour, heartfelt thanks for their excellent advice and editorial assistance with the manuscript. Their attention to detail and specific suggestions were incredibly helpful.

Carol Fenster, a wonderful friend and colleague, deserves an enormous thank you for her expert advice, encouragement and generosity.

Thank you to the many dietitians who provided further information, constructive feedback and/or support, especially – Alexandra Anca, Amy Barr, Pam Cureton, Jenny Dean, Melinda Dennis, Mark Dinga, Nancy Patin Falini, Kelly Fitzpatrick, Jacquelin Gates, Cindy Heroux, Cynthia Kupper, Anne Lee, Mavis Molloy, Carol Rees Parrish, Jackie See, Mary K Sharrett, Lauren Swann, Tricia Thompson and Jeannie Zibrida.

A special thank you to dietitian Tiffany Banow for helping me verify information from hundreds of companies and thousands of products. A challenging and time-consuming job, to say the least.

To the many physicians and scientists for their technical advice and support – Dr. Scott Bean, Dr. Vern Burrows, Dr. Decker Butzner, Dr. Pekka Collin, Dr. Carlo Catassi, Dr. Jeff Dahlberg, Dr. Alessio Fasano, Dr. Peter Green, Dr. Don Kasarda, Dr. Ciaran Kelly, Dr. Joseph Murray, Dr. Michelle Pietzak, Dr. Mohsin Rashid, Dr. Lloyd Rooney, Dr. Cynthia Rudert, Dr. Connie Switzer, Dr. Fred Townley-Smith and Dr. Ralph Warren.

My friend and colleague, Dina Aronson from WellTech Solutions, thank you for the nutritional analysis of the recipes, providing valuable data and designing a great website. You're a technical genius!

To all the gluten-free culinary experts for their sage advice and practical suggestions, especially Heather Butt, Carol Fenster, Connie Sarros and Donna Washburn.

To all those individuals who contributed recipes – Dina Aronson, Heather Butt, Michael and Bev Calihan, Leslie Cerier, Carol Fenster, Bruce Gross, Bette Hagman, Laurel Hutton, Barbara Kliment, Jane Reinhardt-Martin, Vesanto Melina, Amy Perry, Rebecca Reilly, LynnRae Ries, Karen Robertson, Sheri Sanderson, Connie Sarros, Rosie Schwartz, Girma and Ethiopia Sahlu, Jo Stepaniak, Donna Washburn and Meredith Wiking. And to those companies – Amazing Grains Growers Cooperative, Bob's Red Mill, The Birkett Mills, El Peto, The Flax Council of Canada, Northern Quinoa Corporation, Nu World Amaranth, Riese's Canadian Lake Wild Rice, San Pedro Mesquite, Saskatchewan Flax Development Commission, Saskatchewan Pulse Growers and The Teff Company.

I'm grateful to all those in the gluten-free community for their valuable contributions, especially Hertha Deutsch, Association of European Coeliac Societies; Cynthia Kupper, Gluten Intolerance Group; Andrea Levario, American Celiac Disease Alliance; Norma McGough, Coeliac UK; Elaine Monarch, Celiac Disease Foundation; Graham Price, Coeliac Society of Australia; Lani Thompson, Clan Thompson Resources; Peggy Wagener, *Living Without* and Ann Whelan, *Gluten-Free Living*.

To the many staff from various government departments in Canada and the USA, a special thank you for the assistance and information about food standards and labeling regulations.

Thank you to all the food companies that provided detailed information, with special appreciation to Cassidy, Matt and Yvonne (Bob's Red Mill), Elisabeth Carlson (The Teff Company), Peter Felker (Casa deFruta), Bob Hansen (Briess Malt and Ingredient Company), Cindy Kaplan and Scott Mandell (Enjoy Life Foods), Peggy McKeon (Kingsmill Foods), Steve Rice (Authentic Foods), Raj Sukul (Maplegrove Gluten-Free Foods) and Larry and Diane Walters, Susan Walters-Flood (Nu World Amaranth) for their additional support and for digging up hard-to-find information.

To my good friend Glenda Francis for your support and prayers!

Thanks Aunt Carolyn for the many ways in which you helped in the research and reviewing of the book over the years.

Librarians Martina Hahnefeld and Doris Hein, thanks a million for tracking down all those reference articles from around the world.

To Mark Humphreys and Mike Warnecke, special thanks for solving my on-going computer malfunctions.

To Donna Poole, my "strong" massage therapist, for getting rid of all those aches and pains from countless hours at the computer and on the phone.

To Carie Romanuik who deciphered and typed my first hand-written manuscripts for the first book.

Thanks to dietetic student Alex Crerar for reviewing the material for the eighth printing of this book.

A "BIG" thank you to Kathryn for coming to the rescue once again to make the press deadline – I never could have done it without you!

And for the many people whose names I have not mentioned but who also contributed to this book, I say a heartfelt thank you.

TABLE OF CONTENTS

Meet Shelley Case, BSc, RD

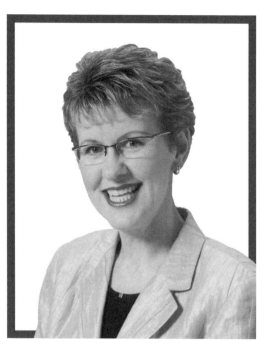

A registered dietitian, Shelley Case is a leading international nutrition expert on celiac disease and the gluten-free diet. She is a member of the Medical Advisory Boards of the Celiac Disease Foundation and Gluten Intolerance Group in the United States and the Professional Advisory Board of the Canadian Celiac Association.

Shelley is a frequent guest on television and radio, including the *NBC Today Show* and *CBC Newsworld*. A popular speaker, she has delivered numerous lectures and workshops at national and regional medical, dietetic, celiac and food industry conferences throughout the USA and Canada, including the National Institutes of Health Consensus Development Conference on Celiac Disease, American Dietetic Association and Dietitians of Canada annual conferences and the Institute of Food Technologists and Natural Products Food Expo Conferences.

She is the author of many articles on celiac disease and the gluten-free diet in leading publications such as *Gastroenterology, Digestive Disease Sciences, Pediatrics, Journal of Human Nutrition and Dietetics, Topics in Clinical Nutrition* and *Today's Dietitian*. In addition, she co-authored the celiac section in the *Manual of Clinical Dietetics (6th edition)* by the American Dietetic Association and Dietitians of Canada, and has contributed to many other publications including textbooks, magazines and other patient education resources. Shelley writes "Ask the Celiac Expert" column for *Allergic Living Magazine*, "Good for You" column at glutenfreeda.com and "Ask Shelley Case" at befreeforme.com

In recognition of Shelley's major contributions to the celiac community and dedication to educating health professionals and individuals with celiac disease in Canada and the United States, she was awarded the Queen Elizabeth Golden Jubilee Medal. Shelley also recently received the Canadian Celiac Association's Honourary Life Member Award.

Shelley earned a Bachelor of Science Degree in Nutrition and Dietetics from the University of Saskatchewan and completed her Dietetic Internship at the Health Sciences Center in Winnipeg, Manitoba. Over the past 29 years, Shelley has helped thousands of people improve their eating habits and manage a variety of disease conditions through good nutrition. Currently, she has her own nutrition consulting company specializing in celiac disease and the gluten-free diet that offers a variety of services to individuals, health organizations and the food industry.

Professionally, Shelley is a member of the Dietitians of Canada, Saskatchewan Dietitians Association and American Dietetic Association, as well as the Nutrition Entrepreneurs, Dietitians in Business and Communications, Food and Culinary Professionals and the Medical Nutrition Practice Groups of the American Dietetic Association. She also serves on the Grain Foods Foundation Scientific Advisory Board, as well as the Advisory Board of *Living Without* magazine and *Today's Diet and Nutrition* magazine.

Very active in her community and church, she has chaired many conferences and special events. Shelley is an accomplished musician who enjoys playing piano and electric keyboard. She lives with her husband and two children in Regina, Saskatchewan, Canada.

PREFACE

In the Beginning

As a new graduate dietitian in 1981, I was excited to finally enter the workforce after five challenging years of university and internship. My passion, which continues to this day, was to be able to help people eat nutritiously and improve their overall health and well-being. In my first job at a large outpatient diabetes and diet education center I was responsible for counseling children and adults with various conditions such as diabetes, heart disease, high blood pressure, obesity, cystic fibrosis, food allergies and gastrointestinal disorders, including celiac disease. I was well prepared to counsel individuals with many different problems, however celiac disease was definitely not one of them! Never having seen anyone with celiac disease during internship, and receiving only minimal information in one nutrition class at university, left me ill-prepared. The day I was to counsel my first patient with celiac disease, I remember scrambling to find any relevant information about the disease itself and especially about the gluten-free diet. The little information I did find was out of date and of little use. Realizing I needed help, I contacted the local celiac support group in Regina, Saskatchewan, which welcomed me and taught me so much about the disease and diet, and provided me with some basic materials for counseling future patients. After attending several meetings, I was asked to be their dietitian advisor. I accepted the position and, over time, my knowledge of the disease and diet grew. Ten years later I was invited to become a member of the Canadian Celiac Association Professional Advisory Board, a position I have held ever since.

The Birth of an Idea

Every patient that I saw with celiac disease always wanted very specific and practical information on food labeling and ingredients; names of gluten-free companies/products and where to find them; recipes; meal planning suggestions; tips for eating out; how to prevent cross-contamination and other gluten-free diet resources. However, such information was usually only available from many different pamphlets, books, manuals and other sources, which meant that the patient had a pile of loose papers to take home after the counseling sessions! In addition to educating patients, I often got calls from other dietitians in the city, and from around the province, seeking information, as they too felt their knowledge of the disease and diet was inadequate. It soon became apparent that there was a real need for a more comprehensive resource, for both health professionals and patients, on celiac disease. This was the birth of the idea for the *Gluten-Free Diet: A Comprehensive Resource Guide*.

Dreams Become a Reality

In 1997 I left a very rewarding career at a hospital to pursue a dream of starting a nutrition consulting business. In 1999 I decided to get serious about turning this gluten-free resource idea into a reality and dedicated the next two years to researching and writing my first book – *Gluten-Free Diet: A Comprehensive Resource Guide*. It was self-published in May 2001. The next big hurdle was letting health professionals and individuals with celiac disease know about the resource. Without the backing of a large publishing house, it required creative promotional strategies on a shoestring budget. As the book became better known, positive feedback from individuals with celiac disease and from dietitians was very encouraging. News about the book continued to spread and more of my consulting time was being devoted to celiac disease. Being the marketing representative, shipper and accountant, as well as author and speaker has given me a new appreciation for the role of authors and publishers, and even more for the importance of accurate up-to-date resources for those with celiac disease.

The Continuing Saga

The gluten-free world continues to grow in both the number of individuals being diagnosed and the products and resources available in the marketplace. These changes have necessitated several revisions to the *Gluten-Free Diet* to include more information to meet this huge demand. I'm thrilled to finally release this expanded edition, packed full of new information, products and resources that I hope will make your gluten-free life easier and healthier.

An Amazing Journey

Twenty-nine years ago I never would have dreamed that I would be a dietitian specializing in celiac disease and the gluten-free diet, let alone be the author of a national best-seller or being interviewed by Matt Lauer on the *NBC Today Show*. Rather ironic for a dietitian from Saskatchewan, the province known as the "bread basket of the world." So, for everyone out there with an idea or dream – pursue it, work hard and never give up. Who knows where you may end up! I'm amazed and truly blessed to have had the opportunity to become involved in such an incredible field, meeting so many wonderful individuals with the disease, along with health professionals and those in industry and government, from the USA and Canada and around the world, who are working so hard to improve the lives of people with celiac disease. The Canadian Celiac Association's motto "Together We're Better" is a worthy ideal. I look forward to working together with you and continuing on this challenging gluten-free journey.

Shelley M. Case, BSc, RD

FOREWORD

The day you were diagnosed with celiac disease and started on a gluten-free diet, your life changed for the better. With a gluten-free diet the damage to the lining of the small bowel begins to heal and intestinal function starts to return to normal. With this healing process comes a renewed sense of health and well-being and an improved quality of life. Strict adherence to a gluten-free diet reduces the risks of developing other illnesses that occur with increased frequency in individuals with untreated celiac disease. The gluten-free diet is the only treatment for celiac disease.

Shelley's book is a valuable resource to help you conquer the challenges of managing and living with a gluten-free diet for life.

Connie M. Switzer, MD, FRCPC, Clinical Professor of Medicine, University of Alberta, Edmonton, Alberta and Chair of the Canadian Celiac Association Professional Advisory Board.

INTRODUCTION TO THE GLUTEN-FREE DIET: A COMPREHENSIVE RESOURCE GUIDE

Gluten-Free Diet – A Comprehensive Resource Guide was written for those with celiac disease or its skin form, dermatitis herpetiformis, who must follow a strict gluten-free diet for life. This book provides practical information, in an easy-to-read format, about celiac disease and the gluten-free diet. It is also a valuable resource for:

✦ Family members and caregivers of those with celiac disease or dermatitis herpetiformis
✦ Dietitians, nutritionists, physicians, nurses and other health practitioners
✦ Educators in health science, food service and culinary programs
✦ Food manufacturers – research and development staff and consumer representatives
✦ Chefs, cooks, servers and other food-service staff
✦ Managers of grocery, health food and specialty food stores

Celiac Disease

The first section of this Guide provides a brief overview of celiac disease and dermatitis herpetiformis, including the prevalence, signs and symptoms, other associated conditions, complications and diagnosis. Recommended references are listed for those needing more detailed information about these conditions.

Foods Allowed

In order to successfully follow a gluten-free diet, it is essential to have a good understanding of which foods and ingredients contain gluten. Unfortunately, there is considerable misinformation published about what constitutes a gluten-free diet. As a result, many individuals are often confused and needlessly avoid certain foods and ingredients, thus limiting the variety in their diet which may lead to nutritional imbalances. The gluten-free diet section contains background information and references on the gluten-free status and safety of numerous foods and ingredients, including the acceptability of oats. The Gluten-Free Diet By Food Groups table is a handy tool that organizes foods and ingredients into three categories – foods allowed, foods to question and foods to avoid. Food labeling regulations in the USA and Canada are reviewed along with a detailed discussion of specific gluten-free labeling regulations and standards in North America, Europe, Australia/New Zealand and the international Codex Alimentarius Commission.

Nutritional Concerns

Specific nutritional concerns such as anemia, bone disease and lactose intolerance are addressed. Recommended amounts of key nutrients (iron, folate, vitamin B_{12}, calcium, vitamin D and fiber) and gluten-free food sources for these nutrients are found in tables throughout this section. Information about nutritious gluten-free grains and seeds and how to incorporate them into the diet is included. Healthy Gluten-Free Dietary Guidelines have been developed which incorporate key components of the new MyPyramid food guidance system in the USA and Canada's Food Guide to Healthy Eating. Comprehensive nutritional composition tables of various gluten-free foods and ingredients are provided at the end of the section.

Meal Planning

This section provides suggestions for meals and snacks along with a number of recipes. Specific tips for improving the nutritional quality of meal plans and a Sample Seven-Day Gluten-Free Menu are also featured.

Gluten-Free Cooking

Information about many different gluten-free flours and starches, substitutions, baking hints and recipes are included in this section. Each recipe includes a nutritional analysis for calories, carbohydrate, dietary fiber, fat, protein, iron, calcium and sodium, which is particularly helpful for individuals who have both celiac disease and type 1 diabetes.

Shopping

Gluten-free shopping tips, a sample shopping list, and how to prevent cross-contamination of gluten-free foods with gluten-containing foods are highlighted in this section. The need for careful reading of ingredients on food labels on a regular basis and contacting the company when in doubt about the gluten-free status of a food is stressed.

The growing demand for gluten-free foods has resulted in an increased number and wide variety of items in many different food and beverage categories. This Guide provides the company name, product name and package size in both grams and ounces for over 3100 products in the following categories: cereals, breads and other baked products, desserts, cookies, crackers, baking mixes, flours, grains and legumes, pastas, entrées and side dishes, soups, snacks, miscellaneous items and dairy and non-dairy substitutes. The company directory section contains an extensive listing of over 270 gluten-free specialty manufacturers, bakeries, stores and distributors in North America and Europe, and whether their products are made in a dedicated gluten-free facility.

Other Resources

A variety of recommended books, cookbooks, magazines, newsletters and other materials are featured in the gluten-free resource section. In addition, celiac research and education centers in the USA and a directory of celiac organizations in the USA, Canada and other countries around the world are listed.

Closing Remarks

The information in this book has been exhaustively researched from a wide variety of sources believed to be reliable and representative of the best current scientific research and opinions on the subject at the time of printing. These sources include health professionals; food scientists; agricultural specialists; culinary experts; medical, dietetic and food science/technology organizations; governmental departments; food manufacturers and associations; and celiac organizations. Information from these sources was obtained through personal communication (telephone, email and/or mail), the internet, and libraries. Textbooks, manuals, books, position papers, journal articles, professional and trade magazines, newsletters and product labels were used as references. The author does not endorse any products or resources in this Guide. Inclusion of brand-name products and resources is strictly for information purposes. Please notify the author if you learn that information in this Guide has changed, so that the changes can be included in future revisions.

Celiac Disease and Dermatitis Herpetiformis

Celiac Disease

Celiac disease, also known as gluten-sensitive enteropathy or celiac sprue, is a chronic autoimmune intestinal disorder. When genetically susceptible individuals consume specific proteins in the grains wheat, rye and barley, which are collectively known as "gluten," the absorptive surface of the small intestine is damaged. This surface contains tiny finger-like projections called villi that become inflamed and flattened (known as villous atrophy) due to the immunologic reaction to gluten, causing malabsorption of nutrients needed for good health. Iron, calcium and folate are key nutrients often affected since they are absorbed in the first part of the small intestine. If the damage progresses further down the small intestinal tract, malabsorption of carbohydrates (especially lactose), fat and fat-soluble vitamins (A, D, E, K), protein and other nutrients may also occur. The development of celiac disease involves a combination of genetic, environmental and immunological factors. Celiac disease can occur at any age, including the elderly, and may be triggered by a gastrointestinal or viral infection, severe stress, surgery or pregnancy.

Continued exposure to gluten can result in vitamin and mineral deficiencies causing conditions such as anemia and osteoporosis; neurological disorders (e.g., ataxia, seizures and neuropathy); and an increased risk for developing other autoimmune disorders (e.g., thyroid disease, type 1 diabetes, connective tissue diseases, Addison's disease) and certain types of cancer, especially gastrointestinal malignancies. Also, there is an increased risk of miscarriage or having a low-birth-weight baby, and infertility in both women and men. For more information about celiac disease, see the references listed on page 18, nutritional concerns on pages 73-75, 91, 92, 97, 101-103, celiac organizations on pages 343-344 and other resources on pages 345-356.

Prevalence

Originally thought to be a rare disorder, celiac disease is now recognized as one of the most common inherited diseases, with a world prevalence estimated at 1:266 people. Recent studies have revealed that celiac disease affects approximately 1% of the U.S. population (1:100 individuals) which is similar to data from European countries.

Symptoms

Celiac disease not only affects the gastrointestinal system but many other systems in the body, resulting in a wide range and severity of symptoms that can vary greatly from one person to another (see page 16). These symptoms may occur singly or in combination in children and adults. Many individuals have "silent celiac disease" (i.e., have no or very subtle symptoms) in spite of gluten sensitivity.

Symptoms of Celiac Disease

- Iron, folate and/or vitamin B_{12} deficiency
- Other vitamin and mineral deficiencies (A, D, E, K, calcium)
- Chronic fatigue and weakness
- Abdominal pain, bloating and gas
- Indigestion/reflux ("heartburn")
- Nausea and vomiting
- Diarrhea, constipation or intermittent diarrhea and/or constipation
- Lactose intolerance
- Weight loss (note that CD can also occur in obese individuals)
- Bone/joint pain
- Easy bruising of the skin
- Tingling (in hands and feet)
- Edema (swelling) of hands and feet
- Migraine headaches
- Depression
- Mouth ulcers (canker sores)
- Menstrual irregularities
- Infertility (in both women and men)
- Recurrent miscarriages
- Elevated liver enzymes

Additional symptoms in children

- Irritability and behavioral changes
- Concentration and learning difficulties
- Failure to thrive (delayed growth and short stature)
- Delayed puberty
- Dental enamel abnormalities

Associated Conditions

Celiac disease can also occur more frequently in a variety of other disorders. Individuals with any of the following conditions and symptoms of celiac disease should be screened for celiac disease:

- Type 1 diabetes
- Other autoimmune disorders (e.g., autoimmune thyroid disease, autoimmune liver disease, Sjögren's syndrome, Addison's disease, alopecia areata)
- Osteoporosis
- Down syndrome
- Turner Syndrome
- Selective IgA deficiency

Diagnosis

The diagnosis of celiac disease is often very difficult because of the broad range of symptoms that can vary from mild to severe or none at all. Individuals are often misdiagnosed with irritable bowel syndrome, lactose intolerance, fibromyalgia, chronic fatigue syndrome or ulcers. Recent studies by Columbia University in New York and the Canadian Celiac Association have reported that many people have suffered with symptoms for more than 10 years and have seen numerous physicians before a correct diagnosis of celiac disease was made.

There are specific blood tests, including IgA endomysial (EMA) and IgA tissue transglutaminase (tTG) antibody tests, to detect celiac disease. Unfortunately these tests are not 100% accurate and some individuals test negative in spite of having celiac disease. Therefore, the only definitive test for diagnosing celiac disease is the small intestinal biopsy. **A gluten-free diet should never be started before the blood tests and biopsy are completed as this can interfere with making an accurate diagnosis.**

Treatment

Once a diagnosis for celiac disease is confirmed, it is essential to follow a strict gluten-free diet for life. Additional vitamin and mineral supplements may be necessary to correct the malnutrition. Some individuals may also need to eliminate lactose until the damaged bowel is healed (see pages 101-102).

Dermatitis Herpetiformis

Dermatitis herpetiformis (DH) is another form of celiac disease. This chronic skin condition is characterized by an intense burning, itchy and blistering rash. The rash is symmetrically distributed and commonly found on the elbows, knees and the buttocks, but can also occur on the back of the neck, upper back, scalp and hairline. Initially, groups of small blisters are formed that soon erupt into small erosions. Most people with DH will also have varying degrees of small intestinal villous atrophy although many will have no bowel complaints. A small percentage may present with bloating, abdominal pain and diarrhea, especially if the bowel involvement is severe, and some individuals may show evidence of malabsorption and malnutrition.

Prevalence

Approximately 10% of individuals with celiac disease have DH with a male to female ratio of 2:1. The age of onset is typically between 25-45 but can also occur in children and older adults.

Diagnosis

Individuals with DH are frequently misdiagnosed with other skin conditions such as eczema, contact dermatitis, allergies, hives, herpes or psoriasis and treated with a variety of topical creams. The only way to correctly diagnose DH is a skin biopsy from unaffected skin adjacent to blisters or erosions. A small intestinal biopsy is not essential if the skin biopsy is positive for DH.

Treatment

Treatment for DH is a **strict gluten-free diet for life**. For some individuals, Dapsone, a drug from the "sulphone family," may be prescribed to reduce the itching. Response to the medication can be dramatic (usually 48-72 hours). However, Dapsone has no effect on the ongoing immune response or intestinal atrophy. Following a strict gluten-free diet will result in:

✦ Improvement in the skin lesions.

✦ Major reduction in drug dosage for those people initially started on Dapsone. After a time, it is often possible to discontinue the drug to control the skin rash. Flare-ups due to inadvertent or intentional gluten consumption may require temporary use of Dapsone.

✦ The gut function will return to normal.

For more information about DH see: http://digestive.niddk.nih.gov/diseases/pubs/dh/index.htm

---

NOTE: Once a diagnosis of celiac disease or dermatitis herpetiformis is confirmed, it is essential to consult with a registered dietitian with expertise in celiac disease and the gluten-free diet for nutritional assessment, diet education, meal planning and assistance with social and emotional adaptation to the new gluten-free lifestyle. Also, joining a celiac support organization for further information and ongoing support is highly recommended.

References

✦ NIH Consensus Development Conference on Celiac Disease
http://consensus.nih.gov/2004/2004celiacdisease118html.htm

✦ Celiac Disease: Proceedings of the NIH Consensus Conference on Celiac Disease. *Gastroenterology* 2005; 128:S1-S141.

✦ Guidelines for the diagnosis and treatment of celiac disease in children: Recommendations of the North American Society for Pediatric Gastroenterology, Hepatology and Nutrition. http://www.naspghan.org/user-assets/Documents/pdf/PositionPapers/celiac_guideline_2004 _jpgn.pdf

✦ Gasbarrini G, Malandrino N, Giorgio V, et al. Celiac disease: What's new about it? *Dig Dis Sci* 2008; 26:121-127.

✦ Green PHR and Cellier C. Celiac Disease. N Engl J Med 2007; 357:1731-1743.

✦ Alaedini A, Green P. Narrative review: celiac disease. Understanding a complex autoimmune disorder. *Ann Intern Med* 2005; 142:289-298.

✦ Green PHR, Jabri B. Celiac disease. *Lancet* 2003; 362:383-391.

✦ Catassi C, Kryszak D, Louis-Jacques O, et al. Detection of celiac disease in primary care: A multicenter case-finding study in North America. *Am J Gastroenterol* 2007; 102:1454-1460.

✦ Fasano A, Berti I, Gerdarduzzi T, et al. Prevalence of celiac disease in at-risk and not-at-risk groups in the United States: A large multicenter study. *Arch Intern Med* 2003; 163:286-292.

✦ Collin P and Reunala. Recognition and management of the cutaneous manifestations of celiac disease: A guide for dermatologists. *Am J Clin Derm* 2003; 4:13-20.

✦ Cranney A, Zarkadas M, Graham I, et al. The Canadian Celiac Health Survey. *Dig Dis Sci* 2007; 52:1087-1095.

✦ Rashid M, Cranney A, Zarkadas M, et al. Celiac disease: Evaluation of the diagnosis and dietary compliance in Canadian children. *Pediatrics* 2005; 116:e754-759. http://pediatrics.aappublications.org/cgi/content/full/116/6/e754?

✦ Zarkadas M, Cranney A, Case S, et al. The impact of a gluten-free diet on adults with coeliac disease: results of a national survey. *J Hum Nutr Dietet* 2006; 19:41-49.

✦ Green PHR, Stavropoulos S, Panagi SG, et al. Characteristics of adult celiac disease in the USA: Results of a National Survey. *Am J Gastroenterol* 2001; 120:636-651.

✦ Lee AR, Newman J. Celiac disease: Impact on quality of life. *J Am Diet Assoc* 2003; 103:1533-1535.

✦ Zarkadas M, Case S. Celiac disease and the gluten-free diet: An overview. *Top Clin Nutr* 2005; 20:127-138.

✦ Lee AR. Celiac disease: Detection and treatment. *Top Clin Nutr* 2005; 20:139-145.

THE GLUTEN-FREE DIET

Gluten Defined

Gluten is the general name for the storage proteins (prolamins) found in wheat, rye and barley. These specific prolamins damage the small intestine in people with celiac disease and dermatitis herpetiformis. The actual names of the toxic prolamins are gliadin in wheat, secalin in rye and hordein in barley. All forms of wheat, rye and barley must be avoided and are outlined in the table on page 20. Although rice contains the prolamin called orzenin and corn contains zein, these prolamins are not toxic to persons with celiac disease. The corn prolamin is sometimes erroneously referred to as "corn gluten" by the food industry, however, it does not need to be restricted on a gluten-free diet.

Oats

Historically, the avenin prolamin in oats was also thought to be toxic based on the early work of Dr. W.K. Dicke and his colleagues in 1953. Since then the safety of oats for individuals with celiac disease has been widely debated. Many studies in Europe and the USA over the past 14 years, in both children and adults with celiac disease, have revealed that consumption of moderate amounts of oats is safe for most people. Early studies done between 1953 and 1976 had major limitations (small in size, did not test the oats for purity and did not evaluate the diet for hidden sources of gluten). Most of the studies followed children for a short period of time (three months or less). It was obvious that this important question needed to be investigated further and two decades later additional studies were conducted to investigate the safety of oats. In spite of improved study design and methodology, these later studies (1995-2008) also had limitations, which are discussed below.

Many of the studies since 1995 that evaluated the safety of oats for people with celiac disease stated they used pure, uncontaminated oats or oats "suitable" for people with celiac disease. However, the descriptions of how the purity of the oats was maintained, from the purity of seed used in planting, to equipment used for planting, harvesting, transporting and processing the oats, is not always clear. In addition, the gluten testing methods were not consistent. Barley is often one of the main contaminating grains in oats and some of the studies used the barley-insensitive omega-gliadin method for testing the gluten content or the purity of the oats.

Some investigators have examined the purity of oat products using the highly sensitive R5 ELISA test that detects wheat, rye and barley. An American study by dietitian Tricia Thompson tested three brands of commercially available oats (12 samples) and found varying levels of gluten contamination. Similar results were reported in two recent studies. Hernando tested 109 oat food samples from Europe, USA and Canada and over 59% were heavily contaminated. Gelinas found 8 out of 12 Canadian commercial oat products were also very contaminated. Cross-contamination has been the major reason why most health professionals and celiac groups have not allowed oats on a gluten-free diet. Fortunately, a number of companies in North America and Europe are currently offering pure, uncontaminated oat products (see pages 285, 289, 294, 296, 297 and 341 for information about purchasing these oat products).

In the research studies on the oat-containing diets, some individuals experienced gastrointestinal symptoms, although these were generally mild and transient in nature. The increased fiber intake from oats was thought to be a major contributing factor to the development of these symptoms. There were several reports of a few highly sensitive individuals with celiac disease who did not tolerate even pure, uncontaminated oats. The mechanism causing this intolerance has not been clearly established. Further long-term research on the incidence of oat intolerance in individuals with celiac disease is needed.

In spite of the limitations in the studies evaluating the safety of oats, a growing number of health professionals, celiac organizations, celiac research centers and other associations around the world allow consumption of moderate amounts of pure, uncontaminated oat products in a gluten-free diet. Some groups restrict oats under certain conditions and a few organizations do not recommend oats in the gluten-free diet. See pages 21-27 for Position Statements/Guidelines on the Use of Oats in Celiac Disease from various organizations. References about oats in celiac disease including Health Canada's review on *Celiac Disease and the Safety of Oats* can be found on pages 28 and 69.

Gluten-Containing Foods & Ingredients To Avoid

Wheat

Atta*
Bulgur
Couscous
Dinkel (also known as spelt)**
Durum**
Einkorn**
Emmer**
Farina Farro or Faro (also known as spelt)**
Fu***
Graham Flour
Hydrolyzed Wheat Protein

Kamut**
Matzoh, Matzoh Meal
Modified Wheat Starch
Seitan****
Semolina
Spelt (also known as farro or faro; dinkel)**
Triticale Wheat Bran
Wheat Flour
Wheat Germ
Wheat Starch

* A fine whole-meal flour made from low-gluten, soft-textured wheat used to make Indian flatbread (also known as chapatti flour)
** Types of wheat
*** A dried gluten product derived from wheat that is sold as thin sheets or thick round cakes. Used as a protein supplement in Asian dishes such as soups and vegetables.
**** A meat-like food derived from wheat gluten used in many vegetarian dishes. Sometimes called "wheat meat."

Barley

Ale*
Barley (Flakes, Flour, Pearl)
Beer*
Brewer's Yeast Lager*

Malt**
Malt Extract/Malt Syrup/Malt Flavoring***
Malt Vinegar
Malted Milk

* Most regular ale, beer and lager are derived from barley which is not gluten-free. However, there are several new varieties of gluten-free beer derived from buckwheat, sorghum and/or rice which are gluten-free. See page 266.
** Malt is an enzyme preparation usually derived from sprouted barley which is not gluten-free. Other cereal grains can also be malted and may or may not be gluten-free depending on the additional ingredients used in the malting process.
*** These terms are used interchangeably to denote a concentrated liquid solution of barley malt that is used as a flavoring agent.

Rye

Rye Bread

Rye Flour

Oats*

Oatmeal
Oat Bran

Oat Flour
Oats

* Celiac organizations in Canada and the USA do not recommend consumption of commercially available oat products as they are often cross-contaminated with wheat and/or barley. However, pure, uncontaminated specialty gluten-free oat products from North America are now available and many organizations allow consumption of moderate amounts of these oats for persons with celiac disease. For more information about the use of oats in celiac disease and where to purchase these products, see pages 19, 21-29, 285, 289, 294, 296, 297 and 341.

Position Statements/Guidelines on the Use of Oats in Celiac Disease from Various Organizations

The position statements and/or guidelines on the use of oats from various celiac, dietetic, medical and other health related organizations are highlighted below. It should be noted that this is not an all-inclusive list. The information was current at the time of printing, however, the various organizations' positions on the use of oats in celiac disease may change based on new research findings.

North American Organizations

Canadian Celiac Association

Professional Advisory Board Position Statement on Oats, Revised August 20, 2007

"The safety of oats in individuals with celiac disease has been extensively investigated. Clinical evidence confirms that consumption of pure, uncontaminated oats is safe in the amount of 50 to 70 grams per day (1/2 - 3/4 cup dry rolled oats) by adults and 20 to 25 grams per day (1/4 cup dry rolled oats) by children with celiac disease. Studies looking at the consumption of oats over five years have confirmed their safety. However, the studies looking at safety of oats in celiac disease have involved a small number of subjects, the oats used were pure, free of gluten contamination and the amount allowed per day was also limited.

In Canada, **pure and uncontaminated*** oats are now being produced. Individuals with celiac disease who wish to add oats or oat products to their diet must ensure that the oats they are eating are free from gluten contamination.

A small number of individuals with celiac disease may not tolerate even pure, uncontaminated oats. To ensure that persons with celiac disease are not intolerant to pure and uncontaminated oats, proper clinical follow-up with the physician is advised when introducing oats to a gluten-free diet.

The Canadian Celiac Association will continue to monitor the scientific developments in the area of oats in celiac disease and will keep its members updated.

* *These oats will meet or exceed the purity standards of Foundation #1 as defined by the Canada Seeds Act or equivalent level of purity obtained by current available methods.* * *
* * *The CCA is currently developing a certification standard for PAVENA™ (pure, uncontaminated oats and oat products)."*

Reference: www.celiac.ca/position_on_oats.php   Accessed July 7, 2008.

Celiac Disease Foundation

Medical Advisory Board Position Statement, January 18, 2006

"The addition of oats to the diet of individuals with celiac disease has been the subject of research studies which indicate that the prolamin avenin (protein fraction) in oats is not toxic. However, it has been shown that commercial oat products can be contaminated with wheat if they are grown, stored, transported or processed in a facility that also processes wheat. For these reasons, the source and processing methods of oats should be thoroughly researched so that the individual can make an informed decision before eating oats.

"Clinical studies suggest that **pure, uncontaminated oats** consumed daily in moderation (1/2 cup dry) can be tolerated by most people with celiac disease. Oats add soluble fiber and added nutrients to the gluten-free diet that may have limited amounts of whole grains.

"The CDF Medical Advisory Board suggests that the celiac individual and their healthcare team discuss the options and consequences together before deciding to introduce oats into their gluten-free diet. If the individual chooses to consume oats, they should have their antibody (IgA and tTGA) levels reviewed annually."

This position has been approved by the Celiac Disease Foundation Medical Advisory Board.

Reference:
Personal communication with Elaine Monarch, Executive Director, Celiac Disease Foundation February 24, 2006 and September 9, 2008.

Celiac Sprue Association (CSA)

"Oats appear to be suitable for some people with celiac disease, but not all. Thus oats are not yet a risk free choice for all people with celiac disease. If choosing to include oats, limit risk by choosing specially handled, uncontaminated oats and consuming no more than 50 g/day. Most physicians advise people, newly diagnosed with celiac disease, to wait until their health is restored before ingesting oats."

To read further statements on oats see the website reference below.

Reference:
www.csaceliacs.org/InfoonOats.php
Accessed on December 5, 2009.

Gluten Intolerance Group of North America (GIG)

Medical Advisory Board Position Statement, October 2005

"Research shows that pure, uncontaminated oats in moderation (½ cup dry) daily are safe for most persons with celiac disease. There is concern by health professionals that most oats are cross-contaminated with glutenous grains. Oats add soluble fiber and added nutrients to the GFD that are otherwise lacking or have limited availability. Some studies indicate that compliance with the GFD is increased when oats are included. Some persons using oats may notice increased abdominal discomfort, gas and stool changes. This may be due to the increased fiber from oats. Introducing oats slowly may decrease this discomfort. Rarely, some persons with celiac disease may have a hypersensitivity to oats. There is insufficient research to suggest this is related to a gluten-like reaction, or an allergic reaction. The GIG Medical Advisory Board suggests you work closely with your health care team before deciding to introduce oats in your diet, and that you have your antibody levels reviewed periodically."

Reference:
GIG Quarterly Newsletter, Fall 2005, Volume 28, pages 4, 5. Email correspondence with Cynthia Kupper, Executive Director on July 16, 2008.

Celiac Center at Beth Israel Deaconess Medical Center (BIDMC), Harvard Medical School

"The role of oats in celiac disease and the gluten-free diet remains controversial. Based on numerous studies conducted with adults and children in Europe and the United States, it appears that the majority of individuals with CD can tolerate oats[1-4].

"In practice, however, oats are often grown or processed with other cereals leading to cross-contamination by wheat, barley or rye. Currently there are also very few known producers of pure gluten-free oats in North America. The American Dietetic Association recommends that those with newly diagnosed celiac disease avoid oats, and that the addition of oats be discussed with the individual's clinician only after the intestine has healed as documented by normalization of blood work and small intestinal biopsy appearance.

"Although oats appear to be safe in the vast majority of individuals with celiac disease, there is evidence that, in some individuals, avenins in oats can trigger an immune response similar to gluten[5-6]. In addition, some people may need to avoid oats due to sensitivities or allergies, similar to other foods, such as nuts or shellfish. For these reasons, close monitoring by a healthcare professional experienced in celiac disease is recommended during introduction of oats into a gluten-free diet.

"Currently, avoiding consumption of oats is recommended by the clinicians of the Celiac Center at BIDMC for newly diagnosed patients until it can be clearly demonstrated that celiac disease is well-controlled. Good control is demonstrated by the complete resolution of symptoms (diarrhea, other symptoms of malabsorption or DH skin rash) and a normal tissue transglutaminase level (IgA tTG). At that point, under physician guidance, the gradual addition of pure oats up to 50 grams/day (a little more than ½ cup rolled oats or ¼ cup steel-cut oats) from a dedicated gluten-free facility may be attempted. Routine follow-up with the patient's gastroenterologist is expected three to six months after the addition of oats into the gluten-free diet.

"We remain optimistic that uncontaminated sources of oats will become more widely available and affordable in this country and can be a safe and useful addition to the gluten-free diet."

Referenced Articles:

1. Storsrud S, Olsson M, Arvidsson Lenner R, Nilsson LA, Nilsson O, Kilander A. Adult coeliac patients do tolerate large amounts of oats. *Eur J Clin Nutr* 2003 Jan;57(1):163-9.

2. Janatuinen EK, Pikkarainen PH, Kemppainen TA, et al. A comparison of diets with and without oats in adults with celiac disease. *N Engl J Med* 1995;333:1033-1037.

3. Hogberg L, Laurin P, Flath-Magnusson K, et al. Oats to children with newly diagnosed coeliac disease: a randomized double blind study. *Gut* 2004; 53:649-654.

4. Janatuinen EK, Pikkarainen PH, Kemppainen TA, et al. Lack of cellular and humoral immunological responses to oats in adults with coeliac disease. *Gut* 2000;46:327-331.

5. Peraaho M, Kaukinen K, Mustalahti K, Vuolteenaho N, Maki M, Laippala P, et al. Effect of an oats-containing gluten-free diet on symptoms and quality of life in coeliac disease. A randomized study. *Scand J Gastroenterol* 2004, Jan;39(1):27-31.

6. Arentz-Hansen H, Fleckenstein B, Molberg O, Scott H, Koning F, Jung G, Roepstorff P, Lundin KE, Sollid LM. The molecular basis for oat intolerance in patients with celiac disease. *PLoS Med* 2004 Oct;1(1):e1. Epub 2004. Oct 19.

Reference:
Email and telephone correspondence with Dr. Ciaran Kelly, Medical Director and Melinda Dennis, MS, RD, LDN, Nutrition Coordinator, Celiac Center on December 9, 2005 and July 10, 2008.

Celiac Disease Center at Columbia University, New York City

"We recommend the use of oats (from companies that claim them to be gluten-free) for people with celiac disease because most (99%) tolerate them fine. Oats add fiber, needed nutrients and diversity to the diet. Advise to gradually introduce oats in small amounts due to the increased fiber intake which may not be tolerated by all patients. Limit consumption to 50 grams per day. Individuals need to be monitored with annual TTG tests. Would advise that oats be commenced after the individual is stable on the GF diet."

Reference:
1. Email correspondence with Dr. Peter Green, Medical Director and Anne Lee, RD, Nutritionist, Celiac Disease Center, Columbia University on December 5, 2005.
2. Email correspondence with Dr. Peter Green on July 14, 2008.

Celiac Clinic, Mayo Clinic

"At Mayo Clinic Rochester, Celiac Clinic, the clinicians discourage ingestion of oats by our patients unless verified gluten-free in their production and free of contamination (by testing) from wheat, rye or barley. Recent studies have demonstrated that several commercial varieties of oats are contaminated with gluten. We do not want to expose our patients to this risk (versus we must warn our patients of this risk). Although the majority of people with celiac disease can tolerate oats, patients who try oats should be monitored closely for reactions. People who do not react to the ingestion of gluten with outward symptoms should be especially wary of trying oats.

Patients whose celiac disease is not well controlled are discouraged from trying oats. We will continue to monitor new information as it pertains to this important issue."

Reference:
Email correspondence with Jackie See, MS, RD, Nutritionist, and Dr. Joe Murray on behalf of the clinicians in the Celiac Disease Clinic, Mayo Clinic Rochester on February 6, 2006 and July 9, 2008.

University of Maryland Center for Celiac Research

"Several studies have been performed showing that oats did not cause any harm to celiac patients. However, concerns still remain, mainly due to two issues: 1) The possibility of cross-contamination of oats with wheat or barley during processing of the grain. This concern is now mitigated by the fact that several companies are dedicating their facilities to oats and, 2) A subgroup of celiac patients has been found to react to the oat prolamin avenin and may suffer intestinal damage. Therfore our current recommendations include omitting oats from the diet of newly diagnosed patient with celiac disease. Once presenting symptoms have resolved and antibody levels have returned to normal, the introduction of pure oats may be tried. We also recommend a follow-up clinic visit and repeat serology testing 6 months after the introduction of oats to the diet."

Reference:
Email and telephone correspondence with Dr. Alessio Fasano, Medical Director, and Pam Cureton, RD, LDN, Dietitian, Center for Celiac Research on December 9, 2005 and July 9, 2008

American Dietetic Association
Evidence Analysis Library® Celiac Disease Project

Evidence Analysis Question:
"How does the inclusion of oats in a dietary pattern for people with celiac disease impact effectiveness and acceptability of the dietary pattern?

"Studies have shown that incorporating oats uncontaminated with wheat, barley or rye, into a gluten-free dietary pattern for people with celiac disease, at intake levels of approximately 50 g dry oats per day, is generally safe and improves compliance. However, many studies report that the introduction of oats may result in gastrointestinal symptoms such as diarrhea and abdominal discomfort. These symptoms tend to be the primary reason for study subject withdrawal. Additional adverse effects that have been reported include dermatitis herpetiformis, villous atrophy and an increased density of intraepithelial lymphocytes, indicating that some persons with celiac disease may be unable to tolerate oats. Since limited research has been conducted on the similarities among those with adverse reactions to oats, further research is needed in this area. Further research is also needed regarding the contamination of oats by wheat, barley and rye". Grade II (fair) rating.

Evidence Based Guidelines: Recommendations Summary

CD: Inclusion of Gluten-Free Oats as Tolerated
The registered dietitian (RD) should advise individuals with celiac disease who enjoy and can tolerate gluten-free oats to gradually include them in their gluten-free dietary pattern. Research on individuals with celiac disease reports that incorporating oats uncontaminated with wheat, barley or rye at intake levels of approximately 50g dry oats per day is generally safe and improves compliance with the gluten-free dietary pattern. In a small number of persons with celiac disease, research reports that oats may cause villous atrophy, an increase in intraepithelial lymphocytes or exacerbate dermatitis herpetiformis. **Rating: Fair** - Conditional

Conditions of Application:

- This recommendation applies to individuals with celiac disease who enjoy and can tolerate gluten-free oats
- Inclusion of oats requires medical supervision
- Gluten-free oats must meet the proposed FDA definition. Oats may be labeled gluten free only if they contain less than 20 parts per million of gluten.
- The introduction of oats may result in gastrointestinal symptoms such as diarrhea and abdominal discomfort. These symptoms may be due to an increase in fiber intake and not be a sign of intolerance to oats.

The above is an excerpt from the ADA Evidence Analysis Library®. To read the entire section that includes the complete list of references see following links below. ADA Evidence Analysis Library available to ADA members and by subscription for non-members.

www.adaevidencelibrary.com
www.adaevidencelibrary.com/topic.cfm?cat = 1471
http://www.adaevidencelibrary.com/template.cfm?template = guide_summary&key = 2103
Accessed December 15, 2009

© American Dietetic Association. Reprinted with permission.
Evidence-based Nutrition Practice Guideline on Celiac Disease published on May 2009 at http://www.adaevidencelibrary.com/topic.cfm?cat = 3726 and copyrighted by the American Dietetic Association.

Dietitians of Canada

Practice-based Evidence in Nutrition (PEN): Celiac Disease Knowledge Pathway

Question: "Is consumption of moderate amounts of uncontaminated oats by adults (50-70 gm/day) and children (20-25 gm/day) safe for people with celiac disease?

"Moderate amounts of pure, uncontaminated oats (50-70 gm/day) can be included in a gluten-free diet for most adults with stable celiac disease. Moderate amounts of pure, uncontaminated oats (20-25 gm/day) can be included for most children with stable celiac disease without apparent adverse effects. People with celiac disease who are extremely sensitive could show intolerance to even uncontaminated oats therefore, they would need regular monitoring and follow-up. Educating people with CD on introduction of pure, uncontaminated oats and how to obtain them is very important. See *Guidelines for Consumption of Pure and Uncontaminated Oats by Individuals with Celiac Disease* by the Professional Advisory Board of the Canadian Celiac Association. Consumption of oats by people with celiac disease is a way to enhance fiber content in their diet which otherwise is often deficient in gluten-free diets. Inclusion of oats in a gluten-free diet enhances the quality and acceptance of the diet."

Reference:
http://www.dieteticsatwork.com/PEN/index.asp
Accessed December 6, 2009.

National Institutes of Health (NIH)

Consensus Development Conference on Celiac Disease, June 28-30, 2004.

"A gluten-free diet is defined as one that excludes wheat, rye and barley. These dietary grains contain the peptides or glutens known to cause celiac disease. Even small quantities of gluten may be harmful. Oats appear to be safe for use by most individuals with celiac disease, but their practical inclusion in a gluten-free diet is limited by potential contamination with gluten during processing."

Reference:
http://consensus.nih.gov/2004/2004CeliacDisease118html.htm
Accessed January 4, 2006.

North American Society for Pediatric Gastroenterology Hepatology and Nutrition (NASPGHAN)

Guideline for the Diagnosis and Treatment of Celiac Disease in Children: Recommendations of the North American Society for Pediatric Gastroenterology, Hepatalogy and Nutrition

"Previously, oats were implicated in the development of villous damage in CD. More recently this has been questioned as both in vivo and in vitro immunologic studies suggest oats are safe (193-199). Despite the accumulating evidence that oats are safe for individuals with CD, there remains some concern about recommending consumption of this grain to CD patients. Contamination of oats with gluten during the harvesting and milling process is known to occur, so unless the purity of the oats can be guaranteed, their safety remains questionable."

Note: To read references 193-199 in the above statement see the full article at the website below.

Reference:
Journal of Pediatric Gastroenterology and Nutrition 40:1-19, 2005 (Quote from page 11).
http://www.naspghan.org/PDF/PositionPapers/celiac_guideline_2004_jpgn.pdf
Accessed December 4, 2005.

International Organizations

Association of European Coeliac Societies (AOECS)

AOECS is an independent, non-profit organization of 33 Coeliac Societies from 29 countries with approximately 270,000 members. The majority of AOECS members do not support labeling oats as "gluten-free" because some individuals with coeliac disease do not tolerate pure, uncontaminated oats as documented in scientific studies. However, most do tolerate moderate amounts of pure, uncontaminated oats but should do so in consultation and under supervision of their gastroenterologist.

In recent years the AOECS has had extensive discussions with the Codex Committee on Nutrition and Foods For Special Dietary Uses regarding the oats issue. We have found a good solution: to keep oats in the definition of gluten-containing cereals but to add a footnote in the new Codex Standard for Foods for Special Dietary Use for Persons Intolerant to Gluten. This Standard was adopted by the Codex Alimentarius Commission on June 30-July 4, 2008 and replaces the Codex Standard for Gluten-Free Foods 118-1981 (see pages 63-64).

In this new Codex Standard oats remain on the list of foods which cannot have a "gluten-free claim". If oats had been declared "gluten-free", the concern would be that individuals with coeliac disease might purchase regular oat products that are heavily contaminated with wheat, rye or barley and potentially consume unlimited, high amounts.

Reference:
Email discussion on August 28, 2008 with Hertha Deutsch, Chair of AOECS Codex Working Group (Labelling and Symbol); AOECS delegate in Codex (FAO/WHO) and President of the Austrian Coeliac Society.

The Coeliac Society of Australia

"The inclusion of oats (even if pure and uncontaminated) is not recommended. It has been shown that approximately 1:5 people with coeliac disease react to oat protein. If there is a compelling reason to consume oats, it may be that a systematic challenge with oats and endoscopic biopsy before and during is the only definitive test for oats sensitivity."

Reference:
Email and telephone correspondence with Graham Price, Technical Officer, The Coeliac Society of Australia on December 5-7, 2005 and July 8, 2008.

Coeliac UK

General Guidelines:

1. Moderate amounts of pure, uncontaminated oats may be consumed by most people with coeliac disease.
2. Introduction of oats can occur once the person is well established on the gluten-free diet and the disease is well controlled.
3. The decision to add oats to the gluten-free diet should be done in consultation with their local health care team.
4. Careful follow-up is necessary to assess tolerance to oat products.

Reference:
Email and telephone correspondence with Norma McGough, BSc., SRD, Dietetic Services Manager, Coeliac UK on November 9, 2005 and July 21, 2008.

Danish Coeliac Society (Dansk Coliaki Forening)

"Research has shown that most people with celiac disease can tolerate oats. It is important to use specially processed clean oats as regular oats are contaminated with gluten-containing grains in the field and/or at the mill. Children and adults should not consume clean oats until their disease is well controlled and the blood tests have normalized. Children should limit oat consumption to 25-50 grams/day, however, there are no restrictions for adults on the amounts of oats per day that can be consumed. It should be noted that if symptoms develop while consuming oats, they should be discontinued."

Reference:
1. Email correspondence with Milena Hasdorf, Secretary, November 10, 2005 and January 17, 2006.
2. "Coeliaki og mad uden gluten" at:
   www.foedevarestyrelsen.dk/fdir/Pub/2005214/rapport.pdf

Finnish Coeliac Society (Suomen Keliakialiitto ry)

"In 1998, the scientific advisory board issued a statement whereby oat-containing gluten-free products were permissible for adults with celiac disease. The statement was extended in 1998 to concern patients with dermatitis herpetiformis and to children in 2000."

Reference:
Quote from the article: Oats can diversify a gluten-free diet in celiac disease and dermatitis herpetiformis by Peraaho, M., et al. *J Am Diet Assoc* 2004; 104:1148-1150.

Oats References

✦ Arentz-Hansen H, Fleckenstein B, Molberg Ø, Scott H, Konding F, Jung G, Roepstorff P, Lundin K, Sollid L. The Molecular basis for oat intolerance in patients with celiac disease. *PLoS Med* 2004; 1:84-92

✦ Dickey W. Making oats safer for patients with coeliac disease. *Eur J Gastroenterol Hepatol* 2008; 20:494-95.

✦ Ellis HJ, Ciclitira PJ. Should coeliac sufferers be allowed their oats? *Eur J Gastroenterol Hepatol* 2008; 20:492-93.

✦ Garsed K, Scott BB. Can oats be taken in a gluten-free diet? A systematic review. *Scand J Gastroenterol* 2007; 42:171-78.

✦ Gélinas P, McKinnon CM, Méndez E. Gluten contamination of cereal foods in Canada. *Int J Food Sci Technol* 2007; 43:1245-52.

✦ Guttormsen V, Løvik A, Bye A, Bratlie J, Mørkrid L, Lundin KEA. No induction of anti-avenin IgA by oats in adult, diet-treated coeliac disease. *Scand J Gastroenterol* 2008; 43:161-65.

✦ Hernando A, Mujico JR, Mena MC, Lombardia M, Méndez E. Measurement of wheat gluten and barley hordeins in contaminated oats from Europe, the United States and Canada by sandwich R5 ELISA. *Eur J Gastroenterol Hepatol* 2008; 20:545-54.

✦ Hardman C, Fry L, TAllatham A, Thomas HJ. Absence of toxicity of avenin in patients with dermatitis herpetiformis. *N Engl J Med* 1999; 340:321.

✦ Health Canada. Celiac disease and the safety of oats: Health Canada's position on the introduction of oats to the diet of individuals diagnosed with celiac disease (CD). 2007 http://www.hc-sc.gc.ca/fn-an/securit/allerg/cel-coe/oats_cd-avoine-eng.php

✦ Högberg L, Laurin P, Fälth-Magnusson K, Grant C, Grodzinsky E, Jansson G, Ascher H, Browaldh L, Hammersjö JA, Lindberg E, Myrdal U, Stenhammar L. Oats to children with newly diagnosed coeliac disease: a randomised double blind study. *Gut* 2004; 53:649-54.

✦ Hoffenberg EJ, Haas J, Drescher A, Barnhurst R, Osberg I, Bao F, Eisenbarth G. A trial of oats in children with newly diagnosed celiac disease. *J Pediatr* 2000; 137:361-66.

✦ Hollén E, Högberg L, Stenhammar L, Fälth-Magnusson K, Magnusson KE. Antibodies to oat prolamines (avenins) in children with coeliac disease. *Scand J Gastroenterol* 2003; 38:742-6.

✦ Hollén E, Holmgren Peterson K, Sundqvist T, et al. Coeliac children on a gluten-free diet with or without oats display equal anti-avenin antibody titres. *Scand J Gastroenterol* 2006; 41:42-47.

✦ Janatuinen EK, Kemppainen TA, Julkunen RJ, Kosma VM, Mäki M, Heikkinen M, Uusitupa MI. No harm from five year ingestion of oats in coeliac disease. *Gut* 2002; 50:332-35.

✦ Janatuinen EK, Kemppainen TA, Pikkarainen PH, Holm KH, Kosma VM, Uusitupa MIJ, Mäki M, Julkunen RJK. Lack of cellular and humoral immunological responses to oats in adults with coeliac disease. *Gut* 2000; 46:327-31.

✦ Janatuinen EK, Pikkarainen PH, Kemppainen TA, Kosma VM, Järvinen RM, Uusitupa MI, Julkunen RJ. A comparison of diets with and without oats in adults with celiac disease. *N Engl J Med* 1995; 333:1033-37.

✦ Kilmartin C, Lynch S, Abuzakouk M, Wieser H, Feighery C. Avenin fails to induce a Th1 response in coeliac tissue following *in vitro* culture. *Gut* 2003; 52:47-52.

✦ Lundin KE, Nilsen EM, Scott HG, Loberg EM, Gjøen A, Bratlie J, Skar V, Mendez E, Løvik A, Kett K. Oats induced villous atrophy in coeliac disease. *Gut* 2003; 52:1649-52.

✦ Peräaho M, Collin P, Kaukinen K, Kekkonen L, Miettinen S, Maki M. Oats can diversify a gluten-free diet in celiac disease and dermatitis herpetiformis. *J Am Diet Assoc* 2004; 104:1148-50.

✦ Peräaho M, Kaukinen K, Mustalahti K, Vuolteenaho N, Mäki M, Laippala P, Collin P. Effect of an oats-containing gluten-free diet on symptoms and quality of life in coeliac disease. A randomized study. *Scand J Gastroenterol* 2004; 39:27-31.

✦ Picarelli A, Di Tola M, Sabbatella L, Gabrielli F, Di Cello T, Anania MC, Mastracchio A, Silano M, De Vincenzi M. Immunologic evidence of no harmful effect of oats in celiac disease. *Am J Clin Nutr* 2001; 74:137-40.

✦ Pulido OM, Gillespie Z, Zarkadas M, et al. Chapter 6 Introduction of oats in the diet of individuals with celiac disease a systematic review. *Adv Food Nutr Res* 2009; 57: 235-85.

✦ Reunala T, Collin P, Holm K, Pikkarainen P, Miettinen A, Vuolteenaho N, Mäki M. Tolerance to oats in dermatitis herpetiformis. *Gut* 1998; 43:490-93.

✦ Schmitz J. Lack of oats toxicity in coeliac disease. *BMJ* 1997; 314:159-60.

✦ Srinivasan U, Leonard N, Jones E, Kasarda DD, Weir DG, O'Farrelly C, Feighery C. Absence of oats toxicity in adult coeliac disease. *BMJ* 1996; 313:1300-1.

✦ Størsrud S, Hulthén LR, Lenner RA. Beneficial effects of oats in the gluten-free diet of adults with special reference to nutrient status, symptoms and subjective experiences. *Br J Nutr* 2003; 90:101-7.

✦ Storsrud S, Olsson M, Arvidsson Lenner R, Nilsson LA, Nilsson O, Kilander A. Adult coeliac patients do tolerate large amounts of oats. *Eur J Clin Nutr* 2003; 57:163-69.

✦ Størsrud S, Yman IM, Lenner RA. Gluten contamination in oat products and products naturally free from gluten. *Eur Food Res Technol* 2003; 217:481-85.

✦ Thompson T. Do oats belong in a gluten-free diet? *J Am Diet Assoc* 1997; 97:1413-6.

✦ Thompson T. Oats and the gluten-free diet. *J Am Diet Assoc* 2003; 103:376-79.

✦ Thompson T. Gluten contamination of commercial oat products in the United States. *N Engl J Med* 2004; 351:2021-2.

✦ Thompson T. Contaminated oats and other gluten-free foods in the United States. *J Am Diet Assoc* 2005; 105:348. Letter in response to: Peräaho et al. Oats can diversify a gluten-free diet in celiac disease and dermatitis herpetiformis. *J Am Diet Assoc* 2004; 104:1148-50. Author reply 348-9.

Hidden Gluten

Gluten is the substance in flour responsible for forming the structure of dough, holding products together and leavening. While the presence of gluten is evident in baked goods (e.g., breads, cookies, cakes, crackers) and pasta, it is often a "hidden ingredient" in many other items such as sauces, marinades, gravies, salad dressings, soups, prepared meats (hamburger patties, deli meats, hot dogs), candy, flavored coffees and teas, as well as some medications and nutritional supplements. For a more comprehensive listing of foods allowed, foods to question, and foods to avoid, see the chart entitled **Gluten-Free Diet By Food Groups** on pages 30-34.

Other Ingredients

It is not uncommon to find a lot of misinformation written about the gluten-free status and safety of a number of ingredients, on the internet, in pamphlets, books, magazines, and from other sources. A list of frequently questioned ingredients, their gluten-free status, additional background information and reputable references, including specific sections of the U.S. *Code of Federal Regulations* (CFR) and *Canadian Food and Drug Regulations* (FDR) for certain ingredients where applicable is found on pages 45-58. Background information and the web links for these regulations are on pages 59-60. Additional information on ingredients is also found in the **Gluten-Free Diet By Food Groups** Table on pages 30-34 and **Gluten-Free Additives and Ingredients** Table on page 44. The Canadian Celiac Association's *Acceptability of Foods and Food Ingredients for the Gluten-Free Diet Pocket Dictionary* and *Gluten-Free Living* magazine are two excellent resources on the status of ingredients (see page 347).

Gluten-Free Diet by Food Groups[1]

Food Category	Foods Allowed[a]	Foods to Question[b]	Foods to Avoid[c]
Milk & Dairy	Milk, cream, most ice cream, buttermilk, plain yogurt, cheese, cream cheese, processed cheese, processed cheese foods, cottage cheese	Flavored yogurt, frozen yogurt, cheese sauces, cheese spreads, seasoned (flavored) shredded cheese or cheese blends	Malted milk, ice cream made with ingredients not allowed
Grains & Starches	**Breads, Baked Products and Other Items:** Made with amaranth, arrowroot, buckwheat, corn bran, corn flour, cornmeal, cornstarch, flax, legume flours (bean, garbanzo or chickpea, Garfava™, lentil, pea), mesquite flour, millet, Montina™ flour (Indian ricegrass), nut flours (almond, chestnut, hazelnut), potato flour, potato starch, pure uncontaminated oat products (oat flour, oat groat, oatmeal)*, quinoa, rice (black, brown, red, white, wild) rice bran, rice flours (brown, glutinous, sweet, white), rice polish, sago, sorghum flour, soy flour, sweet potato flour, tapioca (cassava, manioc), taro, teff * See pages 19-27 for discussion about oats.	Items made with buckwheat flour	Items made with wheat bran, wheat farina, wheat flour, wheat germ, wheat-based semolina, wheat starch**, durum flour, gluten flour, graham flour, atta, bulgur, einkorn, emmer, farro, kamut, spelt, barley, rye, triticale, commercial oat products (oat bran, oat flour, oat groats, oatmeal)*** **Imported foods labeled "gluten-free" made with wheat starch ***See pages 19-27 for discussion about oats.

[1] Table adapted and revised October 2000 by S. Case, M. Molloy and M. Zarakadas from *Celiac Disease Needs a Diet for Life Handbook*, Canadian Celiac Association. Further revisions made by S. Case for *Gluten-Free Diet: A Comprehensive Resource Guide*, May 2001, April 2002, July 2003, May 2004, January 2005, March 2006, September 2008, January 2010 and December 2010.

(a), (b), (c) See pages 35-43 for further background information on foods allowed, foods to question and foods to avoid.

Food Category	Foods Allowed[a]	Foods to Question[b]	Foods to Avoid[c]
Grains & Starches	**Cereals: Hot** Puffed amaranth, cornmeal, cream of buckwheat, cream of rice (brown, white), hominy grits, pure, uncontaminated oatmeal*, quinoa, rice flakes, soy flakes, soy grits *See pages 19-27 for discussion about oats.	Rice and soy pablum	Cereals made from wheat, rye, triticale, barley and commercial oats*** ***See pages 19-27 for discussion about oats.
	Cold: Puffed (amaranth, buckwheat, corn, millet, rice), rice crisps or corn flakes (with no barley malt extract or barley malt flavoring), rice flakes, soy cereals	Rice and corn cereals	Cereals made with added barley malt extract or barley malt flavoring
	Pastas: Macaroni, spaghetti and noodles made from beans, corn, lentils, peas, potato, quinoa, rice, soy, wild rice	Buckwheat pasta	Pastas made from wheat, wheat starch and other ingredients not allowed (e.g., orzo)
	Rice: Plain (e.g., basmati, black, brown, jasmine, red, white, wild)	Seasoned or flavored rice mixes	
	Miscellaneous: Corn tacos, rice tortillas, teff tortillas	Corn tortillas	Wheat flour tacos and tortillas Matzoh, matzoh meal, matzoh balls, couscous, tabouli
	Plain rice crackers, rice cakes & corn cakes	Multi-grain or flavored rice crackers, rice cakes & corn cakes	
	Gluten-free communion wafers	Low gluten communion wafers* *See page 38.	Regular communion wafers

Food Category	Foods Allowed[a]	Foods to Question[b]	Foods to Avoid[c]
Meats & Alternatives	**Meat, Fish, Poultry:** Plain (fresh or frozen)	Deli or luncheon meats (e.g., bologna, salami), wieners, frankfurters, sausages, pâte, meat and sandwich spread, frozen burgers (meat, fish, chicken), meatloaf, ham (ready to cook), dried meats (e.g., beef jerky), seasoned/flavored fish in pouches, imitation fish products (e.g., surimi), meat substitutes, meat product extenders	Canned fish in vegetable broth containing hydrolyzed wheat protein Frozen turkey basted or injected with hydrolyzed wheat protein. Frozen or fresh turkey with bread stuffing Frozen chicken breasts containing chicken broth (made with ingredients not allowed) Meat, poultry or fish breaded in ingredients not allowed
	Eggs: Fresh, liquid, dried or powdered	Flavored egg products (liquid or frozen)	
	Others: Dried beans (e.g., black, garbanzo [also known as chickpea, besan, channa, gram], kidney, navy, pinto, soy, white), dried peas, lentils	Baked beans	
	Plain nuts and seeds (chia, flax, sesame, pumpkin, sunflower)	Seasoned or dry roasted nuts, seasoned pumpkin or sunflower seeds Nut butters (e.g., almond, peanut)	
	Plain tofu	Flavored tofu Tempeh, miso	Fu, Seitan
Fruits & Vegetables	**Fruits:** Fresh, frozen and canned fruits & juices	Dates, fruits with sauces	
	Vegetables: Fresh, frozen and canned vegetables & juices	Vegetables with sauces, French-fried potatoes cooked in oil also used for gluten-containing products, French fries (various shapes)	Scalloped potatoes (containing wheat flour), battered deep-fried vegetables

Food Category	Foods Allowed[a]	Foods to Question[b]	Foods to Avoid[c]
Soups	Homemade broth, gluten-free bouillon cubes, cream soups and stocks made from ingredients allowed	Canned soups, dried soup mixes, soup bases and bouillon cubes	Soups made with ingredients not allowed, bouillon cubes containing hydrolyzed wheat protein
Fats	Butter, margarine, lard, shortening, vegetable oils, salad dressings with allowed ingredients	Salad dressings, suet, baking cooking spray	Salad dressing made with ingredients not allowed.
Desserts	Ice cream, sherbet, whipped toppings, whipping cream, milk puddings, custard, gelatin desserts, cakes, cookies, pies and pastries made with allowed ingredients	Cake icings and frostings	Bread pudding, ice cream made with ingredients not allowed (e.g., cookie crumbs), cakes, cookies, muffins, pies and pastries made with ingredients not allowed
	Gluten-free ice cream cones, wafers and waffles		Ice cream cones, wafers and waffles made with ingredients not allowed
Others	**Sweets:** Honey, jam, jelly, marmalade, corn syrup, maple syrup, molasses, sugar (brown and white), icing sugar (confectioner's)	Honey powder	
	Gluten-free licorice, marshmallows	Hard candies, Smarties®, chocolates, chocolate bars	Licorice and other candies made with ingredients not allowed
	Snack Foods: Plain popcorn, nuts, soy nuts, potato chips, taco (corn) chips	Seasoned (flavored) potato chips, taco (corn) chips, nuts, soy nuts	Potato chips with ingredients not allowed
	Gluten-free pizza		Pizza made with ingredients not allowed

Food Category	Foods Allowed[a]	Foods to Question[b]	Foods to Avoid[c]
Others	**Beverages:** Tea, instant or ground coffee (regular or decaffeinated), cocoa, soft drinks	Flavored and herbal teas, flavored coffees, coffee substitutes, hot chocolate mixes	Cereal and malt-based beverages (e.g., Ovaltine [chocolate malt and malt flavor], Postum)
	Distilled alcoholic beverages (e.g., bourbon, brandy, gin, rum, rye whiskey, scotch whiskey, vodka and liqueurs), wine	Flavored alcoholic beverages (e.g., coolers, ciders, Caesar vodka beverage)	
	Gluten-free beer, ale and lager		Beer, ale and lager derived from barley
	Most non-dairy beverages made from nut, potato, rice & soy		Non-dairy beverages (nut, potato, rice, soy) made with barley malt extract, barley malt flavoring or oats
	Condiments/Sauces: Ketchup, relish, plain prepared mustard, pure mustard flour, herbs, spices, salt, pepper, olives, plain pickles, tomato paste, vinegars (apple cider, balsamic, distilled white, grape or wine, rice, spirit), gluten-free soy sauce, gluten-free teriyaki sauce, other sauces and gravies made with allowed ingredients	Specialty prepared mustards, prepared mustard flour, mustard pickles, worcestershire sauce, salsa, curry paste, seasoning mixes	Malt vinegar, soy sauce (made from wheat), teriyaki sauce (made with soy sauce containing wheat), other sauces and gravies made with wheat flour and/or hydrolyzed wheat protein
	Miscellaneous: Plain cocoa, pure baking chocolate, carob chips and powder, chocolate chips, baking soda, cream of tartar, coconut, monosodium glutamate (MSG), vanilla, pure vanilla extract, artificial (synthetic, imitation) vanilla extract, vanillin, yeast (active dry, autolyzed, baker's, nutritional, torula), xanthan gum, guar gum	Baking powder, wasabi peas	Brewer's yeast

Notes on Foods Allowed

Food Category	Food Products	Notes
Grains	Garfava™ Flour	A specialty flour from garbanzo beans (chickpeas) and fava beans developed by Authentic Foods.
	Mesquite Flour	Made from the ground pods of the mesquite tree.
	Montina™ Flour	Made from Indian ricegrass.
	Quinoa	A small seed of a South American plant that can be cooked and eaten whole or ground into flour or flakes.
	Glutinous Rice Flour	Also known as sweet, sticky or sushi rice flour. Made from a sticky short-grain rice that is higher in starch than brown or white rice. Does not contain any gluten.
	Sago	An edible starch derived from the pith of the stems of a certain variety of palm trees. Usually ground into a powder and used as a thickener or dense flour.
	Tapioca (Cassava, Manioc, Yuca)	A tropical plant that produces a starchy edible root that is peeled and can be boiled, baked or fried. The peeled root can also be dried and washed with water to extract the starch (known as tapioca starch) which can be used to make baked products and tapioca pearls.
	Taro (Dasheen, Eddo)	A tropical plant harvested for its large, starchy tubers which are consumed as a cooked vegetable or made into breads, puddings or Poi (a Polynesian dish).
	Teff	A tiny seed of a grass native to Ethiopia that can be cooked and eaten whole or ground into flour.
	Hominy Grits (Corn Grits)	Corn kernels that are coarsely or finely ground that are cooked and eaten as a hot breakfast cereal or side dish.
	GF Communion Wafers	No-gluten host made from soy and rice flour by Ener-G Foods. These hosts are allowed by most major denominations except the Catholic Church.

Notes on Foods Allowed

Food Category	Food Products	Notes
Meats & Alternatives	Chia	An oilseed of the ancient plant species (Salvia hispanica L.) belonging to the mint family which is grown in Central and South America. Available in a natural brown and white seed, sold as "Chia" and a pure white variety sold under the trademark name "Salba". It is high in omega-3 fatty acids and fiber. The seed should be ground in order to get the maximum benefit of all the nutritional components.
Other	Distilled Alcoholic Beverages	Rye whiskey, scotch whiskey, gin, vodka and bourbon are distilled from a mash of fermented grains. Even though they are derived from a gluten-containing grain, the distillation process removes the gluten from the purified final product. Rum (distilled from sugar cane) and brandy (distilled from wine) are also gluten-free. Liqueurs (also known as cordials) are made from an infusion of a distilled alcoholic beverage and flavoring agents such as nuts, fruits, seeds or cream.
	Gluten-Free Beer, Ale and Lager	Can be made from fermented rice, buckwheat, millet and/or sorghum.
	Plain Prepared Mustard	Made from distilled vinegar, water, mustard seed, salt, spices and flavors.
	Pure Mustard Flour	A powder made from pure ground mustard seed.
	Vinegars	Produced from various ingredients: Balsamic (grapes), cider (apples), rice (rice wine), white distilled (corn, wheat or both), wine (red wine). All these vinegars are gluten-free (including distilled white derived from wheat as the distillation process removes the gluten from the final purified product). Except for malt vinegar (see page 43).
	Vanilla	Pure vanilla and pure vanilla extract are derived from the vanilla bean pods of a climbing orchid grown in tropical locations. The vanilla beans are chopped and soaked in alcohol and water; aged and then filtered. It must contain at least 35% ethyl alcohol by volume. The pure vanilla is bottled or the pure extract can be mixed with sugar and a stabilizer and then bottled.
	Natural Vanilla Flavor	Derived from vanilla beans but contains less than 35% ethyl alcohol. May also contain sugar and a stabilizer.
	Artificial (Imitation, Synthetic) Vanilla-Vanillin Extract/ Flavoring	Made from a by-product of the pulp and paper industry or a coal-tar derivative that is chemically treated to mimic the flavor of vanilla. Also contains alcohol, water, color and a stabilizer.

Notes on Foods Allowed

Food Category	Food Products	Notes
Other	Baker's Yeast	A type of yeast grown on sugar beet molasses. It is available as active dry yeast granules (sold in packets or jars) or compressed yeast (also known as wet yeast, cake yeast or fresh yeast) which must be refrigerated.
	Autolyzed Yeast/ Autolyzed Yeast Extract	A special process that causes yeast to be broken down by its own enzymes resulting in the production of various compounds that can be used as flavoring agents. Autolyzed yeast is almost always derived from baker's yeast.
	Torula Yeast	A yeast grown on wood sugars (a by-product of waste products from the pulp and paper industry). Used as a flavoring agent that has a hickory smoke characteristic.
	Nutritional Yeast	A specific strain of an inactive form of baker's yeast that is grown on a mixture of sugar beet molasses which is fermented, washed, pasteurized and dried at high temperatures. Used as a dietary supplement as it contains protein, fiber, vitamins and minerals. Available in pills, flakes or powder.
	Xanthan Gum	It is produced from the fermentation of corn sugar. This powder is used to thicken sauces and salad dressings, Also used in gluten-free baked products to improve the structure and texture.
	Guar Gum	A gum extracted from the seed of an East Indian plant. Available as a powder that is used as a thickener and stabilizer. Can be substituted for xanthan gum in gluten-free baked products. It is high in fiber and may have a laxative effect if consumed in large amounts.

Notes on Foods to Question

Food Category	Food Products	Notes
Milk & Dairy	Cheese Spreads, Cheese Sauces (e.g., Nacho), Seasoned (flavored) Shredded Cheese or Cheese Blends	May be thickened with wheat flour or wheat starch. Seasonings may contain hydrolyzed wheat protein, wheat flour or wheat starch.
	Flavored Yogurt, Frozen Yogurt	May contain granola, cookie crumbs or wheat bran.
Grains & Starches	Buckwheat Flour	Pure buckwheat flour is gluten-free, however, some buckwheat flour may be mixed with wheat flour.
	Rice & Corn Cereals	May contain barley malt, barley malt extract, barley malt flavoring.
	Buckwheat Pasta	Also called Japanese Soba noodles. Some Soba pasta contains pure buckwheat flour which is gluten-free but others may also contain wheat flour.
	Seasoned or Flavored Rice Mixes	Seasonings may contain hydrolyzed wheat protein, wheat flour or wheat starch or have added soy sauce that contains wheat.
	Multi-grain or Flavored Rice Crackers, Rice Cakes & Corn Cakes	Multi-grain products may contain barley and/or oats. Some contain soy sauce (made from wheat), seasonings containing hydrolyzed wheat protein, wheat flour or wheat starch.
	Corn Tortillas	May contain wheat flour.
	Low-Gluten Communion Wafers	The Catholic Canon Law, code 924.2, requires the presence of some wheat in communion wafers and will not accept the gluten-free hosts made with other grains. A very low-gluten host made with a small amount of specially processed wheat starch is available from the Benedictine Sisters of Perpetual Hope. The level of gluten in these hosts is extremely small (less than 37 micrograms or 0.037 milligrams per wafer). The Italian Celiac Association's scientific committee approved the use of the low gluten host. Many health professionals allow the use of this host. Some recommend consuming only 1/4 of a wafer per week. The decision of whether to use this host should be discussed with your health professional. The hosts can be purchased by contacting 1-800-223-2772 or email: altarbreads@benedictinesisters.org or write to Benedictine Sisters Altar Bread Department, 31970 State Highway P, Cyde, MO, 64432, USA. More information for Catholics with celiac disease can be found at www.catholicceliacs.org

Notes on Foods to Question

Food Category	Food Products	Notes
Meats & Alternatives	Deli/Luncheon Meats, Hot Dogs & Sausages, Dried Meats	May contain fillers made from wheat. Seasonings may contain hydrolyzed wheat protein, wheat flour or wheat starch.
	Meat & Sandwich Spreads	Products such as pâte may contain wheat flour or seasonings containing hydrolyzed wheat protein, wheat flour or wheat starch.
	Frozen Burgers (Meat, Poultry and Fish) and Meatloaf	May contain fillers (wheat flour, wheat starch, bread crumbs). Seasonings may contain hydrolyzed wheat protein, wheat flour or wheat starch.
	Ham (ready to cook)	Glaze may contain hydrolyzed wheat protein, wheat flour or wheat starch.
	Seasoned/Flavored Fish in Pouches	May contain wheat or barley.
	Imitation Fish Products (e.g., Surimi)	Imitation crab/seafood sticks may contain fillers such as wheat starch.
	Meat Substitutes (e.g., vegetarian burgers, sausages, roasts, nuggets, textured vegetable protein)	Often contain hydrolyzed wheat protein, wheat gluten, wheat starch or barley malt.
	Flavored Egg Products (frozen or liquid)	May contain hydrolyzed wheat protein.
	Baked Beans	Some are thickened with wheat flour.
	Seasoned or Dry Roasted Nuts, Pumpkin or Sunflower Seeds	May contain hydrolyzed wheat protein, wheat flour or wheat starch.
	Nut Butters (e.g., almond, peanut)	Most brands are gluten-free, however some specialty brands may contain wheat germ.
	Flavored Tofu	May contain soy sauce (made from wheat) or other seasonings that contain hydrolyzed wheat protein, wheat flour or wheat starch.
	Tempeh	A meat substitute made from fermented soybeans and millet or rice. Often seasoned with soy sauce (made from wheat).
	Miso	A condiment used in Oriental cooking made from fermented soybeans and/or barley, wheat or rice. Wheat or barley are the most common grains used.

Notes on Foods to Question

Food Category	Food Products	Notes
Fruits & Vegetables	Dates	Chopped, diced or extruded dates are packaged with oat flour, dextrose or rice flour. Oat flour or dextrose are the most common sources used.
	French-Fried Potatoes	Often cooked in the same oil as gluten-containing foods (e.g., breaded fish and chicken fingers) resulting in cross-contamination. Some French fries in various shapes may also contain wheat or barley flour.
Soups	Canned Soups, Dried Soup Mixes, Soup Bases & Bouillon Cubes	May contain noodles or barley. Cream soups are often thickened with wheat flour. Seasonings may contain hydrolyzed wheat protein, wheat flour or wheat starch.
Fats	Salad Dressings	May contain wheat flour, malt vinegar or soy sauce (made from wheat). Seasonings may contain hydrolyzed wheat protein, wheat flour or wheat starch.
	Suet	The hard fat around the loins and kidneys of beef and sheep. Flour may be added to packaged suet. Suet can be used to make mincemeat, steamed Christmas pudding and Haggis (a traditional Scottish dish).
	Cooking sprays	Baking cooking spray may contain wheat flour or wheat starch
Desserts	Cake Icing & Frostings	May contain wheat flour or wheat starch.
Sweets	Honey Powder	This commercial powder is used in glazes, seasoning mixes, dry mixes and sauces. May contain wheat flour or wheat starch.
	Hard Candies & Chocolates	May contain barley malt flavoring and/or wheat flour.
	Smarties®	Canadian product contains wheat flour.
	Chocolate Bars	May contain wheat flour or barley malt flavoring.
Snack Foods	Seasoned Potato Chips, Taco (corn) Chips, Nuts, Soy Nuts	Some potato chips contain wheat starch. Seasoning mixes may contain hydrolyzed wheat protein, wheat flour or wheat starch.
Beverages	Flavored or Herbal Teas Flavored Coffees	May contain barley malt flavoring. Some specialty coffees may be prepared with a chocolate chip-like product that contains cookie crumbs.
	Coffee Substitutes	Roasted chicory is the most common coffee substitute and is gluten-free. Other coffee substitutes are derived from wheat, rye, barley and/or malted barley.
	Hot Chocolate Mixes	May contail barley malt or wheat starch.

Notes on Foods to Question

Food Category	Food Products	Notes
Beverages	Flavored Alcoholic Cooler Beverages	May contain barley malt.
	Caesar Vodka Beverage Mix	May contain hydrolyzed wheat protein.
Condiments/ Sauces	Specialty Prepared Mustards	Some brands contain wheat flour.
	Prepared Mustard Flour	Made from ground mustard seed, sugar, salt and spices which are gluten-free. However, some brands also contain wheat flour.
	Mustard Pickles	May contain wheat flour and/or malt vinegar.
	Worcestershire Sauce	May contain malt vinegar.
	Salsa	Some brands contain wheat flour, wheat starch, hydrolyzed wheat protein or malt extract.
	Curry Paste	Made from the pulp of the tamarind pod and a variety of spices. Some curry pastes may also contain wheat flour or wheat starch.
	Baking Powder	Most brands contain cornstarch which is gluten-free. However, some brands contain wheat starch.
	Seasoning Mixes	Some brands contain wheat flour, wheat starch or hydrolyzed wheat protein as the carrier agent.
	Wasabi Peas	Roasted green peas coated in wasabi. Some brands contain wheat flour or wheat starch.

Notes on Foods to Avoid

Food Category	Food Products	Notes
Milk Products	Malted Milk	Contains malt powder derived from malted barley.
Grains	Semolina	A coarsely ground grain (usually made from the refined portion of durum wheat) that can be used to make porridge or pasta.
	Atta	A fine whole-meal flour made from low-gluten, soft texturized wheat used to make Indian flat bread. Also known as chapatti flour.
	Bulgur (Burghul)	Quick-cooking form of whole wheat. Wheat kernels that are parboiled (partially cooked), dried and then cracked. Used in soups, pilafs, stuffing or salad (e.g., Tabouli).
	Einkorn, Emmer, Farro, Kamut, Spelt	Types of wheat. Many "wheat-free" foods are made from these varieties of wheat, especially kamut and spelt. Remeber that "wheat-free" does not always mean "gluten-free."
	Triticale	A cereal grain that is a cross between wheat and rye.
	Orzo	A type of pasta that is the size and shape of rice. Used in soups and as a substitute for rice.
	Matzoh	Unleavened bread made with wheat flour and water that comes in thin sheets. Used primarily during Passover.
	Matzoh Meal	Ground matzoh.
	Matzoh Balls	Dumplings made of matzoh meal which is not gluten-free. However, can be made with potato flour which is gluten-free.
	Couscous	Granules of semolina (made from durum wheat) that are precooked and dried. Cooked couscous is served hot or cold as a dish or salad.
	Tabouli	A salad usually made with bulgur wheat or couscous which are not gluten-free. Can also be made with quinoa which is gluten-free.

Notes on Foods to Avoid

Food Category	Food Products	Notes
Meats & Alternatives	Fu	A dried gluten product derived from wheat that is sold as thin sheets or thick round cakes. Used as a protein supplement in Asian dishes such as soups and vegetables.
	Seitan	A meat-like food derived from wheat gluten used in many vegetarian dishes. Sometimes called "wheat meat."
Other	Licorice	Regular licorice contains wheat flour.
	Cereal & Malted Beverages	Contain malted barley or other grains such as wheat or rye (e.g., Postum, Ovaltine).
	Beer, Ale & Lager	Basic ingredients include malted barley, hops (a type of flower), yeast and water. As this mixture is only fermented and not distilled, it contains varying levels of gluten.
	Potato Chips	Some brands of plain potato chips contain added wheat flour and/or wheat starch.
	Soy Sauce	Many brands are a combination of soy and wheat.
	Malt Vinegar	Made from malted barley. As this vinegar is only fermented and not distilled, it contains varying levels of gluten.
	Brewer's Yeast	A dried inactive yeast that is a bitter by-product of the brewing industry. It is not commonly used as a flavoring agent in foods. ELISA tests are unable to accurately confirm the amount of residual gluten in this type of yeast.

Gluten-Free Additives and Ingredients

Additives

- Acetic Acid
- Adipic Acid
- Benzoic Acid
- BHA
- BHT
- Calcium Disodium EDTA
- Fumaric Acid
- Glucono-delta-lactone
- Lactic Acid
- Lecithin
- Malic Acid
- Mono and diglycerides
- Polysorbate 60; 80
- Propionic Acid
- Propylene Glycol
- Rennet
- Silicon Dioxide
- Sodium Benzoate
- Sodium Metabisulphite
- Sodium Nitrate
- Sodium Nitrite
- Sodium Sulphite
- Sorbate
- Sorbic Acid
- Stearic Acid
- Tartaric Acid
- Titanium Dioxide

Coloring Agents

- Natural Colors [e.g. annatto, caramel color: pg. 57, carotene, beta carotene, paprika]
- Artificial Colors [e.g., tartrazine*, sunset yellow FCF, erythrosine, citrus red No. 2, brilliant blue FCF, fast green FCF, titanium dioxide]

Flavoring Agents**

- Ethyl Maltol
- Maltol
- Monosodium Glutamate (MSG)
- Vanilla
- Vanilla Extract
- Vanilla Flavoring
- Vanillin

Sugars/Sweeteners

- Acesulfame-potassium
- Agave
- Aspartame
- Brown Sugar
- Cane Sugar
- Corn Syrup/Solids
- Dextrose
- Fructose
- Glucose
- Glucose Syrup: pg. 53
- Honey
- Icing Sugar (confectioner's)
- Invert Sugar
- Isomalt
- Lactose
- Maltitol
- Maltitol Syrup
- Maltose
- Mannitol
- Molasses
- Saccharin
- Sorbitol
- Stevia
- Sucralose
- Sucrose
- White Sugar
- Xylitol

Vegetable Gums

- Acacia Gum (Gum Arabic)
- Agar (Agar-Agar)
- Algin (Alginic Acid)
- Carageenan
- Carboxymethylcellulose (Cellulose Gum)
- Carob Bean (Locust Bean)
- Guaiac Gum
- Guar Gum
- Karaya Gum
- Methylcellulose
- Tragacanth Gum
- Xanthan Gum

Miscellaneous

- Ascorbic Acid
- Autolyzed Yeast
- Baker's Yeast
- Beta Carotene
- Cream of Tartar
- Gelatin
- Lecithin
- Maltodextrin: pg. 52
- Modified Food Starches (except wheat starch) pg. 51-52
- Nutritional Yeast
- Papain
- Pectin
- Psyllium
- Starches (except wheat starch) pg. 51
- Torula Yeast

---

* A very small number of individuals may experience an allergic-type reaction to the yellow food color tartrazine, however this is unrelated to gluten.

** For more information on natural and artificial flavorings see pages 45-47.

Note: This is not an all-inclusive listing. For a more comprehensive listing of ingredients see the Canadian Celiac Association's *Pocket Dictionary: Acceptability of Foods and Food Ingredients for the Gluten-Free Diet* on page 347.

HYDROLYZED PLANT PROTEIN OR HYDROLYZED VEGETABLE PROTEIN (HPP OR HVP)

✦ Hydrolyzed plant/vegetable proteins are used as flavoring agents in a wide variety of foods such as soups, sauces, gravies and seasoning mixtures.

✦ Most hydrolyzed plant proteins are made from corn, soy or wheat (or a combination of 2 or 3 plant proteins) but can be made from other protein sources such as peanut.

✦ Hydrolysis involves breaking down the protein by acids or enzymes. Depending on the type of hydrolysis and degree of hydrolysis, the protein is not always completely broken down, resulting in residual protein levels in the final product. It is for this reason that hydrolyzed wheat protein should be avoided.

USA (Code of Federal Regulations)	Sec.102.22 Protein Hydrolysates The common or usual name of a protein hydrolysate shall be specific to the ingredient and shall include the identity of the food source from which the protein was derived (e.g., "Hydrolyzed wheat gluten," "hydrolyzed soy protein"). The names "hydrolyzed protein" and "hydrolyzed vegetable protein" are not acceptable because they do not identify the food source of the protein.
CANADA (Food & Drug Regulations)	B.01.009 (1) #30 Components of ingredients or of classes of ingredients are not required to be shown on a label of foods identified in this section of the Regulations. In this case "Hydrolyzed plant protein" is acceptable and the plant source does not have to be identified. Note: This refers to plant proteins hydrolyzed by methods other than enzymatic (e.g., acid hydrolysis).
	B.01.010 (3) (a) #8 The ingredient or component of an item shall be shown in the list of ingredients by the common name. Hydrolyzed plant protein produced by the enzymatic process must be listed "hydrolyzed" plus the "name of the plant" plus "protein" (e.g., "hydrolyzed soy protein"). Note: At the time of printing this book, recommendations for identifying the plant source of all types of hydrolyzed plant proteins and including it in the common name of the list of ingredients are being considered under the *Enhanced Labelling For Food Allergens and Gluten Sources and Added Sulphites*. (See pages 69-70).

FLAVORINGS

✦ There are several thousand substances that can be used to flavor foods, including those derived from natural sources (e.g., fruits, vegetables, plant materials, spices, meats, fish, poultry, eggs, dairy products and yeast) and artificial sources (e.g., those obtained by chemical synthesis).

✦ Canadian and American food labelling regulations differ in how they define the term flavorings (see pages 46-47).

✦ According to flavor experts from industry and government in Canada and the USA, gluten-containing grains are not commonly used as flavoring agents. However, there are two exceptions:

1. Hydrolyzed wheat, corn and/or soy proteins can be used as "flavors" or "flavor enhancers" in a variety of foods. In Canada and the USA, they must be declared as "hydrolyzed proteins" and not hidden on the label as "flavor" or "natural flavor" [*Food and Drug Regulations* B.01.009 (3) in *Canada and Code of Federal Regulations* Sec. 101.22 (h) (7) in the USA].

2. Barley malt extract/syrup can be used as a flavoring agent and is almost always listed on the label as "barley malt," "barley malt extract" or "barley malt flavoring." Some companies may list it as "flavor (contains barley malt)" and very rarely is it listed as only "flavor" or "natural flavor." See pages 55-56 for more information on barley malt extract/syrup/flavoring.

✦ It would be rare to find a "natural or artificial flavoring" containing gluten because: (a) hydrolyzed wheat protein cannot be hidden under the term "flavor," and (b) barley malt extract or barley malt flavoring is almost always declared as "barley malt extract" or "barley malt flavoring." For this reason, most experts do not restrict natural and artificial flavorings in the gluten-free diet.

USA *(Code of Federal Regulations)*	**Sec.101.22 Foods; labeling of spices, flavorings, colorings and chemical preservatives** **(a) (1) Artificial Flavor or Artificial Flavoring:** Any substance, the function of which is to impart flavor, which is not derived from a spice, fruit or fruit juice, vegetable or vegetable juice, edible yeast, herb, bark, bud, root, leaf or similar plant material, meat, fish, poultry, eggs, dairy products, or fermentation products thereof. Artificial flavor includes the substances listed in Sec. 172.515 (b) and 182.60 [Synthetic flavoring substances and adjuvants] except where these are derived from natural sources. **(a) (3) Natural Flavor or Natural Flavoring:** The essential oil, oleoresin, essence or extractive, protein hydrolysate, distillate, or any product of roasting, heating or enzymolysis, which contains the flavoring constituents derived from a spice, fruit or fruit juice, vegetable or vegetable juice, edible yeast, herb, bark, bud, root, leaf or similar plant material, meat, seafood, poultry, eggs, dairy products, or fermentation products thereof, whose significant function in food is flavoring rather than nutritional. Natural flavors include the natural essence or extractives obtained from plants listed in Sec. 182.10, 182.20, 182.40 and 182.50 and substances listed in 172.510 [natural flavoring substances and natural substances, e.g., include flowers, roots, herbs, leaves.]
	Sec.101.22 Foods; labeling of spices, flavorings, colorings and chemical preservatives **(h) Labeling of a food to which Flavor is added:** (1) Spice, natural flavor and artificial flavor may be declared as "spice", "natural flavor" or "artificial flavor" or any combination thereof. (7) Because protein hydrolysates function in foods as both flavorings and flavor enhancers, no protein hydrolysate used in food for its effects on flavor may be declared simply as "flavor," "natural flavor" or "flavoring." The ingredients shall be declared by its specific common or usual name as provided in Sec. 102.22.

	Sec. 403 (i) (2) Spices, flavorings and colors, when used as ingredients in other foods, are exempt from a declaration of their components, except for "hypoallergenic foods" Sec. 105.62 (see page 66). **Note:** Effective January 1, 2006, the *Food Allergen Labeling and Consumer Protection Act* required the components of flavorings to be declared on the label if they contain any of the top eight allergens which includes wheat but not barley or rye. (See pages 66-67).
CANADA *(Food & Drug Regulations)*	**B.01.010 (3) (b)** The ingredients or components may be shown in the list of ingredients by the common name. **#4 "Flavour"** One or more substances prepared for their flavouring properties and produced from animal or vegetable raw materials or from food constituents derived solely from animal or vegetable raw materials. **#5 "Artificial Flavour," "Imitation Flavour" or "Simulated Flavour"** One or more substances prepared for their flavouring properties and derived in whole or in part from components obtained by chemical synthesis. **#13 "Name of Plant or Animal Source Plus Flavour"** One or more substances the function of which is to impart flavour and that are obtained solely from the plant or animal source after which the flavour is named.
	B.01.009 (2) #2, #3 and #10 Flavouring preparations, artificial flavouring preparations and food flavour-enhancer preparations, when used as ingredients in other foods, are exempt from a declaration of their ingredients or components, except for the ingredients or components listed in B.01.009 (3) and (4).
	B.01.009 (3) Salt, glutamic acid, or its salts, including MSG, hydrolysed plant protein, aspartame, potassium chloride and any ingredient or component that performs a function in, or has any effect on, that food when present in the preparations or mixture listed in B.01.009 (2) must always be shown by their common names in the list of ingredients to which the preparation or mixture is added, as if they were ingredients of that food.
	B.01.009 (4) Peanut oil, hydrogenated peanut oil and modified peanut oil when present in the foods listed in B.01.009 (1) and the preparations and mixtures listed in B.01.009 (2) must always be listed by name in the list of ingredients. **Note:** At the time of printing this book, recommendations for identifying all cereal grains containing gluten when they are present in foods as ingredients or components in the list of ingredients are currently being considered under the *Enhanced Labelling For Food Allergen and Gluten Sources and Added Sulphites*. (See pages 69-70).

Spices, Herbs and Seasonings

✦ A wide variety of spices and herbs are used in foods for flavoring purposes.

✦ Canadian and American regulations have some differences in how they define the terms spices, seasonings and herbs (see pages 49-50).

✦ **Spices, herbs and seeds do not contain gluten.** Although an anti-caking agent may sometimes be added to spices, it is often silicon dioxide, calcium silicate or sodium aluminum silica and NOT wheat flour or wheat starch. Some imitation black peppers contain other ingredients such as buckwheat hulls and ground rice in addition to black pepper. The author has not been able to find any companies using wheat as a filler in imitation pepper or spices.

✦ In general terms "seasonings" are a blend of flavoring agents (e.g., spices, herbs) and an anti-caking agent (e.g., calcium silicate) which are often combined with a carrier agent (e.g., salt, sugar, lactose, whey powder, starches or flours). **The carrier agent in seasoning mixtures in gravy mixes, sauces and snack foods often contain wheat flour or wheat starch.** Seasonings are usually combined with the other dry ingredients in sauces or gravy mixes, however, snack foods are coated with the seasoning mixture, which requires a larger quantity of the carrier agent.

✦ If a seasoning mixture/blend is sold separately as a bottled or packaged seasoning such as Cajun Seasoning, Taco Seasoning Mix, etc., the components of ingredients must be declared. For example:

Cajun Seasoning: Spice (including red pepper), salt, dehydrated vegetables (onion, green bell pepper, celery, garlic, parsley), sugar, hydrogenated soybean and cottonseed oil, calcium silicate, disodium inosinate and guanylate, ascorbic acid, modified cornstarch, extractives of lemon.

Taco Seasoning: Spice (including red pepper), dehydrated onion, salt, garlic powder, hydrolyzed wheat protein, citric acid, yeast extract.

✦ It should be noted that, in Canada, seasoning, spice or herb mixtures, when used as ingredients in other foods are exempt from a declaration of their components (see page 50). Although it is not currently required by regulation, Health Canada strongly urges manufacturers to declare components of ingredients such as seasonings if they contain allergens or gluten sources. Fortunately many companies are voluntarily labeling the components of seasonings when used in other foods. Also, Health Canada has proposed new labeling regulations entitled *Schedule No. 1220- Enhanced Labelling For Food Allergen and Gluten Sources and Added Sulphites* that would make it mandatory to declare allergen and gluten sources if used as components of ingredients (see pages 69-70).

✦ In the USA, effective January 1, 2006, the *Food Allergen Labeling and Consumer Protection Act* required all components of ingredients when used in other foods be declared if they contain any of the top eight allergens. Also, whenever the term "seasoning" is used in the ingredient statement of a meat or poultry product, its components must be identified as a sublist. (Note: meat and poultry product labeling is under the jurisdiction of the USDA {United States Department of Agriculture}. However, if a meat or poultry product is used as an ingredient in relatively small amounts in another food product, it falls under the jurisdiction of FDA {Food and Drug Administration} in the USA).

USA *(Code of Federal Regulations)*	**Sec. 101.22 (2) (a) Spices**
	The term spice means any aromatic vegetable substance in the whole, broken or ground form, except for those substances which have traditionally been regarded as foods, such as onions, garlic and celery; whose significant function in food is seasoning rather than nutritional; that is true to name; and from which no portion of any volatile oil or other flavoring principle has been removed. Spices include the spices listed in sec.182.10 (such as the following: allspice, anise, basil, bay leaves . . .). Paprika, turmeric and saffron or other spices which are also colors, shall be declared as "spice and coloring" unless declared by their common name.
	Sec. 170. Food Additives
	Sec. 170.3 (26) Definitions
	Herbs, seeds, spices, seasonings, blends, extracts and flavorings, including all natural and artificial spices, blends and flavors.
	Sec. 182.10 Spices and Other Natural Seasonings and Flavorings
	Spices and other natural seasonings and flavorings that are generally recognized as safe for their intended use, within the meaning of section 409 of the act, are as follows (83 items are listed by their common name and botanical name).
	Sec. 403 (i) (2)
	Spices, flavorings and colors, when used as ingredients in other foods are exempt from a declaration of their components (except for "hypoallergenic foods" Sec. 105.62 – see page 66).
	Notes: (1) Effective January 1, 2006, the *Food Allergen Labeling and Consumer Protection Act* required the components of spices and seasonings to be declared on the label if they contain any of the top eight allergens which includes wheat but not barley or rye. (See pages 66-67).
	(2) There is no specific definition of the term "seasoning". However, sections 101.22, 170.3 and 182.10 refer to spices that act as a "seasoning agent."

CANADA *(Food & Drug Regulations)*	**B.01.010 (3) (b) #6**
	The ingredients or components may be shown in the list of ingredients by the common name. One or more spices, seasonings or herbs (except salt) can also be called "spices," "seasonings" or "herbs."
	B.01.009 (2) #4 & #5
	Spice mixtures or seasoning or herb mixtures, when used as ingredients in other foods are exempt from a declaration of their components except for those ingredients or components listed in B.01.009 (3) and (4).
	B.01.009 (3)
	Salt, glutamic acid, or its salts, including MSG, hydrolyzed plant protein, aspartame, potassium chloride and any ingredient or component that performs a function in, or has any effect on, that food when present in the preparations or mixture listed in B.01.009 (2) must always be shown by their common names in the list of ingredients to which the preparation or mixture is added, as if they were ingredients of that food.
	B.01.009 (4)
	Peanut oil, hydrogenated peanut oil and modified peanut oil when present in the foods listed in B.01.009 (1) and the preparations and mixtures listed in B.01.009 (2) must always be listed by name in the list of ingredients.
	Note:
	1. There is no specific definition of the term seasoning.
	2. The class name "seasoning" is permitted if a seasoning mixture is added to a food at 2% or less of weight of the final product.
	3. At the time of printing this book, recommendations for identifying all cereal grains containing gluten when they are present in foods as ingredients or components in the list of ingredients are currently being considered under the *Enhanced Labelling For Food Allergen and Gluten Sources and Added Sulphites*. (See pages 69-70).

References

✦ Author's personal communication with the Canadian Flavour Manufacturers Association (CFMA), United States Flavor and Extract Manufacturers Association (FEMA), various manufacturers in Canada and the USA, Canadian Food Inspection Agency (CFIA), Health Canada (HC) and the Food and Drug Administration (FDA).

✦ Tainter D, Grenis A. *Spices and Seasonings in Food Technology Handbook*, John Wiley and Sons, New York, 2001; pages 198-232.

✦ *Gluten-Free Living* magazine. November/December 2000; Vol. 5, No. 6.

STARCHES

✦ Starches are used as a thickening agent; binding agent; and carrier agent (especially in seasonings).

✦ A variety of starches can be used in foods such as corn, waxy maize, potato, milo (sorghum), waxy milo, potato, tapioca, arrowroot, rice, wheat, etc.

✦ The single word "starch" on a food label in Canada and the USA refers to "cornstarch."

✦ When other starches such as potato, tapioca or wheat are used in food products, the source of the starch must be declared.

✦ **Wheat starch must be avoided due to residual gluten levels.**

USA *(Compliance Policy Guideline)*	**CPG Sec. 578.100** There is no standard identity for food starches in the *Code of Federal Regulations*. However the CPG Sec. 578.100 provides guidelines for the labeling of starches. **Sec. 578.100 Starches** The single word "starch" on a food label is considered the common or usual name for starch made from corn; alternatively, the name "cornstarch" may be used. Starches from other sources should be designated by some non-misleading term that indicates the source of such starch, for example, "potato starch", "wheat starch", or "tapioca starch."
CANADA *(Food & Drug Regulations)*	Starches are presently required to be identified by plant source on the food label except cornstarch, which can be called "cornstarch" or just "starch" made from maize. **B.13.011 [S]** cornstarch shall be starch made from maize.

MODIFIED FOOD STARCHES

✦ A common ingredient in foods used as a texture stabilizing agent; thickener or binding agent; anti-caking agent.

✦ A starch that has been chemically modified to alter its physical properties.

✦ Modified food starches can be made from corn, waxy maize, tapioca, potato, wheat or other starches.

✦ In North America, modified corn, waxy maize and potato are the most common sources, with tapioca and wheat used occasionally.

✦ Wheat starch is used more frequently in European countries. A special type of modified wheat starch is used in some European gluten-free products. However, wheat starch is not permitted in food labeled gluten-free in Canada. There is debate within the scientific community as to the safety of gluten-free products using this special type of wheat starch. The concern is that not all traces of protein can be removed during the processing of wheat starch, resulting in various levels of residual gluten. See references on wheat starch on pages 57-58 and background information on pages 61-62. **Further research is necessary to determine what level of gluten is safe for people with celiac disease, including the use of wheat starch.**

USA (Code of Federal Regulations)	Sec. 172.892 Food Starch – Modified
	Regulations for how food starches may be modified. However, there is no requirement for the identification of the name of the plant source of the modified food starch.
	Note: Effective January 1, 2006 the *Food Allergen Labeling and Consumer Protection Act* required the top eight allergens (which includes wheat) to be declared on all product labels. If wheat is used in modified food starch it must be declared on the label as modified wheat starch or modified food starch (wheat).
CANADA (Food & Drug Regulations)	There is no requirement for the identification of the name of the plant source of the modified food starch.
	Note: At the time of printing this book, recommendations for identifying the plant source of all types of starches and modified starches and including them in the list of ingredients are being considered under the *Enhanced Labelling For Food Allergen and Gluten Sources and Added Sulphites*. (See pages 69-70).

MALTODEXTRIN

✦ It is used as an anti-caking and free-flowing agent, formulation aid, processing aid, carrier agent for flavors, bulking agent, stabilizer and thickener, or surface-finishing agent in a wide variety of foods.

✦ Maltodextrin is a purified, concentrated, non-sweet nutritive mixture of saccharide polymers obtained by hydrolysis of edible starch.

✦ Can be derived from different starches such as corn, waxy maize, potato, rice or wheat.

✦ Corn, waxy maize or potato are the most common sources in North America.

✦ Wheat-based maltodextrin is used more frequently in Europe and is now being used in some North American products. **Although maltodextrin may be derived from wheat, it is highly processed and purified (significantly more than modified food starches).** North American and European scientists using the most sensitive, scientifically validated R5 ELISA Tests have found very low levels or no gluten in wheat-based maltodextrin. As this ingredient is added to food products in small quantities, the final product would contain **insignificant levels of gluten**. The European Food Safety Authority (EFSA) has permanently exempted wheat-based maltodextrin and glucose syrup from allergen labeling based on this recent research.

USA (Code of Federal Regulations)	Sec. 184.1444 Maltodextrin
	CAS Reg. No. 9050-36-6. It is a nonsweet nutritive saccharide polymer that consists of D-glucose units linked primarily by [alpha]-1-4 bonds and has a dextrose equivalent (DE) of less than 20. It is prepared as a white powder or concentrated solution by partial hydrolysis of cornstarch, potato starch or rice starch with safe and suitable acids and enzymes.
	Note: FDA also permits the use of other starches including wheat. For example, if wheat is used it must be labeled "wheat maltodextrin".
CANADA (Food & Drug Regulations)	There is no standard for maltodextrin. The Food Chemical Codex is often used as a guide, however, different starches can be used. Food companies are strongly encouraged to indicate the source if it is from the major food allergens such as wheat.

DEXTRIN

✦ It is used as a thickener; colloidal stabilizer; binder or surface finishing agent in cosmetics, medications and industrial applications. Not commonly used in foods.

✦ Dextrin is starch partially hydrolyzed by heat alone or by heating in the presence of suitable food-grade acids and buffers from any of several grain or root-based native (unmodified) starches (e.g., corn, waxy maize, milo, waxy milo, potato, arrowroot, wheat, rice, tapioca, sago, etc.).

✦ Usually made from corn or tapioca, although occasionally it can be derived from wheat.

✦ As dextrin is only partially hydrolyzed, there is residual protein in the final product. **Wheat-based dextrin when used in foods must be avoided due to residual gluten levels.**

USA *(Code of Federal Regulations)*	**Sec. 184.1277 Dextrin** Definition is based on the Food Chemical Codex CAS Reg. 9004-53-9. **Note:** Effective January 1, 2006 the *Food Allergen Labeling and Consumer Protection Act* required the top 8 allergens (which includes wheat) to be declared on all product labels. If wheat is used in dextrin it must be declared as wheat dextrin or dextrin (wheat).
CANADA *(Food & Drug Regulations)*	**Division 18** Although dextrin does not appear in the standards for Sweetening Agents of Division 18, it is considered a food ingredient of this category.

GLUCOSE SYRUP

✦ Used extensively in foods for sweetening, browning, texture-modification, bulking, moisture control and enhancing shelf-life of various foods.

✦ Can be derived from a variety of starches such as corn, tapioca, potato, wheat, sorghum, barley and rice.

✦ Corn is the most common source in North America, whereas wheat starch is more commonly used in Europe.

✦ **Although glucose syrup may be derived from wheat or barley, it is highly processed and purified (significantly more than modified food starches)** in order to separate and remove the protein from the starch mixture. Enzymes (usually fungal or bacterial) are then added to break down the starch to form glucose syrup. Scientists and research centers in Europe, Australia and other countries using the highly sensitive R5 ELISA tests have found very low levels or no gluten in these glucose syrups. As this ingredient is added to food products in small quantities, the final product would contain **insignificant levels of gluten**. The European Food Safety Authority (EFSA) has permanently exempted wheat-based and barley-based glucose syrups from allergen labeling based on this recent research.

USA *(Code of Federal Regulations)*	**Sec. 168.120 Glucose Sirup** a) Glucose sirup is the purified, concentrated, aqueous solution of nutritive saccharides obtained from edible starch. c) The name of the food is "Glucose Sirup". When the food is derived from a specific type of starch, the name may alternatively be "___ sirup", the blank to be filled in with the name of the starch. For example, "corn sirup," "wheat sirup," "tapioca sirup." When the starch is derived from sorghum grain, the alternative name of the food is "sorghum grain sirup." The word "sirup" may also be spelled "syrup."
	Sec. 184.1865 Corn Syrup a) Corn syrup, commonly called "glucose sirup" or "glucose syrup" is obtained by partial hydrolysis of corn starch with safe and suitable acids or enzymes. It may also occur in the dehydrated form (dried glucose sirup). Depending on the degree of hydrolysis, corn syrup may contain, in addition to glucose, maltose and higher saccharides.
CANADA *(Food & Drug Regulations)*	**B.18.016 [S] Glucose or Glucose Syrup** a) shall be the purified concentrated solution of nutritive saccharides obtained from the incomplete hydrolysis by means of acid or enzymes, of starch or a starch-containing substance.
	B.18.017 [S] Glucose Solids or Dried Glucose Syrup a) shall be glucose or glucose syrup from which the water has been partially removed.

Rice Syrup

✦ Consumers and the food industry use this type of glucose syrup as a substitute for sugar, honey or other refined sweeteners. Like other starch-based syrups, rice syrups are used for other functions in addition to sweetening such as browning, texture modification, bulking, controlling moisture and enhancing shelf-life of various foods.

✦ Used in rice drinks, snack bars, cereals, baked goods and other foods.

✦ There are several different types of rice syrups available.

✦ Can be made from brown or white rice and the addition of laboratory-produced enzymes (bacterial or fungal), Koji enzymes (cultured rice made from rice and koji mold spores) or barley malt enzymes. Rice, water and the enzymes are gently heated which causes the starch, protein and fat to be broken down. This mixture is processed and slowly cooked to produce a thick, sweet syrup. Unlike glucose syrups which are derived only from the starch component of grains and are highly processed, rice syrup is derived from the grain (brown rice syrup is from the whole grain including the fiber) and is less processed. As a result, rice syrup, especially brown rice syrup contains a small amount of protein, vitamins and minerals.

✦ **Most rice syrups in North America are gluten-free as they are made using bacterial or fungal enzymes. Occasionally it is made with barley malt enzymes which may contain very low levels of residual gluten.**

✦ Rice syrup is sometimes referred to as "rice malt." However the rice does not undergo the process of germination/sprouting as in malted barley. Instead, the rice is cooked with an enzyme preparation to break down the starch into a syrup.

BARLEY MALT

✦ Used in the production of malted beverages (e.g., beer, ale, lager and malted milk), distilled alcoholic beverages and malt vinegar. May also be used in doughs to increase the fermentation rate and improve baking properties.

✦ Barley malt can be further processed into various extracts/syrups (see below).

✦ Derived from whole-grain barley that has been soaked, germinated (sprouted) and dried.

✦ A very wide variety of malts in many different flavors and colors can be produced by altering the length of time and temperature of the drying process. Brewer's malts contain higher amounts of active enzymes, starches and sugars used for the fermentation process. Specialty malts contain lower amounts of enzymes and sugars available for fermentation and are used more for flavoring agents.

✦ Available as a powder or liquid.

✦ **Contains varying levels of gluten.**

BARLEY MALT EXTRACT/BARLEY MALT SYRUP

✦ These terms are often used interchangeably.

✦ Malt extract/syrup is used by both the brewing and food industries. During the brewing of beer, it is added for specific flavoring and coloring properties. Food companies also use malt extract/syrup in many foods such as cereals and granola, baked products, crackers, cookies and beverages.

✦ Malt extract/syrup is derived from a mixture of malted barley and water that is steeped, mashed, filtered and then evaporated to remove the excess water, resulting in a sweet, viscous liquid containing approximately 75-80% solids. Because malt extract/syrup is made from the whole-grain malted barley, it contains proteins and free amino acids, nutritive carbohydrates, phytochemicals, vitamins and minerals. These constituents increase the nutritional value of malt extract compared to starch-based glucose syrups (e.g., corn, wheat) that are highly processed and void of these nutritional components. It is these nutritional constituents in barley malt extract that account for its fermentation and browning properties.

✦ To reduce the cost of barley malt extract/syrup, some companies use a combination of malted barley and malted corn. However, this must be labeled as "extract of malted barley and corn" and not "malt extract/syrup."

✦ Available as a powder or liquid.

✦ **Contains varying levels of gluten.**

USA *(Code of Federal Regulations)*	**Sec.184.1443a Malt** (a) Malt is an enzyme preparation obtained from barley which has been softened by a series of steeping operations and germinated under controlled conditions. It is a brown, sweet, and viscous liquid or a white to tan powder. Its characterizing enzyme activities are [alpha]-amylase and [beta]-amylase. (c)(1) The ingredient is used as an enzyme as defined in Sec. 170.3(o)(9) of this chapter to hydrolyze starch or starch-derived polysaccharides.
	Sec. 184.1445 Malt Syrup (malt extract) (a) Malt is the product of barley (Hordeum vulgare L.) germinated under controlled conditions. Malt syrup and malt extract are interchangeable terms for a viscous concentrate of water extract of germinated barley grain, with or without added safe preservative. Malt syrup is usually a brown, sweet and viscous liquid containing varying amounts of amylolytic enzymes and plant constituents. Barley is first softened after cleaning by steeping operations and then allowed to germinate under controlled conditions. The germinated grain then undergoes processing, such as drying, grinding, extracting, filtering and evaporating, to produce malt syrup (malt extract) with 75-80% solids or dried malt syrup with higher solids content. The ingredient is used as a flavoring agent and adjuvant as defined in Sec. 170.3(o) (12) of this chapter.
	Compliance Policy Guide 7105.02 Sec. 515.200 Malt Extract; Malt Syrup; Malted Cereal Syrup; Liquid Malt; Dried Malt Policy: The designation "malt extract" and "malt syrup" should be used only for concentrated water infusions of malt, with or without added safe preservative. The terms "malt extract" and "malt syrup" unqualified should be applied only to products prepared from barley. If any other malted grain is used, the extract or syrup may be designated by a specific name such as "extract of malted barley and corn." The term "liquid malt" is considered false and misleading as applied to mixtures of malt extract or malt syrup with corn syrup or other substances which are not normal constituents of malt extract.

BARLEY MALT FLAVORING

✦ Malt flavoring can be made from barley malt extract/syrup; a combination of barley malt extract/syrup and corn syrup; or synthetic ingredients not derived from barley.

✦ Most companies use a combination of barley malt extract/syrup AND corn syrup.

✦ Contains less gluten than barley malt and barley malt extract/syrup as it is usually mixed with corn syrup and is used in smaller amounts than pure barley malt or barley malt extract/syrup. **Nevertheless, it still must also be avoided as it contains varying levels of gluten.** For example, corn and rice cereals with barley malt flavoring have recently been tested and found to contain over 200 ppm (see pages 61-64 on testing of foods in gluten and measurement levels).

CARAMEL COLOR

✦ Used extensively in a wide variety of food and beverages such as baked products and mixes, cereals, snack foods, soups, sauces, gravies, spice blends, processed meat products, soft drinks and alcoholic beverages (e.g., beer, whiskey, rum and liqueurs) as a coloring agent. Can also act as a flavor enhancer.

✦ Produced by carefully controlled heat treatment of food-grade nutritive sweeteners consisting of fructose, dextrose (glucose), invert sugar, sucrose and/or starch hydrolysates and fractions thereof in the presence of food-grade acids, alkalis and/or salts.

✦ There are many types of caramel color on the market ranging from tannish yellow to reddish brown to nearly black with an odor of burnt sugar and a pleasant but slightly bitter taste.

✦ Although gluten-containing ingredients (barley malt syrup and starch hydrolysates) can be used in the production of caramel color, North American companies use corn as it has a longer shelf life and makes a superior product. European companies use glucose syrup derived from wheat starch, however **caramel color is highly processed and contains no gluten**.

USA (Code of Federal Regulations)	Sec. 73.85 Caramel
	(a) Identity. (1) The color additive caramel is the dark-brown liquid or solid material resulting from the carefully controlled heat treatment of the following food-grade carbohydrates: dextrose, invert sugar, lactose, malt sirup, molasses, starch hydrolysates and fractions thereof, sucrose. (2) The food-grade acids, alkalis, and salts listed in this subparagraph may be employed to assist caramelization, in amounts consistent with good manufacturing practice.
	(c) Uses and restrictions. Caramel may be safely used for coloring foods generally, in amounts consistent with good manufacturing practice, except that it may not be used to color foods for which standards of identity have been promulgated under section 401 of the act unless added color is authorized by such standards.

References and Information Sources for Starches, Maltodextrin, Dextrin, Glucose Syrup, Rice Syrup, Barley Malt and Caramel Color

✦ Canadian Celiac Association *Pocket Dictionary: Acceptability of Foods and Food Ingredients for the Gluten-Free Diet* (Second edition) 2005.

✦ Caballero B., Trugo C.L., Finglas P.M., *Encyclopedia of Food Sciences and Nutrition*, Academic Press, Elsevier Science Ltd., 2003

✦ Valdes L, García E, Llorente M, Méndez E. Innovative approach to low-level gluten determination in foods using a novel sandwich enzyme-linked immunosorbent assay protocol. *Eur J Gastroenterol Hepatol* 2003; 15:465-474.

✦ Collin P, Thorell L, Kaukinen K, Mäki M. The safe threshold for gluten contamination in gluten-free products. Can trace amounts be accepted in the treatment of coeliac disease? *Aliment Pharmacol Ther* 2004; 19:1277-1283.

✦ Chartrand L, Russo P, Duhaime A, Seidman E. Wheat starch intolerance in patients with celiac disease. *J Am Diet Assoc* 1997; 97:612-618.

✦ Thompson T. Wheat starch, gliadin, and the gluten-free diet. *J Am Diet Assoc* 2001; 101:1456-1459.

✦ Inclusion of wheat starch-based gluten-free foods in a dietary pattern for people with celiac disease. American Dietetic Association Evidence Analysis Library. Accessed November 25, 2005. www.adaevidencelibrary.com

✦ CAS Reg. No. 9050-36-6 (maltodextrin), CAS Reg. No. 9004-53-8 (dextrin) and CAS Reg. No. 8028-89-5 (caramel color) in the Food Chemical Codex, Fourth Edition, 1996, National Academy Press, Washington, DC, USA

✦ Association des Amidonneeries de Céréales de l'Union Européene. Industry views. Accessed October 12, 2010. http://www.aaf-eu.org/html/viewpoint.php

✦ Association des Amidonneeries de Céréales de l'Union Européene. Communication on EU Allergen Labelling of Wheat Starch and Wheat Starch Derivatives and their Use in Gluten-Free Foods. Accessed October 12, 2010.
http://www.aaf-eu.org/pdf/AAF_02-2009_Communication_on_EU_allergen_labelling.pdf

✦ Opinion of the Scientific Panel on Dietetic Products, Nutrition and Allergies, Wheat-Based Maltodextrin and Glucose Syrups, European Food Safety Authority. EFSA-Q-2004-091 and 092. Accessed December 3, 2009.
http://www.efsa.europa.eu/EFSA/efsa_locale-1178620753812_1178620761603.htm
http://www.efsa.europa.eu/EFSA/efsa_locale-1178620753812_1178620761736.htm

✦ Permanent exemption obtained for "allergen labelling" of wheat-based maltodextrins, glucose syrups, dextrose. Accessed October 12, 2010.
http://www.aaf-eu.org/pdf/Statement_on_permanent_exemption_obtained_for_allergen_labelling_11-2007.pdf

✦ Commission Directive 2007/68/EC of 27 November, 2007 amending Annex IIIa of Directive 2000/13/EC. http://www.aaf-eu.org/pdf/Commission_Directive_2007-68-EC.pdf

✦ Kaukinen K, Salmi T, et al. Clinical trial: gluten microchallenge with wheat-based starch hydrolysates in coeliac disease patients: a randomized double-blind, placebo-controlled study to evaluate safety. *Aliment Pharmacol Ther* 2008; Aug. 17. "Postprint"; doi: llll/j.1365-2036.2008.03832.X

✦ Email correspondence with Dr. Sue Hefle, Associate Professor and Program Co-Director, Food Allergy Research and Resource Program, University of Nebraska, Lincoln, NE.

✦ Email correspondence with G. Rizzetto, Assistant Regulatory Affairs Manager, Association des Amidonneeries de Céréales de l'Union Européene.

✦ Email correspondence with Mr. Philippe Looten, Manager of Quality Assurance, Roquette, Cedex, France.

✦ Email correspondence with Mr. Graham Price, Technical Officer, The Celiac Society of Australia.

✦ Glucose syrup "sweet" for celiacs. *Gluten-Free Living* magazine, 2004; Vol, 9, No. 2.

✦ Telephone and email correspondence with Mr. Bob Hansen, Manager of Technical Services, Briess Malt and Ingredient Company, Chilton, WI. www.briess.com

✦ Gélinas, P. Analysis of gluten-free products. Report prepared for the Fondation Québécoise de la maladie Coeliaque (FQMC) and the Canadian Celiac Assocation. Presented on October 1, 2005 at the Annual Meeting of the FQMC, Saint-Hyacinthe, Québec, Canada. See www.fqmc.org/content/view/334/70/

✦ Kamuf W, Nixon A, Parker L, Barnum GC. Overview of Caramel Colors. *Cereal Foods World*. 2003; 48:64-69.

✦ Telephone correspondence with D.D. Williamson and Co. Inc. on December 5, 2005. Further information also accessed on website at www.caramel.com on September 5, 2008.

✦ Molloy M. What is the difference between caramel colour and caramel flavour? Are they gluten-free? *Canadian Celiac Association Newsletter*, 1997. Winter Edition, page 4.

Labeling of Foods and Food Ingredients

Most countries have specific regulations and guidelines for the labeling of food products. Development, revision and enforcement of these regulations often falls under different jurisdictions within various government departments. The following is a summary of American and Canadian regulations, including web links for more detailed information.

USA

Together, the Food and Drug Administration (FDA) of the United States (U.S.) Department of Health and Human Services and the Food Safety and Inspection Service (FSIS) of the U.S. Department of Agriculture (USDA) have regulatory authority over most of the food supply. In addition, the Alcohol and Tobacco Tax and Trade Bureau, U.S. Department of Treasury, regulates the labeling of wines that contain 7% or more alcohol by volume and all distilled spirits and malt beverages made with malted barley and hops, irrespective of their alcohol content.

The *Federal Food, Drug, and Cosmetic Act* is the major law that provides the Secretary of Health and Human Services the authority to regulate the vast majority of foods marketed in the U.S., excluding those under the jurisdiction of other Federal Departments. The *Federal Meat Inspection Act*, the *Poultry Products Inspection Act* and the *Egg Products Inspection Act* collectively provide the Secretary of Agriculture authority to regulate meat, poultry and processed egg products. When meat, poultry and processed egg products are used as ingredients in relatively small amounts in other food products, those other food products fall under the jurisdiction of FDA. To reduce confusion about jurisdiction, the FSIS and FDA are currently examining this issue and seeking input from various stakeholders in order to develop clear and consistent rules about product categorization and agency jurisdiction.

The FSIS meat, poultry and egg product regulations, along with other labeling policies and guidelines can be accessed at these links:

http://www.fsis.usda.gov/Regulations_&_Policies/Acts_&_Authorizing_Statutes/index.asp
http://www.fsis.usda.gov/Regulations_&_Policies/Ingredients_Guidance/index.asp
http://www.fsis.usda.gov/OPPDE/larc/Policies/Labeling_Policy_Book_082005.pdf
http://www.fsis.usda.gov/about/labeling_&_consumer_protection/index.asp

Title 21 of the *Code of Federal Regulations* (CFR) represents the regulations of the FDA. Title 21 CFR Parts 100-199 contain FDA's food-related regulations and Part 101 contains most of the FDA's food labeling regulations that can be accessed at the following link by scrolling down to find Title 21 *Food and Drugs*:

http://www.access.gpo.gov/cgi-bin/cfrassemble.cgi?title = 200921

In addition to food labeling regulations in 21 CFR the *Food Allergen Labeling and Consumer Protection Act of 2004* (FALCPA), enacted on August 2, 2004, requires the eight major food allergens that are used as ingredients to be declared in plain English terms on the label of all prepackaged foods under FDA's purview. See page 66, as well as Section 203 of FALCPA at the following link for further information:
http://www.cfsan.fda.gov/ ~ dms/alrgact.html

A major food allergen is defined by FALCPA to be one of the following eight foods/food groups or an ingredient that contains a protein derived from them: milk, egg, fish, crustacean shellfish, tree nuts, **wheat**, peanuts and soybeans. FALCPA labeling requirements do not apply to raw agricultural commodities and the law excludes from its definition of a major food allergen: 1) highly refined oils and ingredients defined from them and 2) ingredients exempt under a petition or notification process described in the new law. FDA guidance materials on FALCPA for industry and consumers can also be accessed at FDA's *Food Allergens* website at:
http://www.cfsan.fda.gov/ ~ dms/wh-alrgy.html

Canada

The Food and Drugs Act regulates foods, drugs, cosmetics and medical devices. Health Canada (HC) and the Canadian Food Inspection Agency (CFIA) share administration of the Food and Drugs Act, including the labeling of all foods, meat, poultry and egg products. HC is responsible for establishing policies and regulations relating to the safety and nutritional quality of foods sold in Canada. CFIA is involved in the development of regulations and policies related to food quality and composition standards. The CFIA is also responsible for all food inspection, compliance and enforcement activities of the Food and Drugs Act, Consumer Packaging and Labelling Act, Agriculture and Agri-Food Administrative Monetary Penalties Act, Canada Agricultural Products Act, Feeds Act, Fertilizers Act, Fish Inspection Act, Health of Animals Act, Meat Inspection Act, Plant Breeders' Rights Act, Plant Protection Act and Seeds Act and all of their associated regulations.

Further information about the FDR and CFIA can be found at these links:

http://www.hc-sc.gc.ca/fn-an/legislation/acts-lois/bill-loi_c28-eng.php

http://laws.justice.gc.ca/PDF/Statute/C/C-16.5.pdf

http://www.inspection.gc.ca/english/reg/rege.shtml

Health Canada is proposing to amend the *Food and Drug Regulations* to enhance the labeling of priority allergens, gluten sources and sulphites in foods. For more information see pages 69-71 and the following links:

http://www.hc-sc.gc.ca/fn-an/label-etiquet/allergen/index-eng.php

http://www.hc-sc.gc.ca/fn-an/label-etiquet/allergen/project_1220_info-eng.php

http://www.hc-sc.gc.ca/fn-an/label-etiquet/allergen/guide_ligne_direct_indust-eng.php

http://www.hc-sc.gc.ca/fn-an/label-etiquet/allergen/precaution_label-etiquette-eng.php

http://www.inspection.gc.ca/english/fssa/labeti/allerg/allerge.shtml

Gluten-Free Labeling

There is no single world-wide definition for the term "gluten-free." Some countries have specific gluten-free labeling regulations that identify which foods and ingredients are allowed and not allowed on a gluten-free diet; what terminology and symbols can be used on the product label; and acceptable levels of gluten. Unfortunately these regulations vary considerably from one country to another, resulting in confusion within the celiac community. For example, some European countries and the United Kingdom (U.K.) allow gluten-free foods to be made from gluten-containing ingredients such as wheat starch that has been specially processed to remove significant amounts of gluten (see page 51 on wheat starch). Other countries such as Canada, Australia and Italy do not allow wheat starch to be used in foods labeled as gluten-free.

In the United States (U.S.) there is no specific definition for the term gluten-free and what ingredients cannot be used in products labeled gluten-free. However, to comply with a directive in the *Food Allergen Labeling and Consumer Protection Act of 2004* (FALCPA), the Food and Drug Administration (FDA) was required to issue a proposed rule in August 2006 to define the food-labeling term "gluten-free". The proposed rule was released in January 2007 (see pages 66, 68). The final rule to establish a regulatory definition for the term "gluten-free" was expected in August 2008, however, it has been delayed. The FDA recently shared the following:

"(FDA) will be publishing a final rule to define the food labeling term "gluten-free" sometime after it solicits and considers the public comments it receives on the agency's safety assessment report on gluten exposure in individuals who have celiac disease. FDA's intent to conduct this safety assessment was mentioned in the preamble of the proposed rule. A Federal Register notice will be published to announce the availability of FDA's draft safety assessment report. Because of this intermediate step, it is premature to estimate when the final rule will be published. However, interested individuals may wish to periodically check FDA's website for updates on the safety assessment report and the final rule."

There are two major reasons why it has been very difficult to develop a universal standard for gluten-free:

(1) There is limited scientific data on a safe threshold level of gluten for people with celiac disease. Catassi (see pages 65, 67) evaluated 49 adults with celiac disease who were given 0, 10 or 50 mg of gluten for 3 months. One patient challenged with 10 mg gluten/day developed a clinical relapse. The study concluded "that ingestion of contaminating gluten should be kept lower than 50 mg/d." A *Systematic Review* by Akonberg found that "The amount of tolerable gluten varies among people with coeliac disease. Whilst some patients tolerated an average of 34-36 mg of gluten per day, other patients who consumed about 10 mg of gluten per day developed mucosal abnormalities. Although there is no evidence to suggest a single definitive threshold, a daily gluten intake of < 10 mg is unlikely to cause significant histological abnormalities."

(2) There has been a lack of an accurate, consistently reproducible analytical method that has undergone a multi-laboratory validation for the detection and quantification of gluten in food products. However, this has been recently addressed with the development of the new R5 enzyme-linked immunosorbent assay (ELISA) test (see pages 62, 64, 65).

In spite of the challenges, a number of organizations and countries have developed standards, regulations and/or guidelines for foods labeled as gluten-free. The following is a summary of some of the gluten-free standards and regulations which have been developed internationally and nationally.

Codex Alimentarius Commission

The World Health Organization (WHO) and the Food and Agriculture Organization (FAO) in 1963 formed an international group called the Codex Alimentarius Commission with a mandate to develop internationally agreed upon food standards to ensure fair trade practices. This organization includes representatives from many countries around the world including the U.S., Canada, most European countries, Africa, Asia and Latin America, however, not all participating countries adopt the standards developed by the Commission and many have their own standards and specific regulations.

The Codex Committee on Nutrition and Foods for Special Dietary Uses (CX/NFSDU) developed a *Codex Standard for Gluten-Free Foods* in 1976 which was adopted in 1981. This standard is referred to as Codex Stan 118-1981. In 1983 amendments to the section on labeling of this standard were adopted. Key components of this standard are found on page 62.

The Codex Stan 118-1981 applied to products made from **gluten-containing grains** that were specially processed to remove most of the toxic protein fraction from the starch component. The nitrogen content for this earlier definition was based upon analysis that used an indirect method to determine the protein content of cereals and wheat starch. Section 2.2.2 states that the nitrogen content of the grain used in the product must not exceed 0.05 grams per 100 grams of grain on a dry-matter basis. At the time when this definition was established, the newer ELISA-based methods for detecting and estimating the gluten content of foods were not available. Using earlier methodology, it was estimated that specially prepared wheat starch used in gluten-free foods that met this Codex standard could contain approximately 40-60 mg of gluten per 100 grams, which is equivalent to 20-30 mg gliadin or 200 to 300 ppm (parts per million) gliadin (see page 64).

CODEX STANDARD FOR "GLUTEN-FREE FOODS"
Codex Stan 118-1981 (amended 1983)

1. **Scope**

   1.1 This standard applies to those processed foods which have been specially prepared to meet the dietary needs of persons intolerant to gluten.

   1.2 The standard refers only to the specific provisions related to the special dietary purpose for which these foods are intended.

   1.3 This standard does not apply to foods which in their normal form do not contain gluten.

2. **Description**

   2.1 **Definition**

   Gluten-free food is a food so described:

   (a) consisting of or containing as ingredients such cereals as wheat, triticale, rye, barley or oats, or their constituents, which have been rendered "gluten-free"; or

   (b) in which any ingredients normally present containing "gluten" have been substituted by other ingredients not containing "gluten."

   2.2 **Subsidiary Definition**

   2.2.1 For the purpose of this standard, gluten is defined as those proteins commonly found in wheat, triticale, rye, barley or oats to which some persons are intolerant.

   2.2.2 For the purpose of this standard, gluten-free means that the total nitrogen content of gluten-containing cereal grains used in the product does not exceed 0.05 g per 100 grammes of these grains on a dry matter basis.

3. **Essential Composition and Quality Factors**

   3.1 A *gluten-free food* shall be based on or shall contain:

   (a) gluten-containing cereals such as wheat, triticale, rye, barley or oats or their constituents, which have been rendered "gluten-free": according to Section 2.2.2; or

   (b) ingredients which do not contain gluten in substitution for the ingredients containing gluten which are normally used in food of that kind; or

   (c) any mixture of two or more ingredients as in (a) or (b).

Above is an excerpt from the standard.

There are now more sensitive tests available for analyzing the gluten content of foods. One such method is the highly sensitive and specific R5 ELISA test, developed by Enrique Méndez from Spain, which can detect and quantify the specific prolamins (gliadin in wheat, secalin in rye and hordein in barley) to levels as low as 3.2 ppm gluten. To put this in perspective, 1 slice of white bread (20 grams) contains approximately 2.5 grams of gluten which is equivalent to 125,000 ppm gluten (62,500 ppm gliadin). For information on how to calculate these conversions see pages 64 and 67.

A proposal to revise the *Codex Standard for Gluten-Free Foods* was adopted in 1993. The *Draft Revised Standard for Gluten-Free Foods* was first published in 1998. There were two categories of gluten-free foods proposed: 1) those made from ingredients (not derived from wheat, barley, rye, oats) with a gluten level less than 20 ppm or 2) those made using wheat, rye, barley or [oat] ingredients that had been rendered gluten-free with a gluten level less than 200 ppm. The two proposed gluten levels of 20 ppm and 200 ppm were developed in order to accommodate different views of Codex member countries on the gluten limit in gluten-free foods. Oats were contained in the square brackets [ ] until there was further information and consensus on their use.

Additional changes were made to the *Draft Revised Standard for Gluten-Free Foods* in 2006. In November 2007 the name of the Codex Standard was changed to *Draft Revised Codex Standard for Foods for Special Dietary Use for Persons Intolerant to Gluten* and further changes were also made including definitions, levels of gluten expressed as mg/kg, use of oats, labeling and methods of analysis and sampling. This was at Step 8 of the Procedure which is the final step before being officially adopted. At the 31st session of the Codex Alimentarius Commission in Geneva, Switzerland on June 30-July 4, 2008 the *Draft Revised Codex Standard for Foods for Special Dietary Use for Persons Intolerant to Gluten* was officially adopted. This new Standard was renumbered to "Codex Stan 118-1979". To access this Standard see: **http://www.codexalimentarius.net/web/standard_list.do?lang = en**
http://www.codexalimentarius.net/web/more_info.jsp?id_sta = 291

CODEX STANDARD FOR FOODS FOR SPECIAL DIETARY USE FOR PERSONS INTOLERANT TO GLUTEN
Codex Stan 118-1979

1. **Scope**
   1.1 This standard applies to foods for special dietary uses that have been formulated, processed or prepared to meet the special dietary needs of people intolerant to gluten.
   1.2 Foods for general consumption which by their nature are suitable for use by people with gluten intolerance may indicate such suitability in accordance with the provisions of section 4.3.

2. **Description**
   2.1 **Definition**
   The products covered by this standard are described as follows:
   2.1.1 **Gluten-free foods**
   Gluten-free foods are dietary foods
   a) consisting of or made only from one or more ingredients which do not contain wheat (i.e., all Triticum species, such as durum wheat, spelt, and kamut), rye, barley, oats1 or their crossbred varieties, and the gluten level does not exceed 20 mg/kg in total, based on the food as sold or distributed to the consumer, and/or
   b) consisting of one or more ingredients from wheat (i.e., all Triticum species, such as durum wheat, spelt, and kamut), rye, barley, oats1 or their crossbred varieties, which have been specially processed to remove gluten, and the gluten level does not exceed 20 mg/kg in total, based on the food as sold or distributed to the consumer.
   2.1.2 **Foods specially processed to reduce gluten content to a level above 20 up to 100 mg/kg**
   These foods consist of one or more ingredients from wheat (i.e., all Triticum species, such as durum wheat, spelt, and kamut), rye, barley, oats1 or their crossbred varieties, which have been specially processed to reduce the gluten content to a level above 20 up to 100 mg/kg in total, based on the food as sold or distributed to the consumer. Decisions on the marketing of products described in this section may be determined at the national level.
   2.2 **Subsidiary Definitions**
   2.2.1 **Gluten**
   For the purpose of this standard, "gluten" is defined as a protein fraction from wheat, rye, barley, oats[1] or their crossbred varieties and derivatives thereof, to which some persons are intolerant and that is insoluble in water and 0.5M NaCl.
   2.2.2 **Prolamins**
   Prolamins are defined as the fraction from gluten that can be extracted by 40-70% of ethanol. The prolamin from wheat is gliadin, from rye is secalin, from barley hordein and from oats[1] avenin. It is however an established custom to speak of gluten sensitivity. The prolamin content of gluten is generally taken as 50%.

---

[1] Oats can be tolerated by most but not all people who are intolerant to gluten. Therefore, the allowance of oats that are not contaminated with wheat, rye or barley in foods covered by this standard may be determined at the national level.

3. ESSENTIAL COMPOSITION AND QUALITY FACTORS

3.1 For products referred to in 2.1.1 a) and b), the gluten content shall not exceed 20 mg/kg in the food as sold or distributed to the consumer.

3.2 For products referred to in 2.1.2 the gluten content shall not exceed 100 mg/kg in the food as sold or distributed to the consumer.

3.3 Products covered by this standard substituting important basic foods, should supply approximately the same amount of vitamins and minerals as the original foods they replace.

3.4 The products covered by this standard shall be prepared with special care under Good Manufacturing Practice (GMP) to avoid contamination with gluten.

4. LABELLING

In addition to the general labelling provisions contained in the General Standard for the Labelling of Prepackaged Foods (CODEX STAN 1-1985) and the General Standard for the Labelling of and Claims for Prepackaged Foods for Special Dietary Uses (CODEX STAN 146-1985), and any specific labelling provisions set out in a Codex standard applying to the particular food concerned, the following provisions for the labelling of "gluten-free foods" shall apply:

4.1 The term "gluten-free" shall be printed in the immediate proximity of the name of the product in the case of products described in section 2.1.1.

4.2 The labelling of products described in section 2.1.2 should be determined at the national level. However these products must not be called gluten-free. The labelling terms for such products should indicate the true nature of the food, and shall be printed in the immediate proximity of the name of the product.

4.3 A food which, by its nature, is suitable for use as part of a gluten-free diet, shall not be designated "special dietary", "special dietetic" or any other equivalent term. However, such a food may bear a statement on the label that "this food is by its nature gluten-free" provided that it complies with the essential composition provisions for gluten-free as set out in section 3.1 and provided that such a statement does not mislead the consumer. More detailed rules in order to ensure that the consumer is not misled may be determined at the national level.

5. METHODS OF ANALYSIS AND SAMPLING

5.1 General outline of the methods

- The quantitative determination of gluten in foods and ingredients shall be based on an immunologic method or other method providing at least equal sensitivity and specificity.
- The antibody used should react with the cereal protein fractions that are toxic for persons intolerant to gluten and should not cross-react with other cereal proteins or other constituents of the foods or ingredients.
- Methods used for determination should be validated and calibrated against a certified reference material, if available.
- The detection limit has to be appropriate according to the state of the art and the technical standard. It should be 10 mg gluten/kg or below.
- The qualitative analysis that indicates the presence of gluten shall be based on relevant methods (e.g. ELISA-based methods, DNA methods).

5.2 Method for determination of gluten
Enzyme-linked Immunoassay (ELISA) R5 Mendez Method.

Gluten Equivalents*

mg/100 g	mg/kg	ppm
2	20	20
20	200	200
* 2 mg/100 g = 20 mg/kg = 20 ppm		

References

✦ Codex Alimentarius Reports of CX/NFSDU available at www.codexalimentarius.net

✦ Joint FAO/WHO Food Standards Program. Codex Alimentarius Commission. Codex Standard for "Gluten-Free Foods". Codex Stan 118-1981. Codex Alimentarius. 1994; 4:100-103 http://www.codexalimentarius.net/web/standard_list.do

✦ Joint FAO/WHO Food Standards Program. Report of the 20th Session of the Joint FAO/WHO Codex Committee on Nutrition and Foods for Special Dietary Uses. ALINORM 93/40. June-July, 1993. www.codexalimentarius.net/download/report/246/al93_26e.pdf

✦ Joint FAO/WHO Food Standards Program. Codex Committee on Foods for Special Dietary Uses. Draft revised standard for gluten-free foods. CX/NFSDU 98/4. July, 1998:1-4

✦ Joint FAO/WHO Food Standards Program. Report of the 28th Session of the Joint FAO/WHO Codex Committee on Nutrition and Foods for Special Dietary Uses. ALINORM 07/30/26. October, 2006: 11-13.
www.codexalimentarius.net/download/report/669/al30_26e.pdf

✦ Joint FAO/WHOFood Standards Program. Report of the 29th Session of the Joint FAO/WHO Codex Committee on Nutrition and Foods for Special Dietary Uses. ALINORM 08/31/26. November, 2007: 50-51. www.codexalimentarius.net/download/report/687/al08_26e.pdf

✦ Hekkens, WthJM. The determination of prolamins in gluten-free food. Introductory remarks. *Panminerva Med* 1991; 33:61-64.

✦ Janssen FW. Codex standard for gluten-free products. In: Lohiniemi S, Collin P, Mäki M, eds. *Changing Features of Coeliac Disease*: Tampere, Finland: The Finnish Coeliac Society; 1998: 31-36.

✦ Mäki M, Kaukinen K, Holm K, Collin P. Treatment of coeliac patients with oats and wheat starch. In: Lohiniemi S, Collin P, Mäki M, eds, *Changing Features of Coeliac Disease*: Tampere, Finland: The Finnish Coeliac Society; 1998: 93-96.

✦ Thompson T. Wheat starch, gliadin, and the gluten-free diet. *J Am Diet Assoc* 2001; 101:1456-59.

✦ Valdes, I., Garcia, E., Llorente, M and Mendez, E. Innovative approach to low-level gluten determination in foods using a novel sandwich enzyme-linked immunosorbent assay protocol. *Eur J Gastroenterol Hepatol* 2003, 15:465-74.

✦ Chartrand LJ, Russo PA, Duhaime AG, Seidman EG. Wheat starch intolerance in patients with celiac disease. *J Am Diet Assoc* 1997; 97:612-18.

✦ Garcia E, Llorente M, Hernando A, Kieffer R, Wieser H, Méndez E. Development of a general procedure for complete extraction of gliadins for heat processed and unheated foods. *Eur J Gastroenterol Hepatol* 2005; 17:529-39.

✦ Méndez E, Vela C, Immer U, Janssen FW. Report of a collaborative trial to investigate the performance of the R5 enzyme linked immunoassay to determine gliadin in gluten-free food. *Eur J Gastroenterol Hepatol* 2005; 17:1053-63.

✦ Thompson T, Méndez E. Commercial assays to assess gluten content of gluten-free foods: why they are not created equal. *J Am Diet Assoc* 2008; 108:1682-87.

✦ Hischenhuber C, Crevel R, Jarry B, et al. Review article: safe amounts of gluten for patients with wheat allergy or coeliac disease. *Aliment Pharmacol Ther* 2006; 23:559-75.

✦ Catassi C, Fabiani E, Iacono G, et al. A prospective, double-blind, placebo-controlled trial to establish a safe gluten threshold for patients with celiac disease. *Am J Clin Nutr* 2007; 85:160-66.

✦ Akobeng Ak, Thomas AG. Systematic review: tolerable amount of gluten for people with coeliac disease. *Aliment Pharmacol Ther* 2008; 27:1044-52.

United States

Currently, there is no specific Federal regulation that defines the term "gluten-free," however, FDA interprets this term to mean "no" gluten. In accordance with FDA policy, when manufacturers label a product "gluten-free" that purports to be or is represented to be for special dietary use, manufacturers should adhere to the provisions for hypoallergenic foods specified in 21 CFR 105.62 Hypoallergenic Foods. See **http://edocket.access.gpo.gov//cfr_2008//aprqtr//pdf//21cfr105.62.pdf**

Food Allergen Labeling and Consumer Protection Act of 2004 (FALCPA)

On August 2, 2004, the *Food Allergen Labeling and Consumer Protection Act of 2004* (Title II of Pub.L.108-282) became law. This new legislation requires any ingredients that are or contain one of the eight major food allergens (i.e., peanuts, tree nuts, soy, fish, shellfish, milk, eggs and **wheat** or a protein derived from any of these foods)* to be declared in plain English terms on the labels of all packaged foods under FDA's purview that are labeled on or after January 1, 2006. This includes all conventional foods, dietary supplements, infant formulas and medical foods regulated by the FDA, but excludes meat, poultry and certain egg products regulated by the USDA. FALCPA requirements apply to both products manufactured in the U.S. and those manufactured abroad and imported into the U.S. If one of the major food allergens is used in a product, either as a food or component of an ingredient, the product must be labeled appropriately. Major food allergens used as ingredients in flavorings, colorings, seasoning mixtures and incidental additives must be listed in accordance with these requirements. For example, if a snack food included seasonings containing whey powder and wheat flour, the terms "milk" and "wheat" must be declared on the label of the snack food. However, distilled vinegar derived from wheat would not have to declare wheat on its food label, as the distillation process removes the wheat protein and is not in the final product.

---

* Although wheat is one of the top 8 allergens that must always be declared, the FALCPA labeling requirements do not apply to the other gluten-containing grains (barley and rye). However, many manufacturers are aware of the increasing need for information about the presence of gluten in ingredients and are more frequently declaring the gluten sources on product labels voluntarily.

The FALCPA also mandated the Secretary, in consultation with appropriate experts and stakeholders, to issue a proposed rule to define and permit the use of, the term "gluten-free" on food labels by August 2006, with the final ruling by August 2008. (Note: This final ruling has been delayed [see page 60]).

Update on Gluten-Free Labeling

On behalf of the Secretary of Health and Human Services, the Food and Drug Administration, Center for Food Safety and Applied Nutrition (FDA/CFSAN) consulted with appropriate experts and stakeholders to help the agency develop a proposed regulation to define and permit the voluntary use of the term "gluten-free" on food labels. Two key meetings have been held to date to examine this issue.

FDA/CFSAN Food Advisory Committee on Thresholds for Major Food Allergens & Gluten in Food

The FDA/CFSAN Food Advisory Committee held a meeting July 13-15, 2005 called "Approaches to Establish Thresholds for Major Food Allergens and for Gluten in Food". The meeting on July 14 brought together scientific experts and stakeholders representing Federal government agencies, trade associations, the food industry, consumers and others. A panel of experts listened to presentations on and discussed the characteristics and treatment of celiac disease, the quality of life issues faced by patients and their families, the relationship between gluten proteins in various grains and celiac disease, analytical methods for measuring gluten levels in food, the value and use of prospective and retrospective gluten tolerance studies, and examples of existing national and international definitions of "gluten-free" standards for food labeling.

Two presentations that examined safe gluten threshold levels were given by Dr. Alessio Fasano, Professor of Pediatrics, Medicine & Physiology, and Director of the Mucosal Biology Research Center, affiliated with the Center for Celiac Research at the University of Maryland and Dr. Pekka Collin, Professor from the University of Tampere Medical School in Finland. Dr. Fasano highlighted the preliminary results of the Italian gluten micro-challenge study* that examined the consequences of protracted ingestion of minimal gluten intakes of either 10 or 50 mg/day for 3 months in adults with celiac disease. It revealed that there was a trend towards an increase in inflammatory cells in the villi (called intraepithelial lymphocytes) at 50 mg/day. Based upon the results of this study and Italy's experience with allowing up to 20 ppm in foods marketed as gluten-free in that country, Dr. Fasano suggested that 20 ppm of gluten is a safe threshold for most people with celiac disease who did not exceed a maximum intake of 300 grams of gluten-free products/day which would be equivalent to a total of 6 mg gluten/day. Dr. Collin presented retrospective data suggesting a safe threshold level of gluten to be 100 ppm if the daily gluten-free flour intake was less than 300 grams/day. This would be equivalent to a maximum of 30 mg gluten/day. Based on these two presentations, it appears that there are various gluten tolerance levels in people with celiac disease that may be between 6-30 mg gluten/day. Further research is necessary to determine safe gluten threshold levels and the amounts of gluten-free specialty products that can safely be consumed by the celiac population at large (see page 61, 65).

Daily Gluten Intake Based on Amount of Gluten (in ppm) of Varying Weights of GF Products**

Gluten content in products (expressed as ppm)	Amount of gluten-free foods (in grams) per day			
	50 grams	100 grams	200 grams	300 grams
20 ppm	1 mg	2 mg	4 mg	6 mg
50 ppm	2.5 mg	5 mg	10 mg	15 mg
100 ppm	5 mg	10 mg	20 mg	30 mg
200 ppm	10 mg	20 mg	40 mg	60 mg

Calculation Facts:

20 ppm gluten = 2 mg gluten/100 grams of food

$$\frac{2 \text{ mg gluten}}{100 \text{ grams of food}} = \frac{6 \text{ mg gluten}}{300 \text{ grams of food}}$$

100 ppm = 10 mg gluten/100 grams of food

$$\frac{10 \text{ mg gluten}}{100 \text{ grams of food}} = \frac{30 \text{ mg gluten}}{300 \text{ grams of food}}$$

*The completed study: "A perspective double-blind, placebo-controlled trial to establish a safe gluten threshold for patients with celiac disease" in the *Am J Clin Nutr* 2007 by Catassi et al (see page 65) concluded that "ingestion of contaminating gluten should be kept lower than 50 mg/d in the treatment of CD."

**Adapted from: Collin P, Thorell L, Kaukinen K, Mäki, M. The safe threshold for gluten contamination in gluten-free products: Can trace amounts be accepted in the treatment of coeliac disease? *Aliment Pharmacol Ther* 2004; 19:1277-83.

The entire agenda, speaker presentations, slides and meeting summary can be accessed at: **http://www.fda.gov/ohrms/dockets/ac/cfsan05.html**

FDA/CFSAN Public Meeting on Gluten-Free Food Labeling
The CFSAN held a meeting on August 19, 2005 that included presentations from representatives of Federal government agencies, the food industry, the scientific community and celiac disease groups. The purpose of the meeting was to help FDA gain a better understanding of how manufacturers produce gluten-free foods, the analytical methods used to verify that foods are gluten-free, costs of producing gluten-free foods, and the food-purchasing practices of consumers with celiac disease and their caregivers related to products marketed or labeled "gluten-free" compared to those products without a "gluten-free" designation. In addition to the presentations at the meeting, individuals and groups not able to attend were invited to submit comments to the FDA.

Various links for the Gluten-Free Food Labeling Public Meeting can be found at:

http://www.fda.gov/Food/LabelingNutrition/FoodAllergensLabeling/GuidanceCompliance
RegulatoryInformation/ucm076941.htm

http://www.fda.gov/Food/LabelingNutrition/FoodAllergensLabeling/GuidanceCompliance
RegulatoryInformation/ucm107204.htm

http://www.fda.gov/ohrms/dockets/dockets/05n0279/33.htm

FDA PROPOSED RULE: GLUTEN-FREE LABELING OF FOODS
Federal Register January 23, 2007, Volume 72, Number 14

Summary: The Food and Drug Administration (FDA) is proposing to define the term "gluten-free" for voluntary use in the labeling of foods, to mean that the food does not contain any of the following:

1. An ingredient that is any species of the grains wheat, rye, barley, or a crossbred hybrid of these grains (all noted grains are collectively referred to as "prohibited grains").

2. An ingredient that is derived from a prohibited grain and that has not been processed to remove gluten (e.g., wheat flour).

3. An ingredient that is derived from a prohibited grain and that has been processed to remove gluten (e.g., wheat starch), if the use of that ingredient results in the presence of 20 parts per million (ppm) or more gluten in the food.

4. Or 20 ppm or more gluten.

   A food that bears the claim "gluten-free" or similar claim in its labeling and fails to meet the conditions specified in the proposed definition of "gluten-free" would be deemed misbranded. FDA also is proposing to deem misbranded a food bearing a gluten-free claim in its labeling if the food is inherently free of gluten and if the claim does not refer to all foods of that same type (e.g., "milk, a gluten-free food" or "all milk is gluten-free").

   In addition, a food made from oats that bears a gluten-free claim in its labeling would be deemed misbranded if the claim suggests that all such foods are gluten-free or if 20 ppm or more gluten is present in the food.

   Establishing a definition of the term "gluten-free" and uniform conditions for its use in the labeling of foods is needed to ensure that individuals with celiac disease are not misled and are provided with truthful and accurate information with respect to foods so labeled. This proposed action is in response to the Food Allergen Labeling and Consumer Protection Act of 2004 (FALCPA).

The proposed rule and a related question and answer document are posted under the subheading "Gluten-Free" that can be accessed at:
http://www.fda.gov/Food/LabelingNutrition/FoodLabelingGuidanceRegulatoryInformation/
Topic-SpecificLabelingInformation/default.htm

USA Websites on Food Allergen and Gluten-Free Labeling

Food Allergen Labeling and Consumer Protection Act of 2004 (FALCPA)
http://www.cfsan.fda.gov/ ~ dms/alrgact.html

Information for Consumers: FALCPA Questions and Answers http://www.fda.gov/Food/Labeling
Nutrition/FoodAllergensLabeling/GuidanceComplianceRegulatoryInformation/ucm106890.htm

Guidance for Industry: Questions and Answers Regarding Food Allergens and the FALCPA
http://www.fda.gov/Food/GuidanceComplianceRegulatoryInformation/GuidanceDocuments/
FoodLabelingNutrition/ucm059116.htm

FDA website on Food Allergens   http://www.fda.gov/Food/FoodSafety/FoodAllergens/default.htm

FDA information on Topic Specific Labeling Information
http://www.cfsan.fda.gov/ ~ dms/lab-cat.html

Proposed rule: Gluten-Free Labeling of Foods   http://www.fda.gov/Food/LabelingNutrition/
FoodAllergensLabeling/GuidanceComplianceRegulatoryInformation/ucm077926.htm

FDA Guidance, Compliance & Regulatory Information (on food allergen and gluten-free issues)
**http://www.fda.gov/Food/LabelingNutrition/FoodAllergensLabeling/GuidanceCompliance
RegulatoryInformation/ucm2006884.htm**

Questions and Answers on the Gluten-Free Labeling Proposed Rule   **http://www.fda.gov/Food/Labeling
Nutrition/FoodAllergensLabeling/GuidanceComplianceRegulatoryInformation/ucm111487.htm**

USDA Food Allergen Labeling
**http://www.fsis.usda.gov/Regulations_&_Policies/Labeling_Allergens/index.asp
http://www.fsis.usda.gov/regulations_&_policies/FAQs_for_Notice_45-05/index.asp**

Canada

The *Food and Drug Regulations* (FDR), Division 24 (Foods for Special Dietary Use) regulate foods that have been specially processed or formulated to meet the particular needs of individuals for whom a physical or physiological condition exists. Section B.24.018 of the FDR defines the terms for food labeled as "gluten-free" (see below). This gluten-free regulation has been in effect since 1995. However, due to recent advances in the understanding of celiac disease and the gluten-free diet, including the safety of pure, uncontaminated oats, Health Canada has communicated that the gluten-free regulation needs revising. On May 13, 2010, *Health Canada's Proposed Policy Intent for Revising Canada's Gluten-Free Labelling Requirements* was released for comments from consumers, industry and other stakeholders. For more information see:
www.hc-sc.gc.ca/fn-an/consult/gluten2010/index-eng.php

Food and Drug Regulations, section B.24.018
No person shall label, package, sell or advertise a food in a manner likely to create an impression that it is a gluten-free food unless the food does not contain wheat, including spelt and kamut, or oats, barley, rye or triticale or any part thereof.

Health Canada has also been reviewing the use and the labeling of pure, uncontaminated oats in the gluten-free diet for a number of years. At the time of printing this book, no regulatory provision has been made to allow pure, uncontaminated oats in foods labeled as "gluten-free." Nevertheless, pure, uncontaminated oats are available for sale in Canada. Health Canada has published "Celiac Disease and the Safety of Oats: Health Canada's Position on the Introduction of Oats to the Diet of Individuals Diagnosed with Celiac Disease (CD)" in August 2007. Link to this extensive review can be found at:
http://www.hc-sc.gc.ca/fn-an/securit/allerg/cel-coe/oats_cd-avoine-eng.php

Also, the Canadian Celiac Association's position statement on oats does allow the use of pure, uncontaminated oats in moderate amounts for individuals stabilized on a gluten-free diet (see page 21).

The Canadian Food Inspection Agency monitors various labeling claims. This includes random testing of products to determine compliance with various regulations. The "gluten- free" claim in Canada means free of gluten. CFIA monitors this claim using an ELISA test.

Regulations Amending the Food and Drug Regulations (1220 – *Enhanced Labelling for Food Allergen and Gluten Sources and Added Sulphites*)

After many years of extensive consultation with health professionals, consumer groups and industry, Health Canada in consultation with the Canadian Food Inspection Agency has developed proposed regulatory amendments to the *Food and Drug Regulations* called *Enhanced Labelling For Food Allergen and Gluten Sources and Added Sulphites* (see page 70 for web links). These proposed amendments were published in the *Canada Gazette*, Part 1 on July 26, 2008. A 90-day consultation period, followed by Health Canada's review of the submissions and preparation of the final version of amendments were required before the amendments can be published in the *Canada Gazette*, Part II. Until these regulations are published and become law, Health Canada and the Canadian Food Inspection Agency strongly urge manufacturers to declare on their food labels the major food allergens and gluten sources, and their protein derivatives, and sulphites ≥10ppm, when added as ingredients or components of ingredients.

Fortunately, many Canadian manufacturers have already made significant changes to the labeling of allergens, gluten and sulphites, both in response to Health Canada and Canadian Food Inspection Agency recommendations, as well as consumer demand. Once the final mandatory regulatory amendments are published in the *Canada Gazette*, Part II, manufacturers and importers will have 18 months to implement the new labeling changes.

Highlights of the proposed regulatory amendments affecting the labeling of allergens and gluten include:

1) Declaration of the source of a food allergen or gluten on the label of prepackaged foods, either: a) in the list of ingredients (in parentheses, immediately following the common name of the ingredient or component in which it is present, e.g., wheat) OR b) in a separate statement "Contains:" which would immediately follow the list of ingredients.

2) If more than one component of an ingredient which is exempt from component declaration contains the same priority allergen or gluten source, the name of the specific allergen or gluten source needs to be declared only once in the ingredient list.

3) Any protein, modified protein or protein fraction from the following foods must be declared by their common name when they are added as an ingredient or a component of an ingredient:

   A. Allergens – Specific tree nuts (almonds, Brazil nuts, cashews, hazelnuts, macadamia nuts, pecans, pine nuts, pistachios or walnuts); peanuts; sesame seeds, wheat, triticale, eggs, milk; soybeans, shellfish (named), crustaceans (named); fish (named), mustard.

   B. Gluten – from the grains wheat, including spelt and kamut, barley, rye, triticale or oats.

4) There are some cases when a food ingredient's common or usual name (e.g., durum or semolina) does not identify the presence of the allergen or gluten source by its food source name (e.g., wheat). Therefore, the declaration of the food allergen source or gluten source must be identified in easy to understand terminology.

5) The common name of the plant source of all starches and modified starches must be declared (e.g., wheat starch or modified wheat starch).

6) The common name of the plant source must be identified in all hydrolyzed proteins (e.g., hydrolyzed wheat protein or hydrolyzed soy protein).

7) Standardized alcoholic beverages (e.g., beer and wine) and various standardized vinegars do not require a list of ingredients. However, the source of each food allergen and/or gluten present in the product must be declared on the label in a separate "Contains:" statement.

8) The proposed regulations do not apply to a food allergen or gluten source that is present in a prepackaged food as a result of cross-contamination, as it is outside the scope and intent of this regulatory proposal. This issue is being examined as a separate initiative (e.g., use of "may contain" statements).

The proposed amendments can be found at these links:

http://www.gazette.gc.ca/rp-pr/p1/2008/2008-07-26/html/reg1-eng.html
http://www.hc-sc.gc.ca/fn-an/label-etiquet/allergen/project_1220_info-eng.php
http://www.hc-sc.gc.ca/fn-an/label-etiquet/allergen/allergen-prop-eng.php

Background document: Health Canada urges food manufacturers to label priority food allergens, gluten sources and added sulphites in the pre-publication period of the Food Allergen Labelling Regulatory Amendments
http://www.hc-sc.gc.ca/fn-an/label-etiquet/allergen/project_1220_info-eng.php

Questions and Answers on the New Regulations to Enhance the Labelling of Food Allergens, Gluten Sources and Added Sulphites
http://www.hc-sc.gc.ca/fn-an/label-etiquet/allergen/project_1220_qa_qr-eng.php

Health Canada Reviews and Answers Comments Received on Regulatory Project 1220 – Enhanced Labelling of Food Allergens, Gluten Sources and Added Sulphites
http://www.hc-sc.gc.ca/fn-an/label-etiquet/allergen/proj1220-comment-eng.php

Other information about food allergen labeling:
http://www.hc-sc.gc.ca/fn-an/label-etiquet/allergen/index-eng.php
http://www.hc-sc.gc.ca/fn-an/label-etiquet/allergen/guide_ligne_direct_indust-eng.php
http://www.hc-sc.gc.ca/fn-an/label-etiquet/allergen/project_1220_info-eng.php
http://www.hc-sc.gc.ca/fn-an/label-etiquet/allergen/precaution_label-etiquette-eng.php

Australia/New Zealand

Food Standards Australia New Zealand (FSANZ) is a bi-national independent authority that develops specific food standards for composition and labeling, done in collaboration with the various government agencies and input from stakeholders including industry, consumers and health professionals in both countries. The *Australia New Zealand Food Standard Code* (known as the *Code*) contains various food labeling regulations including specific gluten-free labeling regulations. Standard 1.2.3 clause 4 pertains to the mandatory declaration of certain substances in food when present as an ingredient, component of an ingredient, food additive or processing aid. These include cereals containing gluten and their products, namely, wheat, rye, barley, oats and spelt and their hybridised strains; egg; fish; milk; peanuts; tree nuts; soybeans; sesame seed; fish; crustacea and sulphites. Clause 1 of Standard 1.2.8 defines gluten as "the main protein in wheat, rye, oats, barley, triticale and spelt relevent to the medical conditions, Coeliac disease and dermatitis herpetiformis". Clause 16 parts 2 and 3 of Standard 1.2.8 was amended on October 14, 2004 and states : "A claim to the effect that a food is **"gluten-free"** must not be made in relation to a food unless the food contains no detectable gluten; and no oats or their products; or cereals containing gluten that have been malted, or their products. A claim to the effect that a food has a **"low-gluten"** content must not be made in relation to a food unless the food contains no more than 20 mg gluten per 100 g of the food" (Note that 20 mg gluten/100 grams is equivalent to 200 ppm). These dual gluten labeling definitions were developed in order to accommodate the opposing views of the Australian and New Zealand Coeliac Societies and health professionals. The Australian Celiac Society does not support the "low-gluten" claim and only recommends the "gluten-free" claim, whereas the New Zealand Coeliac Society does endorse the "low-gluten" claim.

FSANZ and the Code can be found at:
http://www.foodstandards.gov.au/
http://www.foodstandards.gov.au/thecode/foodstandardscode/index.cfm

http://www.foodstandards.gov.au/_srcfiles/P264_Gluten_Claims_FAR.pdf#search = %22gluten%20free%20and%20low%20gluten%20%22

European Union

The European Union (EU) is a group of 25 European countries committed to working together by setting up common institutions where they delegate some of their sovereignty so that decisions on specific issues of mutual concern can be made democratically at the EU level. The EU consists of a Parliament of 732 members and a Council of the European Union which consists of ministers from national governments of all 25 EU countries. Both groups have the responsibility of passing laws and making policy decisions. The European Commission (EC) has 25 members (one from each country) and represents the interests of Europe as a whole and is independent of national governments. Proposals for new laws come from the EC such as food safety laws. The Health and Consumer Protection Directorate General is responsible for enforcing the EU laws.

Directive 2000/13/EC of March 20, 2000 regarding labeling, presentation and advertising of foodstuffs was amended by Directive 2003/89/EC on November 10, 2003. This new legislation was passed November 2004 and became mandatory effective November 24, 2005. It requires allergens and their derivatives (cereals containing gluten, fish, crustaceans, egg, peanut, soy, nuts, celery, mustard, sesame seed, sulphites and milk and dairy products including lactose) to always be declared on the food label.

The EC had requested the Scientific Panel on Dietetic Products, Nutrition and Allergies of the European Food Safety Authority (EFSA) to review the evidence supporting the identification of foods, food components and food ingredients which cause food allergies and intolerances. The Panel was also asked to determine, if possible, thresholds that exist and/or identify specific elements (including food processing) that would indicate food components/ingredients are no longer responsible for triggering adverse reactions. Their report entitled "Opinion of the Scientific Panel on Dietetic Products, Nutrition and Allergies on a request from the Commission relating to the evaluation of allergenic foods for labeling purposes" was adopted on February 19, 2004. Food companies were permitted to submit scientific data on ingredients that could be provisionally exempt from declaration by August 25, 2004. The EFSA published its opinions on wheat-based maltodextrins and glucose syrups (derived from wheat starch and barley starch) November 19, 2004. They concluded that these ingredients "are unlikely to cause an adverse reaction in individuals with coeliac disease" and "are not very likely to cause severe allergic reactions in the majority of cereal allergic individuals". As a result, Directive 2005/26/EC of March 21, 2005 established a list of food ingredients and substances that were provisionally excluded from Annex IIIa of Directive 2000/13/EC until November 25, 2007. Based on further studies and commitment by the industry to follow "Code of Good Practice on purification of wheat starch hydrolysates to a maximum of 20 ppm gluten/dry substance as a quality parameter", the EFSA issued a final opinion on June 6, 2007. The EC published Directive 2007/68/EC on November 27, 2007 that permanently exempted wheat-based maltodextrins glucose syrups and dextrose, as well as barley-based glucose syrups, from allergen labeling.

Further information about EU food labeling can be found at these links:

http://europa.eu/legislation_summaries/consumers/product_labelling_and_packaging/l21090_en.htm

http://eur-lex.europa.eu/LexUriServ/LexUriServ.do?uri = OJ:L:2000:109:0029:0042:EN:PDF
(2000/13/EC)
http://eur-lex.europa.eu/LexUriServ/LexUriServ.do?uri = OJ:L:2003:308:0015:0018:EN:PDF
(2003/89/EC)
http://eur-lex.europa.eu/LexUriServ/LexUriServ.do?uri = OJ:L:2005:075:0033:0034:EN:PDF
(2005/26/EC)
http://eur-lex.europa.eu/LexUriServ/LexUriServ.do?uri = OJ:L:2007:310:0011:0014:EN:PDF
(2007/68/EC)

Commision Regulation (EC) No 41/2009 of 20 January 2009 concerning the composition and labelling of foodstuffs suitable for people intolerant to gluten
http://eur-lex.europa.eu/LexUriServ/LexUriServ.do?uri = OJ:L:2009:016:0003:0005:EN:PDF

Opinion of the Scientific Panel on Dietetic Products, Nutrition and Allergies (Feb. 19, 2004)
http://www.efsa.europa.eu/cs/BlobServer/Scientific_Opinion/opinion_nda_04_en1,1.pdf

http://www.efsa.europa.eu/EFSA/efsa_locale-1178620753812_1178620761603.htm
(wheat-based maltodextrin 2004)
http://www.efsa.europa.eu/EFSA/efsa_locale-1178620753812_1178623595050.htm
(wheat-based maltodextrin 2007)
http://www.efsa.europa.eu/EFSA/efsa_locale-1178620753812_1178620761736.htm
(wheat-based glucose syrup 2004)
http://www.efsa.europa.eu/EFSA/efsa_locale-1178620753812_1178623594476.htm
(wheat-based glucose syrup 2007)
http://www.efsa.europa.eu/EFSA/efsa_locale-1178620753812_1178620764953.htm
(glucose syrup from barley starch 2007)

NUTRITION AND THE GLUTEN-FREE DIET

Learning how to eliminate gluten from the diet can be very challenging, as outlined in the previous chapter. Although it is essential to know about specific ingredients and foods that must be avoided or questioned, and those which are allowed, emphasis on the nutritional quality of the gluten-free diet is also important but is frequently overlooked. This section addresses specific dietary concerns, how to use nutritious gluten-free alternatives, guidelines for healthy eating, as well as the nutritional composition of a variety of gluten-free ingredients and foods.

Nutritional Quality of Gluten-Free Foods

Several studies have examined the nutritional composition of gluten-free products. American dietitian Tricia Thompson assessed the thiamin, riboflavin and niacin content of 368 gluten-free products (1999) and evaluated the folate, iron and dietary fiber content of 83 products (2000). These North American gluten-free products included flours, mixes, breads, cereals and pastas. As most were not enriched/fortified and many were made from refined flours and starches, they tended to be lower in nutrients and dietary fiber than whole-grain and refined gluten-containing products that they replace.

Fortunately, food and drug regulations in both the USA and Canada allow gluten-free flours, breads, cereals and pasta products to be enriched at the same level as their gluten-containing counterparts. Many companies are now enriching more of their gluten-free products (e.g., breads, buns, bagels, cereals, pasta) with thiamin, riboflavin, niacin, iron, folate and other nutrients. They are also incorporating healthier ingredients such as amaranth, buckwheat, flax, mesquite, millet, Montina™, quinoa, sorghum and teff into many products. For background information, including the nutritional composition of these gluten-free alternatives, see pages 111-122, 126-128.

Nutritional Status of Individuals on a Gluten-Free Diet

No large-scale studies have been done on the nutritional adequacy of gluten-free diets. Most studies that have investigated food consumption patterns and nutrient intakes of children or adults with celiac disease were small in number, ranging from 26-71 individuals, although an Italian study by Annibale et al. (2001) on the efficacy of a gluten-free diet on the recovery from iron deficiency anemia evaluated 190 adults for 2 years (majority recovered within 6-12 months). Hallert et al. (2002) assessed the vitamin B_6, B_{12} and folate levels in 30 Swedish adults with celiac disease who had been following a gluten-free diet for 8-12 years and found poor vitamin status in half of the patients. Another Italian study by Bardella et al. (2000) of 71 adults with well-controlled celiac disease found that the weight, height and body mass index of males and the weight and body mass index of females were significantly lower than 142 control subjects without celiac disease. Also, in females diagnosed in adulthood, bone mineral content was significantly lower. Mariani et al. (1998) examined the diets of 47 Italian adolescents with celiac disease and discovered low levels of iron (especially in girls), calcium and fiber. A study by De Lorenzo et al. (1999) of 43 Italian adolescents who had been diagnosed with celiac disease, for at least one year or more, found that all had significantly lower body weight, height, fat-free mass, body mass index and bone mineral density than the 30 healthy control subjects.

The diets of 47 adults (39 females and 8 males) in the USA were recently analyzed by Thompson et al. (2005). Recommended amounts of calcium, iron and fiber were consumed by only 32, 44 and 46% of women and 63, 100 and 88% of men, respectively. Many adults, particularly women, did not consume adequate amounts of grain products. The authors concluded that persons with celiac disease should be encouraged to: 1) consume 6-11 servings per day (depending on caloric intake) of gluten-free grain products (emphasis on whole grain or enriched); 2) increase intake of non-grain food sources of thiamin, riboflavin, niacin, folate and iron; 3) consume 3 servings/day of low-fat or non-fat dairy products and 4) consider the use of gluten-free calcium and multivitamin and mineral supplements. Also, individuals with lactose intolerance should consume gluten-free, low lactose/lactose-free dairy products and/or non-dairy sources of calcium.

References

✦ Thompson T. Thiamin, riboflavin, and niacin contents of the gluten-free diet: Is there cause for concern? *J Am Diet Assoc* 1999; 99:858-62.

✦ Thompson T. Folate, iron and dietary fiber contents of the gluten-free diet. *J Am Diet Assoc* 2000; 100:1389-96.

✦ Annibale B, Severi C, Chistolini A, et al. Efficacy of gluten-free diet alone on recovery from iron deficiency anemia in adult celiac patients. *Am J Gastroenterol* 2001; 96:132-37.

✦ Hallert C, Grant C, Grehn S, et al. Evidence of poor vitamin status in coeliac patients on a gluten-free diet for 10 years. *Aliment Pharmacol Ther* 2002; 16:1333-39.

✦ Bardella MT, Fredella C, Prampolini L, et al. Body composition and dietary intakes in adult celiac disease patients consuming a strict gluten-free diet. A*m J Clin Nutr* 2000; 72:937-39.

✦ Mariani P, Viti MG, Montuori M, et al. The gluten-free diet: a nutritional risk factor for adolescents with celiac disease? *J Pediatr Gastroenterol Nutr* 1998; 27:519-23.

✦ De Lorenzo A, Di Campli C, Andreoli A, et al. Assessment of body composition by bioelectrical impedence in adolescent patients with celiac disease. *Am J Gastroenterol* 1999; 94:2951-55.

✦ Thompson T, Dennis M, Higgins LA, et al. Gluten-free diet survey: are Americans with coeliac disease consuming recommended amounts of fibre, iron, calcium and grain foods? *J Hum Nutr Dietet* 2005; 18:163-69.

Specific Nutritional Concerns

Anemia

Definition: This condition results from a deficiency in the size or number of red blood cells or the amount of hemoglobin in these cells. There are many causes of anemia, however, the most common is due to iron, folate or vitamin B_{12} deficiency. In celiac disease damage to the intestinal villi in the area where iron and folate are absorbed frequently results in a deficiency of these nutrients. As the disease progresses, villous atrophy in the lower part of the small intestine (terminal ileum), resulting in vitamin B_{12} malabsorption, can also occur in some individuals. Other reasons for inadequate absorption of B_{12} may be due to small intestinal bacterial overgrowth, low stomach acid levels (caused by the long-term use of gastric acid blocking agents for the treatment of reflux or ulcers) or pernicious anemia (an autoimmune disease that produces antibodies that destroy specific cells in the stomach which contain the Intrinsic Factor (IF) that is necessary for the absorption of B_{12} from foods).

Types of Anemia

Nutrient	Role	Deficiency
Iron	Essential for the production of hemoglobin, a component of red blood cells that carries oxygen throughout the body. Oxygen is used to release energy from the food that is eaten.	Develops slowly after the normal stores of iron in the body have become depleted. Results in a microcytic anemia (decreased number and size of red blood cells due to inadequate levels of hemoglobin). Symptoms include major fatigue, weakness, irritability, pale skin, headache, brittle nails, decreased appetite and increased susceptibility to infections. Can also cause a reduced attention span in children resulting in behavioral and developmental problems.
Folate	This B vitamin is necessary for the production of DNA, the building block of cells and for the formation of red blood cells. It is particularly important during infancy and pregnancy, when new cells are rapidly being formed. Women of child-bearing age who may become pregnant need to consume adequate amounts of folate, especially during the first few months of pregnancy to reduce the risk of neural tube defects such as spina bifida and anencephaly.	A deficiency of folate results in macrocytic megaloblastic anemia which is characterized by very large immature red blood cells. Symptoms are similar to iron deficiency but can also include tinnitus (ringing in the ears), cracked lips, sore tongue and an irregular heart beat and chest pain.
Vitamin B$_{12}$	Essential for the formation and normal growth of red blood cells and synthesis of DNA. Also plays a role in the maintenance of the nervous system. Vitamin B$_{12}$ is involved in the formation of myelin, which is part of the insulating sheath around the nerves.	Develops slowly after the normal stores of vitamin B$_{12}$ in the liver have become depleted (may take up to 3 years). A deficiency of vitamin B$_{12}$ results in macrocytic megaloblastic anemia as above. Symptoms of vitamin B$_{12}$ deficiency are similar to folate deficiency but can also include depression, numbness and tingling of the hands and feet, muscle weakness, lack of coordination and balance problems and confusion. Prolonged vitamin B$_{12}$ deficiency can cause irreversible nerve damage.

Treatment: Once a diagnosis of celiac disease is confirmed and the gluten-free diet is initiated, the villi begin to heal which allows for the absorption of nutrients. Response to the gluten-free diet varies from one individual to another and may take on average from 2-18 months until the nutritional deficiencies are corrected and symptoms resolve. In addition to a strict gluten-free diet, it is important to include foods high in iron, folate and vitamin B_{12}. Nutrition supplements may be required if the deficiency is severe. In the case of pernicious anemia, life-long vitamin B_{12} supplementation (shots, intranasal or oral supplements) are necessary. Discuss with your physician and dietitian about supplementation. More information about iron, folate and vitamin B_{12}, including the dietary reference intakes and sources, can be found on pages 77-91.

IRON

There are two types of iron in foods, heme iron and non-heme iron:

Heme Iron

- ✦ Is more readily absorbed by the body (approximately 23% of heme iron consumed is absorbed).
- ✦ Absorption is not changed by other foods in the diet.
- ✦ Is found only in red meat, fish and poultry.

Non-Heme Iron

- ✦ Is not absorbed as well as heme iron (only 3-8% of non-heme iron consumed is absorbed).
- ✦ Absorption can be increased or decreased by other foods in the diet.
- ✦ Is found in fruits, vegetables, grains and eggs.

How To Maximize Iron Absorption

1. Choose foods with a higher iron content (see pages 78-82).

2. Eat a source of heme iron with non-heme iron at the same meal:
   e.g., • Stir-fried beef, chicken, pork or fish with vegetables (e.g., broccoli) and rice and toasted almonds or sesame seeds.
   • Chili with meat and beans.

3. Vitamin C increases absorption of non-heme iron so combine vitamin C-rich foods with non-heme iron foods at the same meal.
   e.g., • Poached egg and glass of orange juice.
   • Casserole with rice, beans, canned tomatoes or tomato sauce.
   • Spinach salad with strawberries or orange segments.

   * Citrus fruits and juices, kiwi fruit, strawberries, cantaloupe, broccoli, tomatoes, potatoes, green and red peppers and cabbage are good sources of vitamin C.

4. Avoid coffee or tea with meals rich in iron as these beverages contain tannins which interfere with iron absorption. It is better to drink these beverages between meals.

5. If taking iron supplements, consume supplement with vitamin C-rich foods.

Adapted from: *Iron Essential for Good Health* by **Beef Information Centre, Canada**.

DIETARY REFERENCE INTAKES (DRI'S)

For more than 50 years, nutrition experts have produced a set of nutrient and energy standards known as the Recommended Dietary Allowances (RDA's). A new set of standards has been developed called the Dietary Reference Intakes (DRI's) which reflect collaborative efforts of American and Canadian scientists, through a review process overseen by the National Academy of Science's Food and Nutrition Board, Institute of Medicine, National Academies.

The newly established levels for vitamins, minerals, protein, fats, cholesterol, carbohydrate, fiber, and energy levels can be found at this link:
http://www.iom.edu/Home/Global/News%20Announcements/DRI.aspx

Dietary Reference Intake (DRI) for Iron

	Age	Iron (mg/day)
Infants	0-6 months 7-12 months	0.27* 11
Children	1-3 years 4-8 years	7 10
Males	9-13 years 14-18 19-30 31-50 51-70 > 70	8 11 8 8 8 8
Females	9-13 years 14-18 19-30 31-50 51-70 > 70	8 15 18 18 8 8
Pregnancy	< 18 years 19-30 31-50	27 27 27
Lactation	< 18 years 19-30 31-50	10 9 9

* Adequate Intake (AI)

Iron Content of Flours & Starches

Flours & Starches	1 cup (weight in grams)	Iron (mg)
Almond Flour (Almond Meal)	112	4.3
Amaranth Flour	135	10.3
Arrowroot Starch (Arrowroot Starch Flour)	128	0.4
Buckwheat Bran (Farinetta™)	137	13.6
Buckwheat Flour (whole groat)	120	4.9
Chestnut Flour	100	2.4
Cornmeal (Yellow, degermed, enriched)	138	5.7
Corn Bran	76	2.1
Corn Flour (Yellow, whole grain)	117	2.8
Corn Flour (Yellow, degermed, enriched)	138	5.7
Cornstarch	128	0.6
Flax Seed Meal (Ground Flax)	130	7.5
Garbanzo Bean (Chickpea) Flour	120	7.5
Garfava™ Flour (Garbanzo and Fava Bean Flours)	157	7.9
Hazelnut Flour	112	5.3
Mesquite Flour	146	5.1
Millet Flour	120	9.2
Montina™ Flour	150	10.8
Oat Flour (Pure, uncontaminated, GF)	120	7.7
Pea Flour (Yellow)	112	5.4
Potato Flour	160	2.2
Potato Starch	192	2.9
Quinoa Flour	112	10.4
Rice Bran	134	10.3
Rice Flour (Brown)	158	3.1
Rice Flour (Sweet)	120	0.0
Rice Flour (White)	158	0.6
Rice Polish	112	9.0
Sorghum Flour	136	6.0
Soy Flour (defatted)	100	9.2
Soy Flour (full fat)	84	5.4
Tapioca Starch (Tapioca Flour)	120	0.0
Teff Flour	130	8.7

References for the iron values of flours and starches are on page 79.

Iron Content of Grains & Cereals

Grains & Cereals	1 cup (weight in grams)	Iron (mg)
Amaranth	195	14.8
Buckwheat Groats (roasted, dry)	164	4.1
Flax Seed	168	9.6
Millet	200	6.0
Oat Groats (Pure, uncontaminated, GF)	185	11.1
Quinoa	170	15.7
Rice (Brown, long grain)	185	2.7
Rice (White, long grain, parboiled, enriched)	187	9.8
Rice (Wild)	160	3.1
Sorghum	192	8.5
Teff	180	12.1

Iron values for flours, starches and grains are from:

- ✦ USDA Nutrient Data Base for Standard Reference, Release #18.
  http://www.nal.usda.gov/fnic/foodcomp/Data/SR18/sr18.html
  http://www.nal.usda.gov/fnic/foodcomp/search/

- ✦ Almond Flour, Garbanzo Flour, Hazelnut Flour, Potato Starch, Millet Flour, Sorghum Flour, Sweet Rice Flour and Tapioca Starch from Bob's Red Mill, Milwaukie, OR, USA.
  www.bobsredmill.com

- ✦ Buckwheat Bran (Farinetta™) from Minn-Dak Growers, Grand Forks, ND, USA.
  www.minndak.com

- ✦ Garfava™ Flour from Authentic Foods Company, Gardena, CA, USA.
  www.authenticfoods.com

- ✦ Mesquite Flour from research articles. See page 131.

- ✦ Montina™ Flour from Amazing Grains Grower Cooperative, Ronan, MT, USA.
  www.amazinggrains.com

- ✦ Oat Flour and Groats from Cream Hill Estates, La Salle, QC, Canada was analyzed by Silliker Canada Co., Markham, ON, Canada.

- ✦ Pea Flour (Yellow) from Best Cooking Pulses, Portage la Prairie, MB, Canada was analyzed by Silliker Canada Co., Markham, ON, Canada.

- ✦ Rice Bran and Rice Polish from Ener-G Foods, Seattle, WA, USA.
  www.ener-g.com

- ✦ Teff Flour and Grain analyzed by Silliker Canada Co., Markham, ON, Canada.

Iron Content of Meats & Alternatives

Meat, Fish & Poultry	Serving Size	Iron (mg)
Beef Liver (cooked)	3.5 oz.	5.8
Ground Beef (cooked)	3.5 oz.	2.1
Roast Beef (cooked)	3.5 oz.	1.9
Beef Steak (cooked)	3.5 oz.	3.1
Chicken Breast (cooked)	3.5 oz.	1
Clams	9 small or 4 large	3.4
Egg, Whole (cooked)	1 large	0.7
Oysters (canned)	3.5 oz.	6.7
Pork Chop (cooked)	3.5 oz.	1
Pork Tenderloin (cooked)	3.5 oz.	1.4
Salmon (canned, drained, bones)	3.5 oz.	1.1
Sardines (canned in oil)	8 medium	3.5
Shrimp (canned, drained)	3.5 oz.	2.7
Shrimp (fresh, cooked)	3.5 oz.	1.1
Tuna (white, canned, drained)	3.5 oz.	1
Turkey (dark meat, cooked)	3.5 oz.	2.3
Beans, Lentils & Peas		
Cranberry Beans/Romano Beans (cooked)	1 cup	3.7
Garbanzo Beans/Chickpeas (cooked)	1 cup	4.7
Kidney Beans (cooked)	1 cup	5.2
Lentils (cooked)	1 cup	2.6
Navy Beans (cooked)	1 cup	4.5
Pinto Beans (cooked)	1 cup	4.5
Soybeans (cooked)	1 cup	8.8
Split Peas (cooked)	1 cup	2.5
White Beans (cooked)	1 cup	6.6
Nuts & Seeds		
Almonds (whole, blanched)	1 cup	5.4
Brazil Nuts (dried, blanched)	1 cup	4.8
Peanuts	1 cup	6.7
Pecans (halves)	1 cup	2.7
Walnuts, English (shelled, halved)	1 cup	2.9
Pumpkin Seeds (kernels, dried)	1 cup	20.7
Sesame Seeds (kernels, dried, decorticated)	1 cup	11.7
Sunflower Seeds (hulled kernels, dry roasted)	1 cup	4.9

Iron values for meats and alternatives are from:

✦ USDA Nutrient Data Base for Standard Reference, Release #18.
http://www.nal.usda.gov/fnic/foodcomp/Data/SR18/sr18.html
http://www.nal.usda.gov/fnic/foodcomp/search/

Iron Content of Fruits, Vegetables & Miscellaneous

Fruits	Serving Size	Iron (mg)
Apricots (dried)	1 cup	6.1
Prunes (dried)	1 cup	4.2
Prune Juice	1 cup	3
Raisins, seedless	1 cup	3.4
Vegetables		
Acorn Squash (cooked)	1 cup	1.9
Asparagus (cooked)	1 cup	1.3
Broccoli (cooked)	1 cup	1.3
Brussels Sprouts (cooked)	1 cup	1.8
Collards (frozen, cooked)	1 cup	1.9
Green Peas (cooked)	1 cup	2.5
Potato (white, baked with skin)	1 medium	2.7
Spinach (cooked)	1 cup	6.4
Spinach (raw)	1 cup	0.8
Miscellaneous		
Blackstrap Molasses	1 tbsp.	3.3

Iron values for meats and alternatives, fruits, vegetables and miscellaneous are from:

✦ USDA Nutrient Data Base for Standard Reference, Release #18.
http://www.nal.usda.gov/fnic/foodcomp/Data/SR18/sr18.html
http://www.nal.usda.gov/fnic/foodcomp/search/

Iron Content of Specialty Products

Products (enriched with iron)	Serving Size	Iron (mg)
Kinnikinnick Tapioca Rise Sesame Bagel	1 bagel (94 g)	4.9
Enjoy Life Cranapple Crunch Cereal	3/4 cup (52 g)	2.7
Pastato Fortified Spaghetti	2 oz (56 g) dry	2.2
Ener-G Foods Seattle Brown Bread	1 slice (52 g)	1.8
Enjoy Life Cinnamon Raisin Bagel	1 bagel (91 g)	1.8
Glutino Premium Cinnamon & Raisin Bread	1 slice (40 g)	1.1
Ener-G Foods White Rice Bread	1 slice (38 g)	1.1
Kinnikinnick Robin's Honey Brown Bread	1 slice (46 g)	1.0

Iron values for gluten-free specialty products are from package labels and/or company websites.

Iron Content of Specialty Products

Products (naturally occurring iron)	Serving Size	Iron (mg)
BumbleBar Original with Cashew (made with organic sesame seeds, cashews, flax seeds)	1 bar (45 g)	3.6
Sylvan Border Farm Classic Dark Bread Mix (made with brown rice, garbanzo bean, amaranth, white rice and potato starch flours)	1 slice (56 g) prepared	2.7
Perfect 10 Natural Energy Bar Apricot (made with apricots, dates, figs, hazelnuts, pecans, almonds, flax seeds, poppy seeds, sunflower seeds, pumpkin seeds)	1 bar (50 g)	2.2
Ancient Harvest Quinoa Flakes	1/3 cup (34 g) dry	1.8
Bakery On Main Gluten-Free Cranberry Orange Cashew Granola	2 oz (57 g)	1.4
Authentic Foods Pancake & Baking Mix (made with brown rice flour and Garfava™ flour)	1/4 cup (35 g)	1.4
Lärabar Snack Bars (made with dried fruits and nuts)	1 bar (1.8 oz) (51 g)	1.4
Bob's Red Mill GF Mighty Tasty Hot Cereal™ (made with brown rice, corn, sorghum and buckwheat)	1/4 cup (42 g) dry	1.4
Bob's Red Mill Organic Creamy Buckwheat Hot Cereal	1/4 cup (41 g) dry	1.4
Pamela's Amazing Gluten-Free Bread & Flour Mix (made with sorghum flour, tapioca flour, sweet rice flour, brown rice flour, white rice flour, millet flour, rice bran)	1/16 loaf (56 g) prepared	1.1
Mary's Gone Crackers Original Flavor (made with organic brown rice, quinoa, flax seeds, sesame seeds)	15 crackers (30 g)	1.1
The Ruby Range Southwest Pancake Mix (made with white rice flour, mesquite meal, potato starch flour, teff flour, tapioca flour)	2 pancakes (prepared)	0.9
Breads From Anna Yeast-Free Bread Mix (made with tapioca flour, arrowroot flour, chickpea flour, navy bean flour, potato starch, millet, Montina™ flour)	43 grams mix	0.7

Iron values for gluten-free specialty products are from package labels and/or company websites.

FOLATE

The terms folate and folic acid are used interchangeably for this water-soluble B vitamin. Folates are found naturally in a variety of foods, whereas folic acid is the synthetic form used in vitamin and mineral supplements and fortified foods. The FDA announced in March 1996 that the addition of folic acid to enriched flour and other enriched cereal grain products would be permitted and on January 1, 1998 this enrichment policy became mandatory. Following the US decision, Health Canada permitted folic acid fortification of white flour, bread, cereal and pasta in December 1996. It became mandatory November 1998.

It should be noted that in addition to gluten-containing cereal products, a growing number of gluten-free specialty products are now being fortified with vitamins and minerals including folate. The folate content of gluten-free flours, starches and grains, as well as meats/alternatives, fruits, vegetables and gluten-free specialty products are also listed on pages 84-88. The Dietary Reference Intake (DRI) for folate for various age groups is outlined below.

Dietary Reference Intake (DRI) for Folate

	Age	Folate (micrograms)
Infants	0-6 months 7-12 months	65 80
Children	1-3 years 4-8 years	150 200
Males	9-13 years 14-18 19-30 31-50 51-70 > 70	300 400 400 400 400 400
Females	9-13 years 14-18 19-30 31-50 51-70 > 70	300 400* 400* 400* 400 400
Pregnancy	< 18 years 19-30 31-50	600** 600** 600**
Lactation	< 18 years 19-30 31-50	500 500 500

*   In view of evidence linking folate intake with neural tube defects in the fetus, it is recommended that all women capable of becoming pregnant consume 400 micrograms from supplements or fortified foods in addition to intake of food folate from a varied diet.

**   It is assumed that women will continue consuming 400 micrograms from supplements or fortified food until their pregnancy is confirmed and they enter prenatal care, which ordinarily occurs after the end of the periconceptional period – the critical time for formation of the neural tube in the fetus.

Folate Content of Flours & Starches

Flours & Starches	1 cup (weight in grams)	Folate (micrograms)
Almond Flour (Almond Meal)	112	42
Amaranth Flour	135	66
Buckwheat Bran (Farinetta™)	137	41
Chestnut Flour	100	110
Corn Bran	76	3
Corn Flour (Yellow, whole grain)	117	29
Corn Flour (Masa, enriched)	114	266
Corn Flour (Yellow, degermed, unenriched)	126	60
Cornmeal (Yellow, degermed, enriched)	138	322
Cornmeal (Yellow, degermed, unenriched)	138	66
Cornmeal (Yellow, whole grain)	122	30
Flax Seed Meal (Ground Flax)	130	113
Garbanzo Bean (Chickpea) Flour	120	668
Hazelnut Flour	112	127
Mesquite Flour	146	26
Pea Flour (Yellow)	112	15
Potato Flour	160	40
Quinoa Flour	112	55
Rice Bran	134	36
Rice Flour (Brown)	158	25
Rice Flour (White)	158	6
Soy Flour (defatted)	100	305
Soy Flour (full fat)	84	290
Teff Flour	130	97

References for the folate values of flours and starches are on page 85.

Folate Content of Grains & Cereals

Grains & Cereals (raw)	1 cup (weight in grams)	Folate (micrograms)
Amaranth	195	96
Buckwheat Groats (roasted, dry)	164	69
Flax Seed	168	146
Millet	200	170
Quinoa	170	83
Rice (Brown, long grain)	185	37
Rice (White, long grain, parboiled, enriched)	187	481
Rice (Wild)	160	152
Teff	180	135

Folate values for flours, starches and grains are from:

✦ USDA Nutrient Data Base for Standard Reference, Release #18.
http://www.nal.usda.gov/fnic/foodcomp/Data/SR18/sr18.html
http://www.nal.usda.gov/fnic/foodcomp/search/

✦ Almond Flour, Garbanzo Flour, Hazelnut Flour, Potato Starch, Millet Flour, Sorghum Flour, Sweet Rice Flour and Tapioca Starch from Bob's Red Mill, Milwaukie, OR, USA.
www.bobsredmill.com

✦ Buckwheat Bran (Farinetta™) from Minn-Dak Growers, Grand Forks, ND, USA.
www.minndak.com

✦ Garfava™ Flour from Authentic Foods Company, Gardena, CA, USA.
www.authenticfoods.com

✦ Mesquite Flour from research articles. See page 131.

✦ Montina™ Flour from Amazing Grains Grower Cooperative, Ronan, MT, USA.
www.amazinggrains.com

✦ Pea Flour (Yellow) from Best Cooking Pulses, Portage la Prairie, MB, Canada was analyzed by Silliker Canada Co., Markham, ON, Canada.

✦ Rice Bran from Ener-G Foods, Seattle, WA, USA.
www.ener-g.com

✦ Teff Flour and Grain analyzed by Silliker Canada Co., Markham, ON, Canada.

Folate Content of Meats & Alternatives

Meat, Fish, Poultry & Nuts	Serving Size	Folate (micrograms)
Beef Liver (cooked, braised)	100 grams	2563
Chicken Liver (cooked, simmered)	100 grams	578
Egg (whole, raw)	1 large	47
Almonds (whole, blanched)	1 cup	44
Brazil Nuts (dried, unblanched)	1 cup	31
Hazelnuts (filberts)	1 cup	153
Peanuts (dry roasted)	1 cup	350
Pecan (halves)	1 cup	22
Walnuts (English, shelled, halves)	1 cup	98
Beans, Lentils & Peas		
Cranberry (Romano Bean)	1 cup cooked	366
Fava Beans	1 cup cooked	177
Garbanzo Beans (Chickpea)	1 cup cooked	282
Kidney Beans (Red)	1 cup cooked	230
Lentils	1 cup cooked	358
Navy Beans	1 cup cooked	255
Pinto Beans	1 cup cooked	294
Soybeans (Green)	1 cup cooked	200
Soybeans (Mature)	1 cup cooked	93
Split Peas	1 cup cooked	127
White Beans	1 cup cooked	145
Seeds		
Pumpkin Seeds (kernels, dried)	1 cup	80
Sesame Seeds (kernels, dried, decorticated)	1 cup	172
Sunflower Seeds (hulled kernels, dry roasted)	1 cup	303

Folate values for meats and alternatives are from:

✦ USDA Nutrient Data Base for Standard Reference, Release #18.
http://www.nal.usda.gov/fnic/foodcomp/Data/SR18/sr18.html
http://www.nal.usda.gov/fnic/foodcomp/search/

Folate Content of Fruits & Vegetables

Fruits	Serving Size	Folate (micrograms)
Banana	1 medium	242
Cantaloupe Melon	1 cup diced	34
Honeydew Melon	1 cup diced	32
Orange	1 medium	39
Orange Juice (frozen concentrate with 3 parts water)	1 cup	110
Strawberries	1 cup	40
Tomato Juice	1 cup	49
Vegetables		
Asparagus	4 spears cooked	89
Beets	1 cup cooked	136
Broccoli	1 cup cooked	168
Brussels Sprouts	1 cup cooked	157
Chinese Cabbage	1 cup cooked	70
Collards (frozen, chopped)	1 cup cooked	129
Corn (yellow, sweet, cream style, canned)	1 cup cooked	115
Lettuce (romaine)	1 cup cooked	76
Okra (frozen)	1 cup cooked (boiled)	269
Peas (green, frozen)	1 cup cooked	94
Spinach (raw)	1 cup (raw)	58
Spinach	1 cup cooked (boiled)	26

Folate values for fruits and vegetables are from:

✦ USDA Nutrient Data Base for Standard Reference, Release #18.
http://www.nal.usda.gov/fnic/foodcomp/Data/SR18/sr18.html
http://www.nal.usda.gov/fnic/foodcomp/search/

Folate Content of Specialty Products

Products (enriched with folate)	Serving Size	Folate (micrograms)
Enjoy Life Very Berry Snack Bar	1 bar (28 g)	240
Enjoy Life Cranapple Crunch Cereal	3/4 cup (52 g)	140
Enjoy Life Cinnamon Raisin Bagel	1 bagel (91 g)	120
Pastato Fortified Spaghetti	2 oz (56 g) dry	110
Ener-G Foods Seattle Brown Bread	1 slice (52 g)	40
Ener-G Foods White Rice Bread	1 slice (38 g)	32
Kinnikinnick Tapioca Rice Hamburger Bun	1 bun (100 g)	22
Kinnikinnick Tapioca Rice Sesame Bagel	1 bagel (94 g)	15

Folate values are from product labels and/or company websites.

VITAMIN B$_{12}$

Vitamin B$_{12}$, also known as cobalamin, is found only in animal foods such as meat, fish, poultry, eggs and dairy products. Vegetarians who do not consume foods of animal origin must rely on a B$_{12}$ supplement or fortified foods. Vitamin B$_{12}$ supplements are available in 50 to 1,000 microgram tablets or in a special type of nutritional yeast (grown on cane and sugar beet molasses) which is gluten-free (e.g., Red Star® Vegetarian Support Formula™ Nutritional Yeast – 1 tbsp. {8 grams} of flakes = 4 micrograms B$_{12}$, plus other vitamins/minerals including folic acid). Some brands of soy and other non-dairy beverages, veggie "meats" and USA breakfast cereals are fortified with B$_{12}$, however, most vegetarian meat substitutes and regular breakfast cereals contain wheat and are not gluten-free. The vitamin B$_{12}$ content of various foods are listed on page 90. The Dietary Reference Intake (DRI) for vitamin B$_{12}$ for different age groups is outlined below.

Dietary Reference Intake (DRI) for Vitamin B$_{12}$

	Age	Vitamin B$_{12}$ (micrograms/day)
Infants	0-6 months 7-12 months	0.4 0.5
Children	1-3 years 4-8 years	0.9 1.2
Males	9-13 years 14-18 19-30 31-50 51-70 > 70	1.8 2.4 2.4 2.4 2.4* 2.4*
Females	9-13 years 14-18 19-30 31-50 51-70 > 70	1.8 2.4 2.4 2.4 2.4* 2.4*
Pregnancy	< 18 years 19-30 31-50	2.6 2.6 2.6
Lactation	< 18 years 19-30 31-50	2.8 2.8 2.8

* Because 10-30% of older people may malabsorb food-bound B$_{12}$, it is advisable for those older than 50 years to meet their requirement mainly by consuming foods fortified with B$_{12}$ or a supplement containing B$_{12}$.

Vitamin B$_{12}$ Content of Various Foods

Foods	Serving Size	Vitamin B$_{12}$ (micrograms)
Clams (canned, drained)	3 oz	84.06
Beef Liver (cooked, braised)	100 grams	70.66
Chicken Liver (cooked, simmered)	100 grams	16.85
Salmon (sockeye, cooked)	3 oz	4.93
Salmon (pink, canned with bones)	3 oz	3.70
Tuna (light, canned in water, drained)	3 oz	2.54
Ground Beef (85% lean, cooked, broiled)	3 oz	2.24
Lamb (loin, lean, broiled)	3 oz	2.14
Cottage Cheese (low fat/1%)	1 cup	1.42
Yogurt (plain, skim milk)	8 oz	1.38
Soy Beverage (Pacific Foods Ultra, plain)	1 cup	1.50
Milk (low fat/1%)	1 cup	1.07
Egg (whole, raw)	1 extra large	0.75
Mozzarella Cheese (partially skimmed)	1 oz	0.66
Ham (lean, roasted)	3 oz	0.60
Chicken (dark meat, fried)	3 oz	0.28

Vitamin B$_{12}$ values are from:

✦ USDA Nutrient Data Base for Standard Reference, Release #18.
http://www.nal.usda.gov/fnic/foodcomp/Data/SR18/sr18.html
http://www.nal.usda.gov/fnic/foodcomp/search/

References for iron, folate and vitamin B$_{12}$

✦ Haapalahti M, Kulmala P, Karttunen TH, et al. Nutritional status in adolescents and young adults with screen-detected celiac disease. *J Pediatr Gastroenterol Nutr* 2005; 40:566-70.

✦ Ransford RAJ, Hayes M, Palmer M, et al. A controlled prospective screening study of celiac disease presenting as iron deficiency anemia. *J Clin Gastroenterol* 2002; 35:228-33.

✦ Howard MR, Turnbull AJ, Morley P, et al. A prospective study of the prevalence of undiagnosed coeliac disease in laboratory defined iron and folate deficiency. *J Clin Pathol* 2002; 55:754-57.

✦ Murray J. Celiac disease in patients with an affected member, type 1 diabetes, iron deficiency, or osteoporosis. *Gastroenterol* 2005; 128:S52-56.

✦ Annibale B, Severi C, Chistolini A, et al. Efficacy of gluten-free diet alone on recovery from iron deficiency anemia in adult celiac patients. *Am J Gastroenterol* 2001; 96:132-37.

✦ Dietary Reference Intakes (DRI's) from the Food and Nutrition Board, Institute of Medicine, National Academies.
http://www.iom.edu/Home/Global/News%20Announcements/DRI.aspx

✦ Folic acid to fortify US food products to prevent birth defects.
http://www.fda.gov/Food/LabelingNutrition/LabelClaims/QualifiedHealthClaims/GuidanceCompliance/ucm114251.htm

✦ USA Code of Federal Regulations Sec. 172.345 Folic Acid (folacin)
http://www.access.gpo.gov/cgi-bin/cfrassemble.cgi?title = 200521

✦ Canadian Food and Drug Regulations B.13.001, B.13.022, B.13.051, B.13.060 (Folic Acid)
http://laws.justice.gc.ca/eng/C.R.C.-c.870/page-1.html#anchorbo-ga:l_B-gb:l_13

✦ Dahele A, Ghosh S. Vitamin B$_{12}$ deficiency in untreated celiac disease. *Am J Gastroenterol* 2001; 96:745-50.

✦ Dickey W. Low serum vitamin B$_{12}$ is common in coeliac disease and is not due to autoimmune gastritis. *Eur J Gastroenterol Hepatol* 2002; 14:425-27.

BONE DISEASE

A variety of nutrients, especially calcium, vitamin D and phosphorus are necessary for the formation and maintenance of healthy bones and teeth throughout the life-cycle. A deficiency or alteration in the metabolism of these nutrients is common in undiagnosed/untreated celiac disease and can result in conditions such as osteomalacia, osteopenia and osteoporosis (see page 92). Early diagnosis of celiac disease and treatment with a strict gluten-free diet and/or supplementation with specific nutrients and the use of bone-enhancing medications (for those with osteopenia or osteoporosis) can often reverse the bone disease condition or result in a significant improvement in the condition. However, bone mass may not be completely restored to normal levels in individuals with osteoporosis and celiac disease that was diagnosed later in life. Nevertheless it is essential to prevent further deterioration of the bones by following a life-long, nutritious gluten-free diet and consuming adequate amounts of calcium, vitamin D and other nutrients. For more information about calcium, vitamin D and tips for healthy bones in celiac disease see pages 93-100.

Bone Diseases in Celiac Disease

Condition	Description
Osteomalacia	✦ A failure to deposit calcium into newly formed bones causing them to become soft, flexible, and weak.
	✦ Caused by a deficiency of vitamin D, calcium and/or phosphorus due to malabsorption of these nutrients in the small intestine.
	✦ Can occur in children and adults.
	✦ Osteomalacia in children is called rickets. Symptoms can include bone pain, skeletal deformities (e.g., bowlegs, curved spine), dental deformities (e.g., delayed formation of teeth, holes in the enamel, cavities), bone fractures and short stature.
	✦ Symptoms in adults include bone pain, muscle weakness and fractures.
	✦ Treatment with vitamin D and calcium can improve the condition of the bones within several weeks, with complete healing in 6 months for most individuals. In children, the skeletal deformities can often be corrected, however, some may not reach their full growth potential and be short as adults.
Osteopenia	✦ Mild thinning of the bone tissue and bone loss but not as severe as osteoporosis.
	✦ Bone density is between 1 and 2.5 standard deviations (SD) below the normal.
	✦ Increased risk for development of osteoporosis.
	✦ Caused by a deficiency of calcium and vitamin D.
	✦ Treatment with calcium, vitamin D and/or bone enhancing medications.
Osteoporosis	✦ Significant thinning of the bone tissue and loss of bone mass.
	✦ Bone density is 2.5 SD or more below the normal.
	✦ Results in porous, weak and brittle bones that can easily break. Common fracture areas are the spine, hip, ribs and wrist.
	✦ Caused by a variety of factors such as failure to obtain maximum bone density in childhood and adolescence; malabsorption of calcium and vitamin D; an increased production of cytokines (substances produced from the inflammatory process in the small intestine) and the autoimmune process that not only damages the villi of the small intestine but can also attack the bones directly.
	✦ Treatment with calcium, vitamin D and/or bone-enhancing medications.

Tips for Healthy Bones in Celiac Disease

✦ Follow a strict gluten-free diet for life.

✦ Get adequate amounts of calcium and vitamin D (see pages 94-96, 98-99).

✦ Eat a variety of foods to ensure adequate amounts of other nutrients that help build and maintain bone density (see Gluten-Free Dietary Guidelines for Healthy Eating on pages 123-125).

✦ Limit caffeine intake (2-3 cups of coffee, cola or tea/day) and sodium intake from processed foods and table salt as excessive amounts can cause calcium to be lost in the urine.

✦ Stay active. Regular weight-bearing activities such as brisk walking, hiking, stair climbing, dancing, tennis, as well as resistance training with weights can help maintain bone mass. Consult your physician before starting a regular exercise program.

✦ Don't smoke and also limit alcohol intake as these are risk factors for osteoporosis.

CALCIUM

Calcium is the most abundant mineral in the body found in the skeleton, teeth, blood, muscles and the fluid between cells. The majority of calcium (99%) is located in the bones and teeth. Calcium is needed on a daily basis throughout life for many important functions. It is used to build and maintain strong bones and teeth, aids in blood clotting, plays a role in contraction and relaxation of muscles, nerve transmission, regulation of the heartbeat, and secretion of enzymes and hormones. The body has a tightly regulated system to ensure a constant level of calcium within the body fluids and tissues at all times. It does this by absorbing calcium from foods consumed, slowing down the amount of calcium that is lost through the urine and taking calcium from the bones if there are insufficient amounts available from the diet. It is essential that adequate amounts of calcium be consumed and absorbed in order to prevent the loss of calcium from bones.

Milk and milk products are important sources of calcium, as well as phosphorus, magnesium, riboflavin, vitamins A, D, B_{12} and protein. Milk products supply more than 75% of the calcium in the American and Canadian diets. Other foods contain some calcium but most contain smaller amounts or the calcium is in a form that the body absorbs less efficiently. See pages 95-96 for the calcium content of various dairy products and other foods. If an individual is unable to consume enough calcium from dietary sources, a calcium supplement may also be necessary. Discuss with your dietitian or physician about supplementation. The dietary reference intake for calcium for various age groups is outlined below.

Dietary Reference Intake (DRI) for Calcium

	Age	Calcium (mg/day)
Infants	0-6 months 7-12 months	210 270
Children	1-3 years 4-8 years	500 800
Males	9-13 years 14-18 19-30 31-50 51-70 > 70	1300 1300 1000 1000 1200 1200
Females	9-13 years 14-18 19-30 31-50 51-70 > 70	1300 1300 1000 1000 1200 1200
Pregnancy	< 18 years 19-30 31-50	1300 1000 1000
Lactation	< 18 years 19-30 31-50	1300 1000 1000

Calcium Content of Dairy Products

Dairy Products	Serving	Calcium (mg)	Rating
Brie Cheese	2 oz.	92	☆
Buttermilk	1 cup	303	☆☆☆
Camembert Cheese	2 oz.	194	☆☆
Cheese, firm, such as Brick, Cheddar, Colby, Edam and Gouda	2 oz. 1" x 1" x 3"	350	☆☆☆
Cottage Cheese (creamed, 2%, 1%)	½ cup	76	☆
Feta Cheese	2 oz.	255	☆☆
Ice Cream	½ cup	90	☆
Ice Milk	½ cup	138	☆
Milk (whole, 2%, 1%, skim)*	1 cup	315	☆☆☆
Milk (chocolate)	1 cup	301	☆☆☆
Milk Powder (dry)	3 tbsp.	308	☆☆☆
Mozzarella Cheese	2 oz.	287	☆☆☆
Mozzarella Cheese (partly skimmed)	2 oz.	366	☆☆☆
Parmesan Cheese (grated)	3 tbsp.	261	☆☆
Processed Cheese Slices	2 thin	256	☆☆
Processed Cheese Slices	2 regular	384	☆☆☆
Processed Cheese Spread	3 tbsp.	270	☆☆
Ricotta Cheese	¼ cup	135	☆
Ricotta Cheese (partly skimmed)	¼ cup	177	☆☆
Swiss Cheese	2 oz.	480	☆☆☆
Yogurt Drink	1 cup	274	☆☆☆
Yogurt (frozen)	½ cup	147	☆
Yogurt (fruit-flavored)	¾ cup	240	☆☆
Yogurt (plain)	¾ cup	296	☆☆☆

From: *Calcium For Life: Are You on the Right Track*, Dairy Farmers of Canada

Calcium values from: Health Canada, *Canadian Nutrient File*, 1997.

* Add about 100 mg of calcium for calcium-enriched milk

Code:　☆　　– Source of calcium
　　　☆☆　　– Good source of calcium
　　☆☆☆　　– Excellent source of calcium

This rating is established according to Canadian *Food and Drugs Regulations*. It is based on the content of calcium in foods and is not based on the amount of calcium actually absorbed by the body.

Calcium Content of Various Foods

Dairy Products	Serving	Calcium (mg)	Rating
Almonds	1/2 cup	(200)	★★
Baked Beans	1 cup	(163)	★★
Bok Choy (cooked)	1/2 cup	84	★
Brazil Nuts	1/2 cup	130	★
Broccoli (cooked)	1/2 cup	38	
Chickpeas (cooked)	1 cup	85	★
Chili Con Carne	1 cup	(72)	★
Collards (cooked)	1/2 cup	81	★
Dates	1/4 cup	14	
Figs (dried)	3	81	★
Kale (cooked)	1/2 cup	49	
Lentils (cooked)	1 cup	49	
Nuts (mixed)	1/2 cup	51	
Orange	1 medium	56	★
Orange Juice (calcium fortified)	1 cup	300-350	★★★
Prunes (dried, uncooked)	3 medium	12	
Raisins	1/4 cup	21	
Red Kidney Beans (cooked)	1 cup	(52)	
Rice (white or brown, cooked)	1/4 cup	10	
Salmon (pink, canned, with bones)	half a 7.5 oz. can	225	★★
Salmon (sockeye, canned, with bones)	half a 7.5 oz. can	243	★★
Sardines (canned, with bones)	6 medium	275	★★★
Sesame Seeds	1/2 cup	(89)	★
Soybeans (cooked)	1/2 cup	93	★
Soy Beverage	1 cup	10	
Soy Beverage (fortified)	1 cup	312	★★★
Tofu (regular, processed with calcium sulfate)*	1/3 cup	150	★
White Beans (cooked)	1 cup	(170)	★★

The numbers between parentheses ( ) indicate the calcium from these sources is known to be absorbed less efficiently by the body.

* The Calcium content for tofu is an approximation based on products available on the market. Calcium content varies greatly from one brand to the other and can be quite low. Tofu processed with magnesium chloride also contains less calcium.

Code: ★   – Source of calcium
 ★★   – Good source of calcium
 ★★★   – Excellent source of calcium

VITAMIN D

Vitamin D plays an important role in bone health by maintaining normal blood levels of calcium and phosphorus. This fat-soluble vitamin, known as the "sunshine vitamin" is found in a limited number of foods such as fatty fish, fish oils and egg yolk and is added to milk and margarine. Some yogurt and yogurt-based beverages may also be fortified with vitamin D, however, other dairy products including cheese, ice cream, ice milk and frozen yogurt are not fortified. Most non-dairy beverages (made from soy, potato, rice or nuts) are fortified with vitamin D. In the USA, orange juice and other fruit juices, as well as some breakfast cereals may also contain added vitamin D. In Canada, orange juice and or orange/tangerine juice can be enriched with vitamin D. However, breakfast cereals cannot be enriched with vitamin D. See page 99 for the vitamin D content of various foods.

In addition to food sources, vitamin D can also be produced naturally by the body when the skin is exposed to sunlight. Although this can be a major source of vitamin D for some people, several factors can decrease or inhibit this process. For example, sunlight exposure during the winter months for those individuals living at northern latitudes is insufficient to produce significant amounts of vitamin D in the skin. And in the summer months, the use of suntan lotion with a sun protection factor (SPF) of 8 or greater blocks the skin's production of vitamin D. It is essential to regularly use sunscreen to help prevent skin cancer, however, limited sun exposure of the hands, face and arms for 10-15 minutes at least two to three times per week without sunscreen can help meet vitamin D requirements. After 10-15 minutes of sun exposure, sunscreen should be applied.

Another factor is skin pigmentation. Greater amounts of the pigment melanin result in darker skin and reduce the skin's ability to produce vitamin D from exposure to sunlight. Unfortunately, as people age the skin does not produce vitamin D from sunlight exposure as efficiently so older adults need to get their vitamin D from diet and/or supplements. For those individuals with limited sun exposure (e.g., housebound individuals such as the elderly, people living in northern latitudes, individuals who wear robes and head coverings) it is important to consume adequate amounts of vitamin D from food sources and/or supplements. While it is possible for a healthy person under the age of 50 to get the currently recommended amounts of vitamin D from the diet, it is more difficult for someone over 50 years of age to meet their recommendation.

Vitamin D is also available in various supplements. Most multi-vitamin and mineral supplements contain 10 mcg (400 IU) of vitamin D and some calcium supplements have added vitamin D. Vitamin D is also available as a single supplement in doses ranging from 5-25 mcg (200-1000 IU).

The Dietary Reference Intake (DRI) for vitamin D for various age groups is found on page 98. Vitamin D levels may be expressed as International Units (IU) or micrograms. The biological activity of 1 microgram (mcg) of vitamin D is equivalent to 40 IU. It should be noted that some organizations recommend higher levels of vitamin D. The National Osteoporosis Foundation recommends 10-20 mcg (400-800 IU) per day for adults up to age 50 and 20-25 mcg (800-1000 IU) each day for adults over age 50. Osteoporosis Canada recommends 10-25 mcg (400-1000 IU) each day for adults under age 50 and 20-50 mcg (800 - 2000 IU) per day for those 50 years and older. The Canadian Cancer Society recommends 25 mcg (1000 IU) per day during the fall and winter months for adults. Individuals at a higher risk of having low vitamin D levels should take this dose year round. The American Academy of Pediatrics recommend 10 mcg (400 IU) per day for all infants, children and adolescents.

Since people with celiac disease are at higher risk than the general healthy population of having or developing osteoporosis, those who are not consuming vitamin D-rich or fortified foods, or getting regular sun exposure should consult their health care professional about taking vitamin D supplements to ensure adequate intake.

Dietary Reference Intake (DRI) for Vitamin D

	Age	Vitamin D (micrograms/day)*
Infants	0-6 months 7-12 months	5 5
Children	1-3 years 4-8 years	5 5
Males	9-13 years 14-18 19-30 31-50 51-70 > 70	5 5 5 5 10 15
Females	9-13 years 14-18 19-30 31-50 51-70 > 70	5 5 5 5 10 15
Pregnancy	< 18 years 19-30 31-50	5 5 5
Lactation	< 18 years 19-30 31-50	5 5 5

* Expressed as cholecalciferol. 1 microgram of cholecalciferol = 40 IU vitamin D.
Recommended amounts in the absence of adequate exposure to sunlight.

Since the publication of the DRIs for vitamin D in 1997, there has been a large body of research published that indicates that vitamin D needs may be even higher than those listed above. Both US and Canadian governments have had expert panels reviewing the scientific literature to see if the DRI's need to be revised.

At time of printing the DRI's in the table are still relevant. The UL (Upper Intake Levels) for Vitamin D is 50 micrograms both children and adults and for infants it is 25 micrograms.

Sources of Vitamin D

Foods	Serving Size	Vitamin D (IU)
Cod Liver Oil	1 tbsp.	1360
Salmon (sockeye, canned, drained with bones)	3 oz	649
Salmon (cooked)	3$^1/_2$ oz	360
Mackerel (cooked)	3$^1/_2$ oz	345
Tuna (canned in oil, drained)	3 oz	200
Sardines (canned in oil, drained)	1$^3/_4$ oz	250
Milk (low fat/1%)	1 cup	100
Soy Beverage (fortified)	1 cup	100
Orange Juice (fortified with vitamin D)	1 cup	100
Margarine	1 tbsp.	60
Pudding (made with fortified milk)	$^1/_2$ cup	50
Yogurt (fortified with vitamin D)	$^1/_2$ cup	40
Egg (whole, raw)	1 large	18

Vitamin D values are from:

✦ USDA Nutrient Data Base for Standard Reference, Release #18.
http://www.nal.usda.gov/fnic/foodcomp/Data/SR18/sr18.html
http://www.nal.usda.gov/fnic/foodcomp/search/

✦ http://ods.od.nih.gov/factsheets/vitamind.asp

✦ product labels

References for bone diseases, calcium and vitamin D

✦ Stazi AV, Trecca A, Trinti B. Osteoporosis in celiac diseae and in endocrine and reproductive disorders. *World J Gastroenterol* 2008; 14:498-505.

✦ Zanchi C, Di Leo G, Ronfani L, et al. Bone metabolism in celiac disease. *J Pediatr* 2008; 153; 262-65.

✦ Olmos M, Antelo M, Vazquez H, et al. Systematic review and meta-analysis of observational studies on the prevalence of fractures in coeliac disease. *Dig Liver Dis* 2008; 40:46-53.

✦ Ludvigsson JF, Michaelsson K, Ekbom A., Montgomery SM. Coeliac disease and the risk of fractures – a general population-based cohort study. *Aliment Pharmacol Ther* 2007; 25:273-85.

✦ Murray J. Celiac disease in patients with an affected member, type 1 diabetes, iron deficiency, or osteoporosis. *Gastroenterol* 2005; 128:S52-56.

✦ Barera G, Beccio S, Proverbio MC, Mora S. Longitudinal changes in bone metabolism and bone mineral content in children with celiac disease during consumption of a gluten-free diet. *Am J Clin Nutr* 2004; 79:148-54.

✦ Sategna-Guidetti C, Grosso SB, Grosso S, et al. The effects of 1-year gluten withdrawal on bone mass, bone metabolism and nutritional status in newly diagnosed adult coeliac disease patients. *Aliment Pharmacol Ther* 2000; 14:35-43.

✦ Mora S, Barera G, Beccio S, et al. A prospective, longitudinal study of the long-term effect of treatment on bone density in children with celiac disease. *J Pediatr* 2001; 139:473-75.

✦ Meyer D, Stavropolous S, Diamond B, et al. Osteoporosis in a North American adult population with celiac disease. *Am J Gastroenterol* 2001; 96:112-19.

✦ Kalayci AG, Kansu A, Girgin N, et al. Bone mineral density and importance of a gluten-free diet in patients with celiac disease in childhood. *Pediatrics* 2001; 108:E89.

✦ Dietary Reference Intakes from Food and Nutrition Board, Institute of Medicine, National Academies.
http://www.iom.edu/Home/Global/News Announcements/DRI.aspx

✦ National Osteoporosis Foundation:
http://www.nof.org/prevention/calcium_and_VitaminD.htm

✦ Osteoporosis Canada:
http://www.osteoporosis.ca/english/about%20osteoporosis/nutrition/vitamin%20d/default.asp?s=1

✦ Office of Dietary Supplements, National Institutes of Health, Fact Sheets on Calcium and Vitamin D.
http://dietary-supplements.info.nih.gov/factsheets/calcium.asp
http://ods.od.nih.gov/factsheets/vitamind.asp

✦ Medlines Plus, National Library of Medicine, National Institutes of Health.
http://www.nlm.nih.gov/medlineplus/ency/article/000376.htm
http://www.nlm.nih.gov/medlineplus/ency/article/000360.htm

LACTOSE INTOLERANCE

Definition

Milk and milk products contain a natural sugar called lactose. People who are lactose intolerant or, more precisely, who are lactose mal-digesters, lack enough of the enzyme lactase needed to completely digest the lactose into its simple sugars, glucose and galactose. As a result, undigested lactose passes through the intestinal tract, drawing fluid with it. It is then fermented by bacteria in the large intestine producing short-chain fatty acids and gases. Symptoms of lactose intolerance may include some or all of the following: abdominal cramping, bloating, gas, nausea, headache and diarrhea. These symptoms can occur 15-30 minutes or as long as several hours after consuming lactose.

Causes of Lactose Intolerance

Primary lactase deficiency: The level of lactase enzyme activity in some people may gradually fall with age to the point where they no longer tolerate as much as they used to. This type of intolerance affects as many as 70% of the world's population. It is more prevalent in Asians, Africans, Hispanics and North American aboriginals.

Secondary lactase deficiency: This is usually a temporary condition in which the level of lactase has fallen as a result of injury to the gastrointestinal tract in conditions such as celiac disease, inflammatory bowel disease, surgery, infections and with the use of certain drugs.

Dietary Recommendations for Lactose Intolerance

Tolerance to specific levels of lactose varies considerably among individuals. Those with secondary lactose intolerance, as a result of celiac disease, may need to temporarily eliminate lactose until the villi of the small intestine are healed and the lactase enzyme levels are restored to normal. This may take weeks to months depending on individual response. Most individuals with lactose intolerance can digest small amounts of lactose. In addition, many can become less lactose intolerant over time by **gradually** introducing milk products into their diet. Other factors can affect tolerance besides the total lactose content of foods. The following tips can help improve tolerance:

Milk

✦ Drink small amounts of milk throughout the day, ¼ - ½ cup; avoid drinking large amounts at once.

✦ Enjoy milk with meals or snacks; avoid drinking it on an empty stomach.

✦ Try heating the milk; it may be easier to tolerate.

✦ The higher the fat content in the milk, the slower it is digested and more easily tolerated. For example, whole milk may be better tolerated than low-fat or non-fat milk.

✦ Cultured buttermilk and acidophilus milk are usually tolerated to the same degree as plain milk.

Yogurt

Yogurt is often better tolerated than milk. Although yogurt contains lactose, the lactase enzymes in the active cultures digest this lactose. Look for brands that contain "active" or "live" cultures as they are tolerated more easily.

Cheese

✦ Aged, natural cheeses such as Cheddar, Swiss, Parmesan, and mozzarella, are low in lactose. In these cheeses most of the lactose is removed with the whey and the small amount remaining is broken down during the aging process, therefore, most aged cheeses are well tolerated.

✦ Fresh cheeses, such as creamed cottage cheese, ricotta and quark contain varying amounts of lactose.

✦ Dry-curd cottage cheese contains less lactose than creamed cottage cheese.

✦ Processed cheese has a lactose content similar to that of natural, aged cheeses.

✦ Processed cheese food and processed cheese spread often contain added modified milk solids, therefore their lactose content may be higher than plain processed cheese.

✦ Light cheese products also contain modified milk solids that replace milk fat. They tend to be high in lactose.

Special Products

Several products have been specially developed to help in the management of lactose mal-digestion. For more product information see pages 273-278.

✦ **Lactaid Milk** is a brand of lactose-reduced milk available in skim and 2% (in Canada) and fat-free, low-fat, reduced-fat, whole and calcium-fortified (in USA) in the dairy case of grocery stores.

✦ **Lacteeze Milk** is a brand of lactose-reduced milk available in skim, 1% and 2% in shelf stable and refrigerated forms in grocery stores. The lactase enzyme has been added to the milk and 99% of the naturally occurring lactose has been converted to simple, easily digested sugars. Lactose-reduced milk is slightly sweeter than regular milk but it has the same nutritional value and can be used in cooking and baking.

✦ **Dairy-Ease** is a brand of lactose-reduced milk available in fat-free, reduced-fat (2%) and whole milk in the USA in the dairy case of grocery stores.

✦ **Lactaid Tablets*** is a brand of lactase enzymes available in Original (Regular) and Fast Act Extra-Strength (Ultra) caplets or Fast Act Chewable Tablets (vanilla twist flavor).

✦ **Lacteeze Caplets/Tablets*** contain extra-strength natural enzymes that a person takes just before meals or snacks that contain lactose. These mint-flavored tablets are available from most drug stores. Extra-strength tablet (Canada) and Ultra caplet (USA).

✦ **Lacteeze Children's Tablets*** in strawberry flavor are also available in drug stores.

✦ **Lacteeze Enzyme Drops*** contain lactase enzymes that can be added to liquid dairy products making them more easily digestible. Approximately 99% of the lactose is broken down based on the number of drops used (15 drops) per liter. This product is available in drug stores.

✦ **Lactaid Drops*** contain lactase enzymes used to pre-treat liquid dairy products. Add 15 drops per liter. Available in Canada.

✦ **Non-Dairy Beverages** made from nuts, potatoes, rice or soy do not contain any lactose. Look for brands that are gluten-free (i.e., do not contain any barley malt flavoring) and are enriched with calcium, vitamin D and other nutrients (see pages 273-277).

* The nutritional value of dairy products is not changed when you use enzyme drops or tablets.

DIETARY FIBER

Dietary fiber is the part of whole grains, fruits, vegetables, legumes (dried beans, peas and lentils), nuts and seeds that cannot be broken down by the human digestive system. Although fiber is not readily digested, it plays an important role in the body, particularly through its effects on the digestive system. Fiber helps to maintain regular bowel movements. A high-fiber diet can also play a role in the prevention of certain chronic diseases such as coronary artery disease, diabetes, colon cancer and diverticular disease.

Consuming adequate amounts of fiber is especially important for people with celiac disease. Newly diagnosed individuals may have symptoms of diarrhea due to malabsorption caused by gluten damaging the absorptive surface of the small intestine. However, once a gluten-free diet is initiated, the intestinal tract begins to heal and the malabsorption and diarrhea eventually resolve. Some people may then have problems with constipation. This is often due to an inadequate fiber intake as they are no longer able to consume high-fiber gluten-containing foods such as wheat bran and whole-wheat breads and cereals. Many gluten-free foods are made with starches and/or refined flours which are lower in fiber. During refining, the outer layer of the grain which contains most of the fiber is removed, leaving only the starchy inner layer which contains very little fiber.

Dietary Reference Intake (DRI) for Fiber

	Age	Fiber (grams/day)
Infants	0-6 months 7-12 months	ND* ND*
Children	1-3 years 4-8 years	19 25
Males	9-13 years 14-18 19-30 31-50 51-70 > 70	31 38 38 38 30 30
Females	9-13 years 14-18 19-30 31-50 51-70 > 70	26 26 25 25 21 21
Pregnancy	< 18 years 19-30 31-50	28 28 28
Lactation	< 18 years 19-30 31-50	29 29 29

* **ND** – Not determinable due to lack of data of adverse effects in this age group and concern with regard to lack of ability to handle excess amounts. Source of intake should be from food only to prevent high levels of intake.

Reference Source:
Dietary Reference Intakes from the Food and Nutrition Board, Institute of Medicine, National Academies.
http://www.iom.edu/Home/Global/News%20Announcements/DRI.aspx

Healthy Tips to Increase Your Fiber Intake

✦ Gradually increase fiber in the diet (i.e., start with a small amount at a time to prevent major abdominal pain and gas).

✦ Increase consumption of fluids, especially water. Aim for a minimum of 6-10 glasses a day.

✦ Choose a variety of high-fiber gluten-free foods on a regular basis. See pages 105-110.

✦ Choose gluten-free flour mixes or recipes with high-fiber flours and starches (e.g., almond, amaranth, brown rice, buckwheat, hazelnut, legumes [bean and pea flours], mesquite, millet, Montina™, quinoa, sorghum and teff).

✦ Add corn bran, ground flax, mesquite flour, rice bran or rice polish to pancake batter, in hot cereals or baked products.

✦ Extend hamburger patties or meat loaf with ground flax or cooked brown rice, quinoa, amaranth or teff.

✦ Use brown rice, buckwheat, millet, quinoa, teff or wild rice in salads or pilafs.

✦ Add chickpeas (garbanzo beans), kidney beans or other bean varieties to salads or casseroles.

✦ Make soups with lentils or split peas.

✦ Choose high-fiber snacks such as dried fruits, nuts, seeds, popcorn, gluten-free snack bars (with dried fruits, nuts and seeds), raw fruits and vegetables.

✦ Choose whole grain crackers such as Mary's Gone Crackers.

✦ Add dried fruits, nuts or seeds to hot cereal; in salads or stir-fry dishes; in muffin, cookie or bread recipes.

✦ Eat whole fruits or vegetables rather than drinking juice.

✦ Choose higher-fiber pastas such as bean, brown rice, lentil, quinoa, soy or wild rice instead of white rice.

✦ In addition to fiber sources, your physician or dietitian may also recommend a commercial fiber supplement such as Citrucel® (powder), Fibersure® (powder) and Metamucil® (powder and capsules are gluten-free but not the wafers).

Dietary Fiber Content of Flours & Starches

Flours & Starches	1 cup (weight in grams)	Dietary Fiber (grams)
Almond Flour (Almond Meal)	112	14.7
Amaranth Flour	135	12.6
Arrowroot Starch (Arrowroot Starch Flour)	128	4.4
Buckwheat Bran (Farinetta™)	137	22.7
Buckwheat Flour (whole groat)	120	12.0
Cornmeal (Yellow, degermed,enriched)	138	10.2
Corn Bran	76	60.0
Corn Flour (Yellow, whole grain)	117	15.7
Corn Flour (Yellow, degermed, enriched)	138	2.4
Cornstarch	128	1.2
Flax Seed Meal (Ground Flax)	130	35.5
Garbanzo Bean (Chickpea) Flour	120	20.9
Garfava™ Flour (Garbanzo & Fava Bean Flours)	157	12.0
Hazelnut Flour	112	10.9
Mesquite Flour	146	46.1
Millet Flour	120	10.3
Montina™ Flour	150	36.0
Oat Flour (Pure, uncontaminated, GF)	120	11.0
Pea Flour (Yellow)	112	20.6
Potato Flour	160	9.4
Potato Starch	192	0.0
Quinoa Flour	112	6.6
Rice Bran	118	39.0
Rice Flour (Brown)	158	7.3
Rice Flour (Sweet)	120	1.2
Rice Flour (White)	158	3.8
Rice Polish	112	12.0
Sorghum Flour	136	8.6
Soy Flour (defatted)	100	17.5
Soy Flour (full fat)	84	8.1
Tapioca Starch (Tapioca Flour)	120	0.0
Teff Flour	130	8.1

Dietary fiber value references for flours and starches see page 106.

Dietary Fiber Content of Grains & Cereals

Grains & Cereals (raw)	1 cup (weight in grams)	Dietary Fiber (grams)
Amaranth	195	18.1
Buckwheat Groats (roasted, dry)	164	16.9
Flax Seed	168	45.9
Millet	200	17.0
Oat Groats (Pure, uncontaminated, GF)	185	15.2
Quinoa	170	10.0
Rice (Brown, long grain)	185	6.5
Rice (White, long grain, parboiled, enriched)	187	4.1
Rice (Wild)	160	9.9
Sorghum	192	12.1
Teff	180	11.2

Dietary fiber values for flours, starches and grains are from:

✦ USDA Nutrient Data Base for Standard Reference, Release #18.
http://www.nal.usda.gov/fnic/foodcomp/Data/SR18/sr18.html
http://www.nal.usda.gov/fnic/foodcomp/search/

✦ Almond Flour, Garbanzo Flour, Hazelnut Flour, Potato Starch, Millet Flour, Sweet Rice Flour and Tapioca Starch from Bob's Red Mill, Milwaukie, OR, USA.
www.bobsredmill.com

✦ Buckwheat Bran (Farinetta ™) from Minn-Dak Growers, Grand Forks, ND, USA.
www.minndak.com

✦ Garfava ™ Flour from Authentic Foods Company, Gardena, CA, USA.
www.authenticfoods.com

✦ Mesquite Flour from research articles. See page 131.

✦ Montina™ Flour from Amazing Grains Grower Cooperative, Ronan, MT, USA.
www.amazinggrains.com

✦ Oat Flour and Groats from Cream Hill Estates, La Salle, QC, Canada was analyzed by Silliker Canada Co., Markham, ON, Canada

✦ Pea Flour (Yellow) from Best Cooking Pulses, Portage la Prairie, MB, Canada (www.bestcookingpulses.com) was analyzed by Silliker Canada Co., Markham, ON, Canada.

✦ Rice Bran and Rice Polish from Ener-G Foods, Seattle, WA, USA.
www.ener-g.com

✦ Sorghum Flour from research articles. See page 131.

✦ Teff Flour and Grain analyzed by Silliker Canada Co., Markham, ON, Canada.

Dietary Fiber Content of Beans, Lentils, Peas, Nuts & Seeds

Beans, Lentils & Peas (cooked)	1 cup (weight in grams)	Dietary Fiber (grams)
Cranberry Beans (Romano)	177	17.7
Fava Beans (Broad Beans)	170	9.2
Garbanzo Beans (Chickpeas)	164	12.5
Kidney Beans	177	13.1
Lentils	198	15.6
Navy Beans	182	11.7
Pinto Beans	171	14.7
Soybeans	172	10.3
Split Peas	196	16.3
White Beans	179	11.3
Nuts & Seeds		
Almonds (whole, blanched)	145	15.1
Brazil Nuts (dried, blanched)	140	7.6
Peanuts	146	12.4
Pecans (halves)	108	10.4
Walnuts (English, shelled halves)	100	6.7
Pumpkin Seeds (kernels, dried)	138	5.4
Sesame Seeds (kernels, dried, decorticated)	150	17.4
Sunflower Seeds (hulled kernels, dry roasted)	128	14.2

Dietary fiber values for beans, lentils, peas, nuts and seeds are from:

✦ USDA Nutrient Data Base for Standard Reference, Release #18.
http://www.nal.usda.gov/fnic/foodcomp/Data/SR18/sr18.html
http://www.nal.usda.gov/fnic/foodcomp/search/

Dietary Fiber Content of Fruits

Fruits	Serving Size	Dietary Fiber (grams)
Apple	1 medium	3.7
Applesauce (unsweetened)	1 cup	2.9
Apricots (dried)	1/2 cup	5.9
Apricots (fresh)	2	1.7
Banana	1 medium	2.8
Blackberries	1 cup	7.6
Blueberries	1 cup	3.9
Boysenberries (frozen)	1 cup	5.1
Cherries (sweet, raw)	20	3.2
Cranberries (whole)	1 cup	4.0
Figs (dried)	2	4.6
Grapes (seedless)	20	1.0
Kiwi	1 medium	2.6
Mango	1 whole	3.7
Nectarine	1 medium	2.2
Orange	1 medium	3.1
Peach	1 medium	2.0
Pear	1 medium	4.0
Pineapple (diced, raw)	1 cup	1.9
Plums	2 small	2.0
Prunes (dried)	2	1.2
Raisins	1 cup	6.6
Raspberries	1 cup	8.4
Rhubarb (cooked)	1 cup	4.8
Strawberries	1 cup	3.5

Dietary fiber values of fruits are from:

✦ USDA Nutrient Data Base for Standard Reference, Release #18.
http://www.nal.usda.gov/fnic/foodcomp/Data/SR18/sr18.html
http://www.nal.usda.gov/fnic/foodcomp/search/

Dietary Fiber Content of Vegetables

Vegetables	Serving Size	Dietary Fiber (grams)
Asparagus (cooked)	1 cup	2.9
Beans, Green (cooked)	1 cup	8.0
Beets (cooked)	1 cup	3.4
Broccoli (cooked)	1 cup	4.5
Brussels Sprouts (cooked)	1 cup	4.0
Cabbage (cooked)	1 cup	3.5
Carrots (cooked)	1 cup	5.1
Cauliflower (cooked)	1 cup	3.3
Corn (cooked)	1 cup	4.6
Celery	11" stalk	1.1
Eggplant (cooked)	1 cup	2.5
Lettuce, Iceberg (shredded)	1 cup	0.8
Lettuce, Romaine (shredded)	1 cup	1.0
Mushrooms (cooked)	1 cup	3.4
Okra (cooked)	1 cup	4.0
Onions (cooked)	1 cup	2.9
Parsnips (cooked)	1 cup	6.2
Peas, Green (cooked)	1 cup	8.8
Peppers, Sweet, Green (chopped)	1 cup	2.7
Potato (baked with skin)	1 medium	4.8
Pumpkin (canned)	1/2 cup	3.5
Radish (sliced)	1 cup	1.9
Snow Peas (cooked)	1 cup	4.5
Spinach (cooked)	1 cup	4.3
Sweet Potato (baked with skin)	1 medium	3.4
Squash, Acorn (cooked)	1 cup	9.0
Turnips (cooked)	1 cup	3.1
Tomatoes	1 medium	1.4
Zucchini (cooked)	1 cup	2.5

Dietary fiber values for vegetables are from:

✦ USDA Nutrient Data Base for Standard Reference, Release #18.
http://www.nal.usda.gov/fnic/foodcomp/Data/SR18/sr18.html
http://www.nal.usda.gov/fnic/foodcomp/search/

Dietary Fiber Content of Specialty Foods

Products	Serving Size	Fiber (grams)
Leda Nutrition Leda Apricot Bar (made with gluten-free flour mix [chickpea, corn, tapioca, rice], dried apricots, sultanas, dates, brown rice syrup, fruit concentrate, inulin, coconut, fructose, sodium bicarbonate, flavor)	1 bar (85 g)	8.5
Ener-G Foods Seattle Brown Bread (made with Hi-Maize cornstarch, rice flour, yellow corn flour, Montina™ flour and potato flours)	1 slice (52 g)	6.0
Lärabar Snack Bars Ginger Snap (made with dates, almonds, pecans)	1 bar (51 g)	5.0
BumbleBar Original with Cashew (made with organic sesame seeds, cashews, flax seeds)	1 bar (45 g)	4.0
Perfect 10 Natural Energy Bar Apricot (made with apricots, dates, figs, hazelnuts, pecans, almonds, flax seeds, poppy seeds, sunflower seeds, pumpkin seeds)	1 bar (50 g)	4.0
Bob's Red Mill GF Mighty Tasty Hot Cereal (made with brown rice, corn, sorghum and buckwheat)	¼ cup (42 g)	4.0
Bob's Red Mill Organic Creamy Buckwheat Hot Cereal	¼ cup (41 g)	3.0
Andean Dream Quinoa Macaroni (made with organic rice and quinoa flours)	2 oz. (56 g)	3.0
La Tortilla Factory Gluten-Free Ivory Teff Wrap (made with tapioca flour, teff flour, millet flour)	1 wrap (66 g)	3.0
Mary's Gone Crackers Original Flavor (made with organic brown rice, quinoa, flax seeds, sesame seeds)	15 crackers (30 g)	3.0
Ancient Harvest Quinoa Flakes	⅓ cup (34 g) dry	2.6
Sylvan Border Farm Classic Dark Bread Mix (made with brown rice, garbanzo bean, amaranth, white rice and potato starch flours)	1 slice (56 g)	2.0
Authentic Foods Pancake & Baking Mix (made with brown rice flour and Garfava™ flour)	¼ cup (35 g)	2.0
Breads From Anna Yeast-Free Bread Mix (made with tapioca flour, arrowroot flour, chickpea flour, navy bean flour, potato starch, millet, Montina™ flour)	43 grams	2.0

Dietary fiber values for gluten-free specialty foods are from package labels and/or company websites.

Nutritious Gluten-Free Alternatives

In many countries around the world, gluten-containing grains, especially wheat, are major staples in the diet. Having to completely eliminate wheat, barley and rye from the diet is definitely challenging but the good news is that there are many healthy gluten-free alternatives available. These include amaranth, buckwheat, corn, Indian ricegrass (Montina™), flax, legumes (dried beans, peas and lentils), mesquite, millet, nuts, quinoa, rice, sorghum, teff and wild rice. These may be sold whole, milled into flour, flakes or grits, puffed, and/or incorporated into pasta, cereals, crackers and other gluten-free specialty products. Some of the more unique gluten-free alternatives are highlighted below. For additional information on how to use these alternatives see the gluten-free meal planning and cooking sections on pages 141-153.

AMARANTH

Amaranth is a broad-leafed plant which produces florets containing thousands of tiny grain-like, tan-colored seeds. Although it is used as a grain, it is not an actual grain but a member of the *Amaranthaceae* family, which is a relative of pigweed. This healthy seed has been used as a staple by many ancient civilizations around the world. Amaranth seeds can be used in a wide variety of ways.

Whole-Grain Amaranth
- ✦ It has a robust nutty flavor.
- ✦ In a heavy-bottomed saucepan with a tight-fitting lid, bring 1 cup of amaranth and 2 cups of liquid (e.g., water, gluten-free soup broth or fruit juice) to a boil and simmer for about 20-25 minutes, or until all the liquid is absorbed. Turn off the heat and let stand, covered, for 5 minutes. Makes about 2 cups. Serve as a side dish to replace potatoes or rice.
- ✦ Can be: mixed with beans for a main dish; added to rice and cooked together for a unique flavor; used to thicken soup or stew.
- ✦ For a hot cereal, cook in fruit juice or water and add chopped dried fruits and nuts.

Amaranth Flour
- ✦ Best combined with other gluten-free flours to make pancakes, flat breads and other baked goods. To enhance the nutritional quality of baked-product recipes, replace 1/4 - 1/3 of gluten-free flours with amaranth flour.
- ✦ Can be used for thickening gravy.

Toasted Amaranth Bran Flour
- ✦ It has a mild, toasty nutty flavor that is very good in quick breads and cookies.
- ✦ Replacement quantities similar to amaranth flour.

Amaranth Starch
- ✦ Can be used as a thickener for puddings, soups and sauces.

Amaranth Bread Crumbs
- ✦ Made from amaranth and tapioca starch.

Puffed Amaranth

✦ Can be used as a hot cereal for infants or adults. Mix desired amount of warm liquid with puffed amaranth and stir.

✦ Add to baked products (e.g., cookies, granola bars); combine with spices for a stuffing or side dish; use as a breading for meat, .fish or poultry.

✦ Also available as "Side Serves" which are savory flavored puffed amaranth that can be cooked and used as a substitute for rice pilaf.

Amaranth Cold Cereals

✦ Plain or flavored "Snaps" and "O's" cold cereals.

Amaranth Snack and Crackers

✦ Available in a variety of flavors.

Amaranth Pre-Gel Powder

✦ Used as a nutrition supplement in pancakes, puddings, soups, sauces and beverages such as smoothies.

Nutritional Information

✦ Amaranth is very high in protein, fiber, iron, magnesium, phosphorus, potassium, zinc and calcium. It is also a source of B vitamins. See pages 126-128 for nutrient composition.

Amaranth Recipes

✦ See pages 159-160, 175, 177,181.

References:

✦ Background information from Nu-World Amaranth publications. www.nuworldfoods.com

BUCKWHEAT

Buckwheat is thought to have originated in China. The largest producers of buckwheat today are China, Japan, Russia and North America, although it is also grown in Europe, India, Australia and South America. Buckwheat is botanically classified as a fruit, not a cereal grain, and is of the Polygonaceae family, which is closely related to rhubarb. Buckwheat is triangular in shape and has a black shell. The outer shell is removed (hulled) and the kernel inside is known as a groat. These groats are available in several different forms.

Roasted Groats

✦ Roasting gives the buckwheat kernels a distinctive, nutty flavor.

✦ Roasted groats are called "kasha" and are packaged in four granulations (whole, coarse, medium and fine).

✦ Can be steamed, boiled or baked and served "as is" with seasoning; added to soups and stews for thickening and flavor; used as a stuffing.

✦ In a heavy-bottomed saucepan with a tight-fitting lid, bring 1 cup of groats and 2 cups of liquid (e.g., water, gluten-free soup broth or fruit juice) to a boil and simmer for about 10-12 minutes, or until all the liquid is absorbed. Turn off the heat and let stand, covered, for 5 minutes. Makes about 2 cups.

Unroasted Groats

Whole – cooked and used as a side dish to replace potatoes or rice; as a stuffing for poultry; mixed with fruit and milk as a breakfast cereal. Cook according to roasted groat directions on page 112.

Ground – into grits and often labeled as "cream of buckwheat." Can be cooked and eaten as a hot cereal.

Ground – into flour:

✦ Dark flour has a stronger, distinctive flavor as it contains a higher percentage of finely milled particles of buckwheat hulls and is higher in fiber and nutrients

✦ Light flour has a mild, mellow flavor as it contains fewer buckwheat hulls.

✦ These flours can be added to pancakes, breads and muffins. Use nuts and spices to enhance the flavor of baked goods containing buckwheat flour.

✦ The flour is also used to make Japanese "Soba" noodles. They can be made from 100% pure buckwheat flour which is gluten-free. However, Soba noodles are often made with a combination of pure buckwheat flour and wheat flour and are not gluten-free.

✦ Be aware that some companies sell a buckwheat flour or pancake mix that is a combination of pure buckwheat flour and wheat flour, so be sure to look for 100% pure buckwheat flour.

Buckwheat Bran (Farinetta™)

✦ Is from the outer layer of the buckwheat groat and is high in fiber, protein, iron, riboflavin, niacin and numerous beneficial phytochemicals. Farinetta™ is licensed and trademarked by Minn-Dak Growers, Ltd.

✦ Can be used in pancake and muffin recipes or added to chili or casseroles.

Nutritional Information

✦ Buckwheat provides a good source of high-quality protein in the plant kingdom. It is high in magnesium, zinc, phosphorus, potassium, niacin, riboflavin, vitamin B6 and fiber. It is also a source of iron. See pages 126-128 for nutrient composition.

Buckwheat Recipes

✦ See pages 160, 184, 192, 197.

References:

✦ Background information from the following company publications and websites:

1. The Birkett Mills
   www.thebirkettmills.com

2. Minn-Dak Growers, Ltd.
   www.minndak.com

3. Canadian Special Crops Association
   www.specialcrops.mb.ca/crops/buckwheat.html

Flax

Flax is a member of the *Linaceae* family and is widely grown across the Canadian prairies and northern USA. This flat, oval seed has a pointed tip and is about the size of a sesame seed. Some varieties of flax are grown for human food consumption while other varieties are used to produce fiber for industrial purposes (e.g., linoleum flooring, linen clothing). The brown and yellow flax seeds grown for human consumption are very similar in their nutritional composition. Flax is available as an oil, whole seed or ground flax seed (also known as milled flax seed). Grinding ensures that all seeds are broken up, enabling the nutrients present to be absorbed by the body. Ground flax seed can be purchased in vacuum-sealed packages on store shelves or in plastic bags found in the refrigeration section. Whole flax seed can also be ground in a coffee grinder, food processor or blender to the consistency of finely ground coffee.

Storage and Handling

✦ Whole flax seed can be stored at room temperature for up to one year.

✦ Ground flax seed should be stored in a sealed opaque container in the refrigerator or freezer. For optimum freshness, it is best to grind flax seed as you need it, since the natural fats in flax seed go rancid quickly if left exposed to heat or air.

✦ Flax oil is very perishable and should be kept refrigerated in an opaque container.

Using Flax

✦ Flax oil is best used in cold foods such as fruit smoothies and s's. It is not recommended for frying as it breaks down when exposed to high temperatures. The oil can also be drizzled over cooked gluten-free pasta.

✦ Whole flax seed and ground flax seed have a light, nutty flavor which becomes more robust when the flax is roasted. Whole and ground flax seed can be used in a wide variety of foods such as muffins, breads, pancakes, waffles, cookies, fruit cobblers, hot cereals, casseroles, meat loaf, burgers, stew, spaghetti sauce, rice dishes and salads. Mix ground flax in fruit smoothies, pudding, cottage cheese, ice cream, yogurt and frozen yogurt.

✦ Substitute ¼ cup of ground flax in recipes containing rice bran. It will give a better texture and is less heavy.

✦ When adding ground flax to a recipe extra liquid must be added (e.g., for every 3 tbsp. of flax add 1 tbsp. liquid).

✦ Baked goods containing ground flax have a chewier texture and tend to brown more rapidly so the temperature may need to be reduced.

✦ **Flax can be used as an egg replacer.** To replace 1 egg, soak 1 tsp. of ground flax in ¼ cup boiling water for 5 minutes. Cool before using. Works best in cookie and snack bar recipes.

Nutritional Information

Flax has been consumed throughout history for its nutritional and health benefits. It is rich in alpha-linolenic acid (an essential omega-3 fatty acid), fiber (soluble and insoluble) and plant lignans. These components play a role in the maintenance and improvement of general health. Flax helps promote bowel regularity due to its very high fiber content. It may also help protect against coronary heart disease, as well as breast and colon cancer.

In addition, autoimmune diseases, like many other chronic diseases, are a disease of inflammation, and flax is being studied for its positive role in immune and inflammatory reactions.

✦ Flax oil is high in omega-3 fatty acids but does not contain any fiber and lignans (a type of phytochemical). Note: some flax oils add lignans back after the oil is extracted from the seed.

✦ Whole flax seeds are an excellent source of fiber. In order to gain all the benefits of flax seed, including the omega-3 fatty acids, lignans, protein, vitamins and minerals, it is important to grind the whole flax seed. This improves the bioavailability of the these components.

✦ Flax is very high in iron, magnesium, zinc, calcium, phosphorus, potassium, thiamin, niacin, vitamin B_6 and protein. It is a source of other B vitamins and other nutrients. See pages 126-128 for nutrient composition.

Recipes

✦ See pages 173-174, 177, 182, 198, 199.

References

✦ Background information and excerpts taken from the following company publications and websites:
   1. Flax Council of Canada – www.flaxcouncil.ca
   2. Saskatchewan Flax Development Commission – www.saskflax.com

✦ There are many research articles on the beneficial effects of flax that can be found at the Flax Council of Canada site.

MESQUITE

Mesquite is the North American name for a woody leguminous plant of the genus *Prosopis*. There are over 45 species native to arid and semi-arid regions of North and South America, Africa and southern Asia, ranging from eight-foot shrubs to sixty-foot tall trees. The wood chips of the tree are dried and used to impart the unique mesquite flavor to grilled foods.

These trees contain bean pods that come in different sizes, depending on the specific variety of mesquite tree, and are harvested for a variety of purposes. In some countries, the pods are processed into a syrup, jelly, tea or coffee. The entire pod can also be ground into a coarse, mealy flour that has a cinnamon-mocha aroma and sweet, chocolate, molasses-like flavor with a hint of caramel. Alternatively, a combination of milling and sieving techniques using only the pulp of the bean pod can be used to produce a finer flour (80-100 mesh) that has a sweeter and more concentrated aroma and flavor than the flour from the whole bean pod. The light tan-colored mesquite flour has been a dietary staple for indigenous people for centuries. Mesquite flour has recently been introduced to the North American market and can be used as a baking ingredient or flavoring agent in many foods. It can be combined with other gluten-free flours to make pancakes and baked products such as breads, muffins, cakes, cookies, pie crusts and brownies or it can also be added to hot cereal (e.g., cream of brown or white rice), meat dishes, soups and gravies.

Nutrition Information

✦ The nutritional composition of the mesquite flour varies considerably depending on the variety of mesquite plant, the soil type in which it is grown, and whether the whole pod or the pulp of the pod is used.

✦ The whole-pod flour is higher in protein and calcium than the flour made only from the pulp. However, both types of flours are very high in fiber and are also a source of iron, magnesium, calcium, thiamin, niacin and vitamin B_6. See pages 126-128 for nutrient composition.

Recipes

✦ See pages 172, 183.

References

✦ Background information from:
1. Felker P. Mesquite Flour: New Life for an Ancient Staple. Gastronomica. 2005; 5 (2): 85-89.
   www.ucpress.edu
2. Email and telephone correspondence with Peter Felker. Contact:
   peter_felker@hotmail.com
3. Email and telephone correspondence with Kathryn Ehrhorn, San Pedro Mesquite Company.
4. Email and telephone correspondence Jim Byrd, Cocina deVega, Inc..
   www.cocinadevega.com
5. Casa deFruta Company
   www.casadefruta.com
6. See page 131 for additional research articles on mesquite.

MILLET

The term millet refers to various grasses that grow in semi-arid regions of the world. The six species of major importance are proso, finger, foxtail, barnyard, browntop and pearl. Most millet species are used for animal or bird seed, however, pearl and finger millets are used for human food consumption. Millet is closely related to corn and belongs to the *Gramineae* family. It is primarily used as a food crop in Africa, Asia and India. Millet seed is very small, round in shape and can be yellow, white, gray or red. The most common variety found in North America is the light yellow millet that has a slight corn-like, sweet nutty flavor. Millet is hulled and the inner seed is available as whole seed, coarsely ground into grits or finely ground into flour.

Whole-Grain Millet

✦ Can be cooked in water or broth and eaten alone as a cereal, as a side-dish such as pilaf, or used for poultry stuffing or as a salad.

✦ Rinse the millet seed in cold water and drain. In a heavy-bottomed saucepan with a tight fitting lid, bring 1 cup of millet and $2^{1}/_{2}$ cups of liquid to a boil and simmer for about 20 minutes, or until all the liquid is absorbed. Turn off the heat and let stand, covered, for 5 minutes. Makes about $3^{1}/_{2}$ cups.

Puffed Millet

✦ Use as a cold cereal or crush it for a breading.

Millet Flour

✦ Similar in texture to rice flour and produces a delicate, dry crumb with a pale yellow color in baked products.

✦ Best combined with other gluten-free flours.

✦ Can become rancid easily, therefore, purchase in small amounts or grind millet in a grain mill and use as needed. Store in a tightly covered container in the refrigerator or freezer.

Nutritional Information

✦ Millet is a good source of easily digestible protein. It is also a source of thiamin, riboflavin, niacin, vitamin B_6, folate, fiber, iron, magnesium and zinc. See pages 126-128 for nutrient composition.

Millet Recipes

✦ See pages 159, 186, 191.

References:

✦ Background information from:
1. http://www.hort.purdue.edu/newcrop/afcm/millet.html
2. http://www.cgiar.org/impact/research/millet.html
3. http://www.nap.edu/books/0309049903/html/39.html

MONTINA™ (INDIAN RICEGRASS)

Indian ricegrass (IRG), is a perennial, native bunch grass from the family *Achnatherum hymenoides*, but is not related to rice. It acquired the Indian portion of its name from the fact that the Native Americans had used the small black seeds of the grass as a staple that was ground into flour for a flat bread. It grows wild from southern Manitoba, Canada to higher elevations in southern California. In the early 1990s, Montana State University (MSU) conducted extensive research on IRG and determined that this fairly drought-resistant, hardy plant was very nutritious and also gluten-free. Amazing Grains Grower Cooperative was formed as a result of collaboration between MSU, government and others to grow and market IRG and registered the trade name Montina™ for IRG products. Amazing Grains has 56 producer/members in six states that have over 4,000 acres planted to IRG. It is milled, processed and packaged in a dedicated gluten-free facility. All Montina™ products and their ingredients are tested for gluten using the ELISA test before entering the production facility.

Montina™ is sold in two forms.

Montina™ Pure Baking Supplement (100% Montina™ Flour)

✦ A light brown-gray-colored flour that has a sweet, nutty, almost "wheat-like" flavor.
✦ Best combined with other gluten-free flours. Can substitute 25% Montina™ for one of the primary flours in baked products.

Montina™ All Purpose Baking Flour Blend

✦ This is a blend of white rice flour, tapioca flour and Montina™ flour.
✦ In most cases can be used cup for cup to exchange for any flour. This is not a complete mix and will require xanthan gum and other ingredients in baked recipes. Can be used in breads, muffins, pancakes and waffles, as well as a thickener in stews and gravies.

Nutritional Information

✦ Montina™ is very high in protein, fiber and iron. It is also a source of calcium. Its complete nutritional composition profile is unknown as it has not been analyzed for other nutrients. See pages 126-128 for nutrient composition.

Montina™ Recipes
✦ See pages 162, 167, 172, 200.

References:
✦ Background information and excerpts taken from Amazing Grains Grower Cooperative publications.
www.amazinggrains.com

QUINOA

Quinoa (pronounced "keen-wah") has been consumed for thousands of years in South America and was a staple of the Incas, who called it "the mother grain." It is not actually a grain but the seed of a broad-leafed plant from the *Chenopodiaceae* family which is a close relative of the weed, lamb's quarters. There are hundreds of varieties of quinoa, ranging in color from white to red and purple to black. Many varieties are now grown in North America. The plant stalks grow three to six feet high, containing clusters of seeds near the top of the stalk. The seed looks like a cross between sesame seed and millet. Quinoa seeds are naturally covered with saponin, an extremely bitter resinlike substance which protects it from birds and insects. To be edible the saponin must be removed. Some companies specially process the quinoa to remove this bitter coating, making it pan-ready and fast cooking. Quinoa is sold in several forms.

Quinoa Seed
✦ Can be used as a side dish instead of potatoes or rice or in salads, pilafs, stuffings, casseroles and puddings, as well as a thickener for soups, chili and stews.

✦ Rinse the quinoa in cold water and drain. In a heavy-bottomed saucepan with a tight-fitting lid, bring 1 cup of quinoa and 2 cups of liquid to a boil and simmer for about 15 minutes, or until all the liquid is absorbed. Turn off the heat and let stand, covered, for 5 minutes. Makes about 3 cups.

✦ Can also be cooked in the microwave using a round 2-quart microwave-safe casserole or bowl. Combine 1 cup quinoa and 1½ cups water, cover loosely with plastic wrap and microwave on high for about 10-12 minutes, or until most of the water is absorbed. Remove from microwave, stir once and let stand, covered, for 5 minutes before serving.

Quinoa Flakes
✦ Can be eaten as an instant hot breakfast cereal. Add ⅓ cup of flakes to 1 cup of boiling water and boil for 1½-2 minutes, stirring frequently. Remove from heat and allow to cool. Add chopped nuts and dried fruits and sprinkle with brown sugar. Can also be cooked in the microwave. Combine flakes and water in a medium-to-large microwave-safe bowl and microwave on high for 2-2½ minutes. Stir before serving.

✦ Available in plain and various flavors (contains flaked quinoa, dried fruits, nuts or seeds, sugar and spices).

✦ Substitute quinoa flakes for up to ⅓ of the gluten-free flour in a cookie, muffin or bread recipe.

✦ Can also be added to pancakes and waffles.

Quinoa Flour

- ✦ A tan-colored flour with a slightly nutty, strong flavor so best combined with other gluten-free flours.
- ✦ Can be used in a variety of baked items, especially in highly spiced or flavored products.

Quinoa Pasta

- ✦ Quinoa is combined with corn or rice and is available in a variety of shapes.
- ✦ Cooks in 5-9 minutes.

Nutritional Information

Quinoa contains more high-quality protein than any other grain or cereal. The quality of this protein compares very closely to that of dried skimmed milk. Quinoa is high in iron, magnesium, phosphorus and zinc. It is also a source of calcium, B vitamins and dietary fiber. See pages 126-128 for nutrient composition.

Quinoa Recipes

- ✦ See pages 160, 180, 186-187, 190.

References:

- ✦ Background information from:
  1. Northern Quinoa Corporation
     www.quinoa.com
  2. Quinoa Corporation
     www.quinoa.net

SORGHUM

Sorghum, also referred to as milo, is a member of the *Gramineae* family. This major cereal grain grows in hot, semi-arid tropical and dry temperate areas of the world, including the USA, Mexico, Africa, India and China. The round red or white seeds are slightly smaller than peppercorns. New food-grade varieties of sorghum have been developed in the USA. These sorghums have a hard white grain that is free of any bitter flavors or dark colors often associated with non-food grade sorghums. As a result of these characteristics, whole or decorticated kernels of white or tan sorghums can be flaked, puffed and micronized, and used in a wide range of food products such as cereals, granola bars, snack foods, baked products and beverages, including beer. Sorghum is available as a whole grain or can be milled into flour and grits.

Whole-Grain Sorghum

- ✦ Soak the grain overnight in water. Drain and combine 1 cup sorghum with about 2½-3 cups of water in a heavy-bottomed saucepan with a tight-fitting lid. Bring to a boil, reduce heat and simmer, covered, for about 30-45 minutes. Turn off heat and let stand 5-10 minutes. Drain any excess water. Combine with herbs and/or spices and use as a side dish such as pilaf or in casseroles, stuffings, salad, as well as a thickener for soups and chili.
- ✦ Can be used as an alternative for rice in puddings.

Sorghum Grits

✦ Can be prepared as a hot cereal served with dried fruits, nuts, sweetener and a dash of cinnamon and/or vanilla.

Sorghum Flour

✦ This light tan-colored flour has a slightly nutty, earthy flavor.

✦ A combination of sorghum flour and other gluten-free flours, especially bean flour or amaranth flour works well as sorghum's bland flavor and light color does not alter the taste of baked products.

Nutritional Information

✦ Sorghum is high in phosphorus and potassium. It is also a source of fiber, protein, thiamin, niacin, vitamin B_6, magnesium, zinc and iron. See pages 126-128 for nutrient composition.

Sorghum Recipes

✦ See pages 158-159, 166, 169, 177, 179, 200.

References:

✦ Background information from:
    1. Email correspondence with Dr. Lloyd Rooney, Cereal Quality Laboratory, Soil and Crop Science Department, Texas A & M University, College Station, TX.
    2. Email and telephone correspondence with Dr. Jeff Dahlberg, PhD, Research Director, National Sorghum Producers, Lubbock, TX.
    www.sorghumgrowers.com
    3. Email and telephone correspondence with Dr. Scott Bean, Research Chemist, United States Department of Agriculture-Agriculture Research Service, Manhattan, KS.
    4. See page 131 for additional research article on sorghum.

TEFF

Teff, or tef, a grass native to Ethiopia, belongs to the *Poaceae* family. It is also grown in India, Australia and Northwestern USA. Teff is the smallest of all grains in the world (about 100-150 teff grains equal the size of 1 wheat kernel). The teff grains range from milky white to almost black. In Ethiopia, white, red and brown are the most common types while the USA grows brown and ivory types. Teff has a unique nutty, mild molasses-like flavor and is sold both as a whole grain and as a flour. This major cereal crop in Ethiopia is ground into flour and fermented 1-3 days to make "Injera," a sour-dough-type flat bread that is moist and chewy. Authentic Injera is usually made from pure teff flour, however, many North American restaurants use a combination of teff flour and wheat flour or barley flour which is not gluten-free. Injera is traditionally consumed with "wot," a spicy sauce or stew made of meat or ground legumes.

Whole-Grain Teff

✦ Add 1/2-1 tbsp. teff grain to a serving of gluten-free hot cereal (e.g., cream of brown or white rice cereal) while cooking.

✦ In a heavy-bottomed saucepan with a tight-fitting lid, bring 2 cups of lightly salted water to a boil and then add 1/2 cup teff grain. Cover and simmer 15-20 minutes, or until water is absorbed, stirring occasionally. Use as a side dish instead of potato or rice. For a breakfast cereal, add honey or brown sugar, raisins, nuts, chopped fruit and/or cinnamon for flavor.

✦ Cook teff with other gluten-free grains such as brown rice, buckwheat groats (kasha) or millet. Use 3 parts water or gluten-free broth to 1 part grains. Simmer for about 20 minutes, or until all the water is absorbed.

✦ Mix cooked teff with seeds, beans or tofu and garlic, herbs and onions to make a vegetarian burger.

✦ Use as a thickener for soups, stews and gravies. For stews or soups, add uncooked teff grain to the pot 30 minutes before serving or add cooked teff to the pot 10 minutes before serving.

Teff Flour

✦ Combine with other gluten-free flours in baked products, especially dark breads and cakes such as brownies, chocolate cake and gingerbread, as well as in muffin and cookie recipes. Can use 25-50% teff flour in the total flour blend. For pancakes, use 100% teff flour or a combination of teff and other gluten-free flours.

Nutritional Information

✦ Teff seeds are more nutritious than the major cereal grains (e.g., wheat, barley and corn) for several reasons: (1) the small seed size means the germ and bran (the outer portions where nutrients are concentrated) account for a higher proportion of the seed compared to other grains, and (2) the entire whole-grain teff seed is used. Teff is high in calcium, iron, magnesium, thiamin and zinc. It is also a good source of fiber, protein and B vitamins. See pages 126-128 for nutrient composition.

Teff Recipes

✦ See pages 160, 164, 171, 189.

References:

✦ Background information from:
1. The Teff Company
www.teffco.com
2. www.hort.purdue.edu/newcrop/proceedings1993/V2-231.html
3. http://www.nap.edu/books/0309049903/html/215.html
4. See page 131 for an additional research article on teff.

Wild Rice

Wild rice, an aquatic grass indigenous to North America, grows extensively in shallow lakes and streams. Despite its name, it is not a member of the rice family but is from the *Zizania* family. Most wild rice grown in northern Saskatchewan and Manitoba, Canada, is "OCIA" certified organic. Wild rice has a distinct, nut-like, roasted flavor that is enjoyable by itself or combined with other ingredients. It is sold plain, mixed with other rices, as a flour or made into pasta.

Handling and Preparation

✦ Wash wild rice in a wire strainer and run cold water over it.

✦ In a heavy-bottomed saucepan, with a tight-fitting lid, combine 4 cups of water with 1 cup of wild rice. Bring to a boil and then simmer approximately 40-60 minutes, until the rice kernels have burst their shells and fluffed out. The volume of rice increases up to 4 times (i.e., 1 cup raw rice = 4 cups cooked rice).

✦ Cooked rice can be used in casseroles, salads or side dishes. It can also be combined with white or brown rice. Leftover cooked rice can be kept in the refrigerator for 1 week or frozen (it remains in excellent condition upon thawing). Cool rice before freezing.

Nutritional Information

✦ Wild rice is a source of fiber, protein, niacin, magnesium, phosphorus, potassium and zinc. See pages 126-128 for nutrient composition.

Wild Rice Recipes

✦ See pages 185, 190, 193.

References:

✦ Background information from Riese's Canadian Lake Wild Rice publications. www.wildlakerice.com

Gluten-Free Dietary Guidelines for Healthy Eating

The United States Department of Agriculture (USDA) MyPyramid food guidance system and Canada's Food Guide to Healthy Eating are practical tools to help individuals make wise food choices. These tools differ somewhat with regard to the types of foods that are in specific groups, their serving size and recommended number of servings per day for each food group. However, the total amount per day for each group is based on factors such as age, body size, activity level and sex. For specific information about these tools and how to apply them to your individual needs see these links:

USA : www.mypyramid.gov
CANADA: http://www.hc-sc.gc.ca/fn-an/food-guide-aliment/index-eng.php

The following chart has incorporated many of the key components of the American and Canadian tools with adaptations for the gluten-free diet. The symbol GF denotes gluten-free.

Food Group	Examples	Healthy Tips & Nutrition Facts
Grain Products	GF grain alternatives (e.g., amaranth, buckwheat, cornmeal, millet, Montina™, oats [pure, uncontaminated, gluten-free: see pages 19-29, 210, 211, 254, 256, 285, 289, 294, 296, 297], quinoa, rice [black, brown, red or white], sorghum, teff, wild rice).	1. Choose GF whole grains* more often (e.g.,amaranth, buckwheat, cornmeal [whole grain–not degermed], millet, oats [pure, uncontaminated, gluten-free], quinoa, rice [black, brown, red], sorghum, teff, wild rice).
	GF breads, rolls, bagels, muffins	2. Choose enriched GF products more often. Not all GF breads, flours, cereals and pastas are enriched with iron and B vitamins and are often lower in fiber as many are made from refined flours and starches.
	GF ready-to-eat cold cereals	
	GF hot cereals (e.g., amaranth, cornmeal, cream of buckwheat or brown rice or white rice, hominy, oatmeal [pure, uncontaminated, gluten-free], quinoa, rice flakes; soy flakes, soy grits).	3. Choose breads, rolls, bagels, muffins, cereals and pasta from flours and starches that are higher in fiber, protein and vitamins and minerals (e.g., amaranth, brown rice, buckwheat, flax, legumes, mesquite, millet, Montina™, oats [pure, uncontaminated, gluten-free], quinoa, sorghum, teff and wild rice).
	GF pasta (e.g., bean, 100% buckwheat, corn, pea, potato, quinoa/corn, quinoa/rice, soy, rice [brown, white, wild])	
	GF corn or rice tortillas	
	GF pancake or waffles	
	Popcorn	

* Whole grains contain the entire grain seed (usually called the kernel) and consist of three parts – the bran, germ and endosperm. Refined grains have most of the bran and some of the germ removed which results in the loss of dietary fiber, vitamins/minerals and other nutritional components.

Food Group	Examples	Healthy Tips & Nutrition Facts
Fruits	Fresh, frozen or canned fruits and fruit juices	1. To get more fiber, choose fruit instead of juice.
	Dried fruits	2. Choose unsweetened frozen fruit or canned fruit in 100% fruit juice or water.
		3. Choose orange-colored fruits (e.g., apricot, cantaloupe, orange, mango, nectarine, peach, red or pink grapefruit) more often as they are high in vitamins, minerals and phytochemicals (naturally occurring healthy compounds).
		4. Choose 100% fruit juice rather than fruit beverages which contain less juice and more added sugar.
		5. Some juices (e.g., orange) are enriched with calcium and/or vitamin D. (Vitamin D can be added to juice in the U.S. but not Canada).
Vegetables	Fresh, frozen or canned vegetables and vegetable juices	1. Choose dark green and yellow/orange vegetables (e.g., broccoli, carrot, pumpkin, romaine lettuce, squash, sweet potato) more often as they are high in vitamins, minerals and phytochemicals.
	Dry bean, peas and lentils*	
Milk Products	Milk (fluid and dried powdered)	1. Choose lower-fat milk products more often.
	Milk (lactose-free, lactose-reduced)	2. Milk and some yogurt products are enriched with vitamin D which is a key nutrient that aids in the absorption of calcium. Cheese, ice cream, commercial pudding cups and some yogurts are not enriched with vitamin D.
	Cheese	
	Yogurt and yogurt-based beverages	
	Milk-based desserts (e.g., puddings made with milk, ice cream, frozen yogurt, ice milk)	3. Many brands of non-dairy beverages (e.g., nut, potato, rice, soy) and some orange/other fruit juices may be enriched with calcium and/or vitamin D but may not provide the other nutrients found in milk products.
		4. For individuals with lactose intolerance see pages 101-102.

* In MyPyramid these can be counted either as vegetables or in the meat and alternatives group.

Food Group	Examples	Healthy Tips & Nutrition Facts
Meats, Beans and Alternatives	Meats, poultry, fish, shellfish, eggs	1. Choose leaner meats and poultry as well as legumes more often.
	Legumes (dried beans, peas & lentils)	2. Flax seeds and walnuts, along with some fish (e.g., herring, salmon, trout) are high in omega-3 fatty acids which play a positive role in heart health.
	Nuts and seeds	
	GF tofu, GF tempeh, GF texturized vegetable protein, GF veggie burgers	3. Some seeds and nuts (almonds, hazelnuts, sunflower) are good sources of vitamin E.
Oils*	Oils (e.g., canola, coconut, corn, cottonseed, olive, palm kernel, peanut, safflower, sesame seed, walnut)	1. All oils and fats are a mixture of unsaturated fatty acids and saturated fatty acids.
	Food naturally high in oils (e.g., avocado, flax, nuts, olives, some fish)	2. Most oils (except coconut and palm kernel) contain more monounsaturated and polyunsaturated fatty acids.
	Solid fats (butter, beef fat [tallow, suet], chicken fat, pork fat [lard], stick margarine, shortening)	3. Solid fats and coconut and palm kernel oils contain more saturated fatty acids and/or trans fats than unsaturated oils.
	Foods high in solid fats (e.g., many cheeses, cream, well-marbled cuts of meat, regular ground beef, bacon, poultry skin)	4. Limit solid fats and coconut and palm kernel oils as saturated fats and trans fats raise LDL (bad) cholesterol levels in the blood which are a factor in coronary heart disease.

* This group is in MyPyramid. Canada's Food Guide does not specifically include this group.

NUTRIENT COMPOSITION OF GLUTEN-FREE GRAINS, FLOURS, STARCHES, GUMS, LEGUMES, NUTS & SEEDS

FOOD ITEM	Weight in Grams (1 cup)	Vitamins					Minerals				PROTEIN	CARBO-HYDRATES	DIETARY FIBER
		B₁ Thiamin mg	B₂ Riboflavin mg	B₃ Niacin mg	B₆ Pyridoxine mg	Folate mcg	Calcium mg	Iron mg	Magnesium mg	Zinc mg	grams	grams	grams
GRAINS, FLOURS & STARCHES													
Almond Flour (Almond Meal)	112	0.17	0.70	3.5	0.12	42	289	4.3	338	3.7	23.6	21	14.7
Amaranth Seed	195	0.16	0.41	2.5	0.44	96	298	14.8	519	6.2	28.2	129	18.1
Amaranth Flour	135	0.11	0.28	1.7	0.30	66	207	10.3	359	4.3	19.5	89	12.6
Arrowroot Starch (Arrowroot Starch Flour)	128	0.00	0.00	0.0	0.01	9	51	0.4	4	0.1	0.4	113	4.4
Buckwheat Bran (Farinetta™)	137	0.14	0.58	9.6	0.29	41	104	13.6	878	12.2	49	71	22.7
Buckwheat Groats (roasted, dry)	164	0.37	0.44	8.4	0.58	69	28	4.1	362	4.0	19.2	123	16.9
Buckwheat Groats (roasted, cooked)	168	0.07	0.07	1.6	0.13	24	12	1.3	86	1.0	5.7	34	4.5
Buckwheat Flour (whole groat)	120	0.50	0.23	7.4	0.70	65	49	4.9	301	3.7	15.1	85	12
Chestnut Flour	100	0.35	0.05	0.9	0.67	110	64	2.4	74	0.4	5.0	78	NA
Corn Bran (crude)	76	0.01	0.08	2.1	0.12	3	32	2.1	49	1.2	6.4	65	60
Corn Flour – Yellow (whole grain)	117	0.29	0.09	2.2	0.43	29	8	2.8	109	2.0	8.1	90	15.7
Corn Flour – Yellow (Masa, enriched)	114	1.63	0.86	11.2	0.42	266	161	8.2	125	2.0	10.7	87	NA
Cornmeal – Yellow (degermed, unenriched)	126	0.09	0.07	3.4	0.12	60	3	1.2	23	0.5	7.0	104	2.4
Cornmeal – Yellow (degermed, enriched)	138	0.99	0.56	6.9	0.36	322	7	5.7	55	1.0	11.7	107	10.2
Cornmeal – Yellow (degermed, unenriched)	138	0.19	0.07	1.4	0.36	66	7	1.5	55	1.0	11.7	107	10.2
Cornmeal – Yellow (whole-grain)	122	0.47	0.25	4.4	0.37	30	7	4.2	155	2.2	9.9	94	8.9
Cornstarch	128	0.00	0.00	0.0	0.00	0	3	0.6	4	0.1	0.3	117	1.2
Flax Seed	168	2.76	0.27	5.2	0.80	146	428	9.6	659	7.3	30.7	49	45.9
Flax Seed Meal (Ground Flax)	130	2.14	0.21	4.0	0.62	113	332	7.5	510	5.6	23.8	38	35.5
Garbanzo Bean (Chickpea) Flour	120	0.58	0.25	1.8	0.64	668	126	7.5	138	4.1	23.2	73	20.9
Garfava™ Flour	157	NA	NA	NA	NA	NA	104	7.9	NA	NA	34.9	92	12
Hazelnut Flour	112	0.72	0.12	20.2	0.63	127	128	5.3	183	2.7	16.7	19	10.9
Mesquite Flour	146	0.28	0.09	4.5	0.34	26	196	5.1	125	3.1	11.8	122	46.1
Millet (raw)	200	0.84	0.58	9.4	0.77	170	16	6.0	228	3.4	22.0	146	17
Millet (cooked)	174	0.18	0.14	2.3	0.19	33	5	1.1	77	1.6	6.1	41	2.3
Millet Flour	120	0.76	0.48	2.8	NA	NA	NA	9.2	NA	NA	13.7	89	10.3
Montina™ Flour	150	NA	NA	NA	NA	NA	83	10.8	NA	NA	25.5	105	36

Food Item	Weight in Grams (1 cup)	Vitamins					Minerals				Protein	Carbo-hydrates	Dietary Fiber
		B₁ Thiamin mg	B₂ Riboflavin mg	B₃ Niacin mg	B₆ Pyridoxine mg	Folate mcg	Calcium mg	Iron mg	Magnesium mg	Zinc mg	grams	grams	grams
Oat Groats	185	1.22	0.20	1.85	NA	NA	104	11.1	NA	NA	27.5	121	15.2
Rolled Oats	105	0.69	0.12	1.05	NA	NA	59	6.3	NA	NA	15.6	69	8.6
Oat Flour	120	0.80	0.13	1.56	NA	NA	66	7.7	NA	NA	17.8	79	11.0
Pea Flour – Yellow	112	0.73	0.15	3.02	0.12	15	90	5.4	144	3.9	24.7	71	20.6
Potato Flour	160	0.37	0.08	5.6	1.23	40	104	2.2	104	0.9	11.0	133	9.4
Potato Starch	192	0.00	0.00	0.00	NA	NA	19	2.9	NA	NA	0.2	158	0.0
Quinoa Grain (raw)	170	0.34	0.67	5.0	0.38	83	102	15.7	357	5.6	22.3	117	10.0
Quinoa Flour	112	0.22	0.44	3.3	0.25	55	67	10.4	235	3.7	14.7	77	6.6
Rice Bran	134	3.60	0.38	62.8	4.25	36	54	10.3	974	7.4	19.4	68	39
Rice Polish	112	1.50	0.14	20	NA	NA	NA	9.0	NA	NA	12	76	12
Rice, Brown – raw (long grain)	185	0.74	0.17	9.4	0.94	37	43	2.7	265	3.7	14.7	143	6.5
Rice, Brown – cooked (long grain)	195	0.19	0.05	3.0	0.28	8	20	0.8	84	1.2	5.0	45	3.5
Rice Flour – Brown	158	0.70	0.13	10.0	1.2	25	17	3.1	177	3.9	11.4	121	7.3
Rice Flour – Sweet	120	NA	NA	NA	NA	NA	20	0.0	NA	NA	10.1	95	1.2
Rice Flour – White	158	0.22	0.03	4.1	0.69	6	16	0.6	55	1.3	9.4	127	3.8
Rice, White – raw (long grain, parboiled, enr.)	187	1.3	0.08	9.6	0.85	481	103	9.8	50	1.9	15.2	150	4.1
Rice, White – ckd. (long grain, parboiled, enr.)	158	0.34	0.03	3.6	0.25	128	30	2.9	14	0.6	4.6	41	1.4
Rice, Wild – raw	160	0.18	0.42	10.8	0.63	152	34	3.1	283	9.5	23.6	120	9.9
Rice, Wild – cooked	164	0.09	0.14	2.1	0.22	43	5	1.0	53	2.2	6.5	35	3.0
Sorghum Grain	192	0.46	0.27	5.6	1.13	38	54	8.5	365	3.0	21.7	143	12.1
Sorghum Flour	136	0.32	0.20	4.0	0.79	27	38	6.0	256	2.1	15.4	102	8.6
Soy Flour (full-fat)	84	0.49	0.97	3.6	0.39	290	173	5.4	360	3.3	29.0	30	8.0
Soy Flour (defatted)	100	0.70	0.25	2.6	0.57	305	241	9.2	290	2.5	47.0	38	17.5
Tapioca Starch (Tapioca Flour)	120	0.00	0.00	0	0.00	0	0	0	0	0	0.0	119	0.0
Teff Grain	180	0.70	0.20	2.7	NA	135	331	12.1	342	8.8	21.8	130	11.2
Teff Flour	130	0.51	0.14	1.9	NA	97	239	8.7	247	12.2	15.7	94	8.7
Gluten-Containing Flours													
Wheat Bran	58	0.30	0.34	7.9	0.76	46	42	6.1	354	4.2	9.0	37	24.8
Whole-Wheat Flour	120	0.54	0.26	7.6	0.41	53	41	4.7	166	3.5	16.4	87	14.6
White Flour, All-Purpose (enriched)	125	0.98	0.62	7.4	0.06	229	19	5.8	28	0.9	12.9	95	3.4

NA = Not available   ckd. = cooked   enr. = enriched

FOOD ITEM	Weight in Grams (1 cup)	Vitamins					Minerals				PROTEIN	CARBO-HYDRATES	DIETARY FIBER
		B₁ Thiamin mg	B₂ Riboflavin mg	B₃ Niacin mg	B₆ Pyridoxine mg	Folate mcg	Calcium mg	Iron mg	Magnesium mg	Zinc mg	grams	grams	grams
GUMS													
Guar Gum (1 tbsp.)	7	0.00	0.00	0.0	0.00	0	3	0.1	NA	NA	0.2	6	6.1
Xanthan Gum (1 tbsp.)	9	NA	NA	NA	NA	NA	3	0.1	NA	NA	0.5	7	6.8
BEANS, LENTILS & PEAS (COOKED)													
Black Beans	172	0.42	0.10	0.9	0.12	256	46	3.6	120	1.9	15.2	41	15.0
Cranberry (Romano Bean)	177	0.37	0.12	0.9	0.14	366	88	3.7	88	2.0	16.5	43	17.7
Fava (Broad Bean)	170	0.17	0.15	1.2	0.12	177	61	2.6	73	1.7	12.9	33	9.2
Garbanzo (Chickpea)	164	0.19	0.10	0.9	0.23	282	80	4.7	79	2.5	14.5	45	12.5
Kidney Beans – Red	177	0.29	0.10	1.0	0.2	230	50	5.2	80	1.9	15.4	40	13.1
Lentils	198	0.34	0.15	2.1	0.35	358	38	6.6	71	2.5	17.9	40	15.6
Navy Beans	182	0.43	0.12	1.2	0.25	255	126	4.3	96	1.9	15.0	47	19.1
Pinto Beans	171	0.33	0.11	0.5	0.39	294	79	3.6	86	1.7	15.4	45	14.7
Soybeans (mature)	172	0.27	0.49	0.7	0.4	93	175	8.8	148	2.0	28.6	17	10.3
Split Peas	196	0.37	0.11	1.7	0.1	127	27	2.5	71	2.0	16.4	41	16.3
White Beans	179	0.21	0.08	0.3	0.17	144	161	6.6	113	2.5	17.4	45	11.3
NUTS													
Almonds (whole, blanched)	145	0.29	0.81	5.3	0.17	44	313	5.4	399	4.5	31.8	29	15.1
Brazil Nuts (dried, unblanched)	140	0.86	0.05	0.4	0.14	31	224	3.4	526	5.7	20.1	17	10.5
Hazelnuts (Filberts)	135	0.87	0.15	2.4	0.76	153	154	6.3	220	3.3	20.2	23	13.1
Peanuts (dry roasted)	146	0.64	0.14	19.7	0.37	212	79	3.3	257	4.8	34.6	31	11.7
Pecans (halves)	99	0.65	0.13	1.2	0.21	22	69	2.5	120	4.5	9.1	14	9.5
Walnuts – English (shelled, halves)	100	0.34	0.15	1.1	0.54	98	98	2.9	158	3.1	15.2	14	6.7
SEEDS													
Pumpkin Seeds (kernels, dried)	138	0.29	0.44	2.4	0.31	80	59	20.7	738	10.3	33.9	25	5.4
Sesame Seeds (kernels, dried, decorticated)	150	1.05	0.14	8.7	0.60	172	90	9.5	518	10.1	30.7	18	17.4
Sunflower seeds (hulled kernels, dry roasted)	128	0.14	0.32	9.0	1.0	303	90	4.9	165	6.8	24.7	31	14.2

NA = Not available

Nutrient Composition Background Information

✦ Nutrient composition values can vary considerably depending on factors such as:
  • the specific variety, growing conditions and processing of the grain, legume, nut or seed.
  • the coarseness of the grind of the grain and sifting process used to produce the flour.
  • individual laboratory analytical methods and testing equipment used for nutrient analysis.

✦ The weights in grams for 1 cup of the items in the chart on pages 126-128 are from the following sources:

1. **USDA Nutrient Data Base for Standard Reference, Release #18.**
   http://www.nal.usda.gov/fnic/foodcomp/Data/SR18/sr18.html
   http://www.nal.usda.gov/fnic/foodcomp/search/
   • Amaranth seed, arrowroot starch, buckwheat (flour and groats), corn bran, corn flours, cornmeals, cornstarch, flax seed, millet seed, potato flour, quinoa seed, rice (brown, white, wild), rice flours (brown and white), sorghum grain, soy flours and wheat (bran and flours).

2. **Bob's Red Mill**
   • Almond meal, garbanzo flour, guar gum, hazelnut flour, millet flour, potato starch, rice flour (sweet), sorghum flour, tapioca starch, teff grain, xanthan gum.

3. **Ener-G Foods**
   • Rice bran and rice polish.

4. **Amazing Grains**
   • Montina™ flour

5. **Authentic Foods**
   • Garfava™ flour

6. **Dowd and Rogers**
   • Chestnut flour

7. **Minn-Dak Growers, Ltd.**
   • Buckwheat bran (Farinetta™)

8. **Nu-World Amaranth**
   • Amaranth flour

9. **The Teff Company**
   • Teff (grain and flour)

10. **Saskatchewan Flax Development Commission**
    • Flax Seed Meal (Ground Flax)

11. **Best Cooking Pulses**
    • Pea flour (Yellow)

12. **Peter Felker and Casa deFruta Company**
    • Mesquite flour

13. **Cream Hill Estates**
    • Oat flour, oat groats, rolled oats

✦　Nutrient composition values for the grains, flours, starches, gums, beans, nuts and seeds are from:

1. **USDA Nutrient Data Base for Standard Reference, Release #18.**
   http://www.nal.usda.gov/fnic/foodcomp/Data/SR18/sr18.html
   http://www.nal.usda.gov/fnic/foodcomp/search/
   - Amaranth seed, amaranth flour (calculated based on 135 grams of amaranth seed), arrowroot starch, buckwheat (flour and groats), chestnut flour (calculated from 100 grams chestnuts), corn bran, corn flours, cornmeals, cornstarch, flax seed, flax seed meal (calculated based on 130 grams of flax seed), guar gum, millet, potato flour, quinoa seed, quinoa flour (calculated from 112 grams of quinoa seed), rice (brown, white and wild), rice flour (brown and white), sorghum flour (fiber value calculated from 136 grams of sorghum grain), sorghum grain (except folate, magnesium, zinc and vitamin B_6 – see reference on page 131), soy flours, wheat (bran and flours), xanthan gum.
   - Beans, nuts and seeds.

2. **Bob's Red Mill**
   - Almond flour/meal, garbanzo flour, guar gum, hazelnut flour, millet flour, potato starch, rice flour (sweet), sorghum flour (except fiber value – see USDA reference above), tapioca starch, teff flour (calculated from 130 grams of teff grain: folate, iron, zinc, magnesium and fiber – see page 131), teff grain (except folate, iron, zinc, magnesium and fiber – see references on page 131), xanthan gum.

3. **Ener-G Foods**
   - Rice bran and rice polish.

4. **Amazing Grains**
   - Montina™ flour.

5. **Authentic Foods**
   - Garfava™ flour.

6. **Minn-Dak Growers, Ltd.**
   - Buckwheat bran (except fiber and protein – see references on page 131).

7. **Cream Hill Estates**
   - Oat flour, oat groats, rolled oats.

8. **Best Cooking Pulses**
   - Pea flour (yellow)

   BCP Portage, 124 - 10th St. NE, Portage la Prairie, MB, Canada R1N 1B5
   Phone: 204-857-4451   Fax: 204-239-6885
   www.bestcookingpulses.com

Additional References:

A) **Buckwheat Bran** (protein and fiber values)
    Steadman KJ, Burgoon MS, Lewis BA, et al. Buckwheat seed milling fractions: Description, macronutrient composition and dietary fibre. *J of Cereal Sciences* 2001; 33:271-78.

B) **Sorghum Grain** (folate, magnesium, zinc and vitamin B_6)
    Waniska RD and Rooney LL. 2000. Structure and chemistry of the sorghum caryopsis. In CW Smith and RA Frederiksen (eds). *Sorghum: Origin, history, technology, and production.* John Wiley and Sons, Inc., New York, NY.

C) **Mesquite Flour** (nutritional composition values were derived by averaging data from the research articles below)
    1. Becker R and Grosjean OK. A compositional study of pods of two varieties of mesquite (Prosopis glandulosa, P. velutina). *J Agric Food Chem* 1980; 28:22-25.

    2. Felker P, Grados N, Cruz G, et al. Economic assessment of production of flour from Prosopis alba and P. pallida pods for human food applications. *J Arid Environ* 2003; 53:517-28.

    3. Saunders RM, Becker R, Meyer D, et al. Identification of commercial milling techniques to produce high sugar, high fiber, high protein and high galactomannan gum fractions from Prosopis pods. *Forest Ecology Management* 1986; 16:169-80.

    4. Grados N and Cruz G. New approaches to industrialization of algarrobo (Prosopis pallida) pods in Peru. http://www.udep.edu.pe/upadi/prosopis/s3ctxt.pdf

    5. Prokopuik D. 2005. Sucedáneo del café a partir de algarroba de Prosopis alba Griseb. (Coffee substitute from the pods of Prosopis alba Griseb). Tesis Doctoral (PhD Thesis). Registro N°2183. Universidad Politécnica deValencia, Espana.

    6. Meyer D. 1984. Processing, utilization and economics of mesquite pods as a raw material for the food industry. Swiss Federal Institute of Technology, PhD Thesis Diss. ETH 7688.

D) **Teff Flour** and **Teff Grain** (folate, iron and fiber values)
    Analzyed December 14, 2005 by Silliker Canada Co., 90 Gough Road, Unit 4, Markham, ON, Canada, L3R 5V5.

E) **Teff Flour** and **Teff Grain** (magnesium and zinc values)
    Mengesha M. Chemical composition of teff compared with that of wheat, barley and grain sorghum. *Econ Bot* 1966; 20:268-73.

Iron Content of Flours & Starches
(highest to lowest)

Flours & Starches (1 cup)	Iron (mg)
Buckwheat Bran (Farinetta™)	13.6
Montina™ Flour	10.8
Quinoa Flour	10.4
Amaranth Flour	10.3
Rice Bran	10.3
Soy Flour (defatted)	9.2
Millet Flour	9.2
Rice Polish	9.0
Teff Flour	8.7
Garfava™ Flour	7.9
Oat Flour (Pure, uncontaminated, GF)	7.7
Flax Seed Meal (Ground Flax)	7.5
Garbanzo Bean (Chickpea) Flour	7.5
Pea Flour (Yellow)	5.4
Sorghum Flour	6.0
Corn Flour (Yellow, degermed, enriched)	5.7
Cornmeal (Yellow, degermed, enriched)	5.7
Soy Flour (full fat)	5.4
Hazelnut Flour	5.3
Mesquite Flour	5.1
Buckwheat Flour (whole groat)	4.9
Almond Flour (Almond Meal)	4.3
Rice Flour (Brown)	3.1
Potato Starch	2.9
Corn Flour (Yellow, whole grain)	2.8
Chestnut Flour	2.4
Potato Flour	2.2
Corn Bran	2.1
Cornmeal (Yellow, degermed, unenriched)	1.5
Corn Flour (Yellow, degermed, unenriched)	1.2
Rice Flour (White)	0.6
Cornstarch	0.6
Arrowroot Starch (Arrowroot Starch Flour)	0.4
Rice Flour (Sweet)	0.0
Tapioca Starch (Tapioca Flour)	0.0

Iron Content of Seeds & Grains
(highest to lowest)

Seeds & Grains (raw) (1 cup)	Iron (mg)
Pumpkin Seeds (kernels, dried)	20.7
Quinoa	15.7
Amaranth	14.8
Teff	12.1
Oat Groats (Pure, uncontaminated, GF)	11.1
Rice (White, long grain, parboiled, enriched)	9.8
Flax Seed	9.6
Sesame Seeds (kernels, dried, decorticated)	9.5
Sorghum	8.5
Millet	6.0
Sunflower Seeds (hulled kernels, dry roasted	4.9
Buckwheat Groats (roasted, dry)	4.1
Wild Rice	3.1
Rice (Brown, long grain)	2.7

Folate Content of Seeds & Grains
(highest to lowest)

Seeds & Grains (raw) (1 cup)	Folate (micrograms)
Rice (White, long grain, parboiled, enriched)	481
Sunflower Seeds (hulled kernels, dry roasted)	303
Sesame Seeds (kernels, dried, decorticated)	172
Millet	170
Wild Rice	152
Flax Seed	146
Teff	135
Amaranth	96
Quinoa	83
Pumpkin Seeds (kernels, dried)	80
Buckwheat Groats (roasted, dry)	69
Rice (Brown, long grain)	37

Folate Content of Flours & Starches
(highest to lowest)

Flours & Starches (1 cup)	Folate (micrograms)
Garbanzo Bean (Chickpea) Flour	668
Cornmeal (Yellow, degermed, unenriched)	322
Soy Flour (defatted)	305
Soy Flour (full fat)	290
Corn Flour (Masa, enriched)	266
Hazelnut Flour	127
Flax Seed Meal (Ground Flax)	113
Chestnut Flour	110
Teff Flour	97
Amaranth Flour	66
Cornmeal (Yellow, degermed, unenriched)	66
Corn Flour (Yellow, degermed, unenriched)	60
Quinoa Flour	55
Almond Flour (Almond Meal)	42
Buckwheat Bran (Farinetta™)	41
Potato Flour	40
Cornmeal (Yellow, whole grain)	30
Corn Flour (Yellow, whole grain)	29
Sorghum Flour	27
Mesquite Flour	26
Rice Flour (Brown)	25
Pea Flour (Yellow)	15
Rice Flour (White)	6
Corn Bran	3

Calcium Content of Flours & Starches
(highest to lowest)

Flours & Starches (1 cup)	Calcium (mg)
Flax Seed Meal (Ground Flax)	332
Almond Flour (Almond Meal)	289
Soy Flour (defatted)	241
Teff Flour	239
Amaranth Flour	207
Mesquite Flour	196
Soy Flour (full fat)	173
Corn Flour (Masa, enriched)	161
Hazelnut Flour	128
Garbanzo Bean (Chickpea) Flour	126
Garfava™ Flour	104
Buckwheat Bran (Farinetta™)	104
Potato Flour	104
Montina™ Flour	83
Quinoa Flour	67
Oat Flour (Pure, uncontaminated, GF)	66

Calcium Content of Seeds & Grains
(highest to lowest)

Seeds & Grains (raw) (1 cup)	Calcium (mg)
Flax Seed	428
Teff	331
Amaranth	298
Oat Groats (Pure, uncontaminated, GF)	104
Rice (White, long grain, parboiled, enriched)	103
Quinoa	102
Sesame Seeds	90
Sunflower Seeds	90
Pumpkin Seeds (kernels, dried)	59
Sorghum	54
Rice (Brown, long grain)	43
Wild Rice	34
Millet	16

* The bioavailability (ability of the body to absorb the nutrient) of calcium from many of these sources is unknown. Nevertheless, they also contain a variety of nutrients and dietary fiber that are important for good health.

Fiber Content of Flours & Starches
(highest to lowest)

Flours & Starches (1 cup)	Fiber (grams)
Corn Bran	60.0
Mesquite Flour	46.1
Rice Bran	39.0
Montina™ Flour	36.0
Flax Seed Meal (Ground Flax)	35.5
Buckwheat Bran (Farinetta™)	22.7
Garbanzo Bean (Chickpea) Flour	20.9
Soy Flour (defatted)	17.5
Corn Flour (Yellow, whole grain)	15.7
Almond Flour (Almond Meal)	14.7
Amaranth Flour	12.6
Buckwheat Flour (whole groat)	12.0
Garfava™ Flour	12.0
Rice Polish	12.0
Pea Flour (Yellow)	20.6
Oat Flour (Pure, uncontaminated, GF)	11.0
Hazelnut Flour	10.9
Millet Flour	10.3
Cornmeal (Yellow, degermed, enriched)	10.2
Potato Flour	9.4
Sorghum Flour	8.6
Soy Flour (full fat)	8.1
Teff Flour	8.1
Rice Flour (Brown)	7.3
Quinoa Flour	6.6
Arrowroot Starch (Arrowroot Starch Flour)	4.4
Rice Flour (White)	3.8
Corn Flour (Yellow, degermed, enriched)	2.4
Rice Flour (Sweet)	1.2
Cornstarch	1.2
Potato Starch	0.0
Tapioca Starch (Tapioca Flour)	0.0

Fiber Content of Seeds & Grains
(highest to lowest)

Seeds & Grains (raw) (1 cup)	Fiber (grams)
Flax Seed	45.9
Amaranth	18.1
Sesame Seeds (kernels, dried, decorticated)	17.4
Millet	17.0
Buckwheat Groats (roasted, dry)	16.9
Oat Groats (Pure, uncontaminated, GF)	15.2
Sunflower Seeds (hulled kernels, dry roasted)	14.2
Sorghum	12.1
Teff	11.2
Quinoa	10.0
Wild Rice	9.9
Rice (Brown, long grain)	6.5
Pumpkin Seeds (kernels, dried)	5.4
Rice (White, long grain, parboiled, enriched)	4.1

Protein Content of Seeds & Grains
(highest to lowest)

Seeds & Grains (raw) (1 cup)	Protein (grams)
Flax Seed	30.7
Amaranth	28.2
Wild Rice	23.6
Oat Groats (Pure, uncontaminated, GF)	27.5
Quinoa	23.3
Millet	22.0
Teff	21.8
Sorghum	21.7
Buckwheat Groats (roasted, dry)	19.2
Sesame Seeds (kernels, dried, decorticated)	17.4
Rice (White, long grain, parboiled, enriched)	15.2
Rice (Brown, long grain)	14.7
Sunflower Seeds (hulled kernels, dry roasted)	14.2
Pumpkin Seeds (kernels, dried)	5.4

Protein Content of Flours & Starches
(highest to lowest)

Flours & Starches (1 cup)	Protein (grams)
Buckwheat Bran (Farinetta™)	49.0
Soy Flour (defatted)	47.0
Garfava™ Flour	34.9
Pea Flour (Yellow)	24.7
Soy Flour (full fat)	29.0
Montina™ Flour	25.5
Flax Seed Meal (Ground Flax)	23.8
Almond Flour	23.6
Garbanzo Bean (Chickpea) Flour	23.2
Amaranth Flour (Almond Meal)	19.5
Rice Bran	19.4
Oat Flour (Pure, uncontaminated, GF)	17.8
Hazelnut Flour	16.7
Teff Flour	15.7
Sorghum Flour	15.4
Buckwheat Flour (whole groat)	15.1
Quinoa Flour	14.7
Millet Flour	13.7
Rice Polish	12.0
Mesquite Flour	11.8
Cornmeal (Yellow, degermed, enriched)	11.7
Rice Flour (Brown)	11.4
Potato Flour	11.0
Corn Flour (Yellow, whole grain)	10.7
Rice Flour (Sweet)	10.1
Cornmeal (Yellow, whole grain)	9.9
Rice Flour (White)	9.4
Corn Bran	6.4
Chestnut Flour	5.0
Arrowroot Starch (Arrowroot Starch Flour)	0.4
Cornstarch	0.3
Potato Starch	0.2
Tapioca Starch (Tapioca Flour)	0.0

Carbohydrate Content of Flours & Starches
(highest to lowest)

Flours & Starches (1 cup)	Carbohydrate (grams)
Potato Starch	158
Potato Flour	133
Rice Flour (White)	127
Mesquite Flour	122
Rice Flour (Brown)	121
Tapioca Starch (Tapioca Flour)	119
Cornstarch	117
Arrowroot Starch (Arrowroot Starch Flour)	113
Cornmeal (Yellow, degermed, enriched or unenriched)	107
Montina™ Flour	105
Corn Flour (Yellow, degermed, enriched)	104
Sorghum Flour	102
Rice Flour (Sweet)	95
Teff Flour	94
Garfava™ Flour	92
Corn Flour (Yellow, whole grain)	90
Millet Flour	89
Amaranth Flour	89
Buckwheat Flour (whole groat)	85
Oat Flour (Pure, uncontaminated, GF)	79
Chestnut Flour	78
Quinoa Flour	77
Rice Polish	76
Pea Flour (Yellow)	71
Garbanzo Bean (Chickpea) Flour	73
Buckwheat Bran (Farinetta™)	71
Rice Bran	68
Corn Bran	65
Soy Flour (defatted)	38
Flax Seed Meal (Ground Flax)	38
Soy Flour (full fat)	30
Almond Flour	21
Hazelnut Flour	19

Protein Content of Seeds & Grains
(highest to lowest)

Seeds & Grains (raw) (1 cup)	Carbohydrate (grams)
Rice (White, long grain, parboiled, enriched)	150
Millet	146
Sorghum	143
Rice (Brown, long grain)	143
Teff	130
Amaranth	129
Buckwheat Groats (roasted, dry)	123
Oat Groats (Pure, uncontaminated, GF)	121
Wild Rice	120
Quinoa	117
Flax Seed	49
Sunflower Seeds (hulled kernels, dry roasted)	31
Pumpkin Seeds (kernels, dried)	25
Sesame Seeds (kernels, dried, decorticated)	18

GLUTEN-FREE MEAL PLANNING

Getting Started

Successful gluten-free meal planning requires a positive attitude, a little creativity and learning how to make substitutions for some ingredients and food items in favorite recipes and menu items. Fortunately, many foods are naturally gluten-free, including plain meats, fish, poultry, eggs, milk, cheese, yogurt, legumes (dried beans, lentils and peas), nuts, seeds, fruits, vegetables, and grain alternatives such as amaranth, buckwheat, corn, flax, millet, quinoa, rice, sorghum and teff. In addition, there are numerous gluten-free specialty products (e.g., pasta, breads and baked goods, cereals, sauces, soups) that can be substituted for traditional gluten-containing items (see pages 210-278).

Plan simple meals and snacks with plain foods in the beginning so you don't become overwhelmed with the new gluten-free lifestyle. Once you have mastered the basics gradually incorporate new items and try more complex dishes with multiple ingredients. To save time and energy, prepare gluten-free recipe and menu items that everyone can eat rather than having to "cook twice." Other family members can supplement their meal plan with gluten-containing bread or dessert items if desired.

Gluten-Free (GF) Meal-Planning Ideas

The following ideas for breakfast, lunch, dinner and snacks, including some of the recipes and gluten-free specialty products found in this book, can be used as a starting point to create your own favorite meals and snacks.

Breakfast

✦   GF cold cereal (see pages 210-212), sliced fresh fruit, milk*.

✦   GF Granola (see recipes on pages 174-175) and milk*.

✦   Hot cereal (white or yellow cornmeal, cream of white or brown rice, cream of buckwheat, quinoa or teff) with chopped dates, apricots or raisins, cinnamon, brown sugar and milk*.

✦   Shelley's High-Fiber Hot Cereal (see page 173), dried fruits, brown sugar and milk*.

✦   GF toast and yogurt with fruit**, chopped nuts, coconut or ground flax.

✦   GF toasted bread, bun, bagel or English muffin with cream cheese and fruit** or peanut butter and jam or honey, milk* or juice.

✦   GF muffin (see pages 168-170), fresh fruit** and yogurt.

✦   GF French toast (warm bread in microwave first to improve absorption of the egg mixture), fruit** and syrup.

✦   GF freezer waffles, fruit** and syrup and a glass of milk*.

✦   GF pancakes (use a GF mix or make your own, see pages 171-172), with fruit** and syrup.

✦   GF toasted bread and poached egg.

✦   Omelet (chopped green or red peppers, onion, shredded cheese) and leftover fried potatoes.

✦   Fruit smoothie (skim milk powder*, fresh or frozen fruit**, honey or sugar, ground flax, water, crushed ice).

*   GF non-dairy substitutes (e.g., almond, potato, rice or soy beverages) can replace milk.

**   Fruits (e.g., canned crushed pineapple or peach slices, fresh or frozen strawberries or blueberries, applesauce and a sprinkle of cinnamon, sliced bananas or kiwis).

Sandwich Tips

Gluten-Free breads can become dry and crumbly so here are a few tips:

✦ When you buy rice bread, slice (if not sliced) and freeze immediately, placing waxed paper between slices so you can remove one at a time. Seal in a plastic bag.

✦ Toasting bread improves flavor and keeps it from crumbling.

✦ Make a sandwich on lightly toasted bread and freeze it for lunch the next day.

✦ Consider buying a bread machine, as homemade gluten-free breads are much fresher and more economical than ready-made breads.

✦ Try open-face sandwiches and put them under a broiler. (e.g., tuna or pure crab meat with shredded cheese; toasted cheese, tomato and bacon).

Lunch

✦ Homemade soups (vegetable, chicken, corn chowder, salmon chowder, cream of potato, lentil, pea, etc.) and a GF muffin or bagel with melted cheese.

✦ GF soup (see pages 266-270) and GF bread sticks, brushed with melted butter and garlic powder and heated in the oven.

✦ Toasted GF cheese bread or GF grilled cheese sandwich with canned or homemade GF soup.

✦ Egg salad on toasted GF bagel and fresh fruit.

✦ GF bagel with turkey, lettuce, tomato, cucumbers, sprouts and avocado; baby carrots and fresh fruit.

✦ Fettuccini Alfredo (GF pasta, butter or margarine, garlic powder, Parmesan cheese, milk) and salad.

✦ GF pasta with homemade cheese sauce or GF Tomato Pasta Sauce (in jars or homemade) and salad.

✦ GF crackers, hummus (chickpeas, sesame seed oil, garlic), raw vegetables and fresh fruit.

✦ Wild Rice and Vegetable Casserole (see page 193).

✦ GF Pasta and Cheese Dinner, raw vegetables and dip (GF salad dressing).

✦ Quinoa salad (see page 187) and glass of juice.

✦ Canned GF baked beans, coleslaw and homemade corn bread or Montina™ Vegetable Skillet Bread (see page 167).

✦ Green salad with added meat, chicken, canned shrimp, tuna or salmon and GF bun.

✦ GF pasta salad with chicken, GF ham or canned shrimp, tuna or crab and fresh fruit.

✦ Spinach salad with sunflower seeds, chickpeas, feta cheese, strawberries and GF rice crackers.

✦ Stuffed baked potato (cheese and GF ham or broccoli and cheese) – make ahead, freeze and heat in microwave.

✦ Black Bean Chili (see page 194) served over a baked potato or toasted GF bun, top with grated cheese.

✦ Pizza (use GF crust mix [see pages 238-252] or GF prebaked frozen crust, GF pizza sauce, grated cheese, chopped green peppers, mushrooms, onions, GF ham or salami). For recipe, see page 163.

✦ GF hot dog bun and GF wiener or sausage, raw vegetables.

✦ Rice cakes with peanut butter and banana; melted cheese; egg, salmon or tuna salad.

✦ Moroccan Salad (see page 186) and GF roll or bread.

✦ Eggs scrambled in the microwave or an omelet with GF toast.

✦ GF pancakes, waffles or French toast (see breakfast ideas) and GF sausages.

✦ Leftovers (casseroles, chili, stew, meat and potatoes, chicken and rice).

✦ Precooked rice (stored and frozen to heat later) with shredded cheese and leftover meat or chicken and vegetables.

✦ Soft corn tortillas made into "wraps," stuffed with: (A) cooked mung bean noodles or rice noodles, meat or shrimp with vegetables (e.g., sprouts, tomatoes, cucumber, green pepper) drizzled with a mixture of GF soy sauce, honey, ginger and garlic powder **OR** (B) kernel corn with cooked rice and pesto sauce, add cooked ground beef, fresh vegetables, and top with salsa and yogurt or shredded cheese.

Dinner

✦ Rice, hamburger and tomato casserole with grated cheese.

✦ GF lasagne and salad.

✦ Shish Kebobs served over rice.

✦ GF pasta (see pages 256-260) with homemade cheese sauce or GF pasta sauce (in jars or homemade) and salad.

✦ Moroccan Millet (see page 191) and salad.

✦ Creamed salmon or tuna with green peas served on GF toast.

✦ Cabbage rolls or Lentil Leaf Rolls (see page 195).

✦ Homemade beef stew (thickened with GF starch) and GF bread.

✦ Chili con Carne, GF cornbread or corn chips and raw vegetables.

✦ Steak, baked potato, vegetables and a salad.

✦ Baked chicken* or fish*, rice or GF pasta, cooked vegetables and/or salad.
    * Crunchy Coating: crushed potato or tortilla chips, crushed GF cereal, nuts, rice bread crumbs or cornmeal. Also, see page 199 for Cajun Flax Coating recipe.

✦ Lentil stew and GF toasted cheese bread.

✦ GF tacos or tortillas – ground beef, GF taco seasoning, grated cheese, chopped lettuce and tomatoes, GF salsa and sour cream in corn tortilla or served over tortilla chips.

✦ Stir-fry beef, pork, chicken or seafood and vegetables, (GF soy sauce, arrowroot or tapioca starch, garlic and ginger, mixed with water to make a sauce) served over rice with toasted almonds and/or sesame seeds.

✦ Barbecue chicken, pork chops or fish (GF barbecue sauce) with rice pilaf (white, brown or wild) or Quinoa and Wild Rice Pilaf (see page 190) and vegetables.

✦ Lentil Pizza Squares (see page 196) and tossed salad.

✦ GF pizza (see lunch) and salad.

✦ Roast chicken or turkey with dressing (GF bread crumbs), mashed potatoes, gravy (thickened with GF starch) and vegetables.

✦ Sweet and sour meatballs served over rice with stir-fried vegetables.

✦ Oven-Fried Chicken (see page 198), baked potato, cooked vegetables or salad.

✦ Turkey meatballs with Lemon Sauce (see page 197), rice or kasha and cooked vegetables.

✦ Roast pork, applesauce, mashed potatoes, gravy (thickened with GF starch) and vegetables.

✦ Meatloaf (GF rice cereal, GF instant mashed potatoes, GF bread crumbs or crushed corn chips or potato chips and egg, herbs or spices), baked potato and tossed salad.

✦ Beef or chicken kabobs and millet, quinoa or buckwheat pilaf with nuts and dried fruits, and steamed vegetables.

✦ Poached or broiled salmon, brown and/or wild rice and green beans with slivered almonds.

✦ Hamburger patty or grilled chicken breast, corn on the cob, coleslaw and watermelon.

✦ Hearty Vegetarian Kasha Casserole (see page 192) and GF roll.

✦ Savory Pot Pie (see page 200) and salad.

Snacks

✦ Fresh or canned fruit.

✦ Fruit juice.

✦ Dried fruit (e.g., raisins, apricots, cranberries, blueberries, mangoes, apples).

✦ Pumpkin or sunflower seeds (plain or GF flavored).

✦ Nuts (plain).

✦ Dried fruit and nut mixtures.

✦ Soy nuts (plain or GF flavored) or corn nuts (plain).

✦ GF Granola (see pages 174, 175, 210-212).

✦ Celery sticks with peanut butter and raisins OR cream cheese.

✦ Raw vegetables and dip (made with yogurt/herbs or GF salad dressing).

✦ Popcorn.

✦ GF pretzels (see page 236).

✦ Plain corn tortilla chips, salsa, grated cheese and sour cream.

✦ GF flavored mini or large rice cakes (see pages 234, 235).

✦ Banana Seed Bread (see page 166).

✦ Apple Date Bread (see page 165).

✦ GF crackers (see pages 233, 234) with hummus.

✦ GF rice cakes or GF bagel with cream cheese and apple slices.

✦ GF rice cakes with peanut butter and jelly, honey or sliced bananas.

✦ GF snack bars (see pages 230-232).

✦ Fig Bars (see page 176) or Carrot Apple Energy Bars (see page 177).

✦ GF muffins (see pages 168-170) and cheese cubes.

✦ String cheese or cheese slices on GF rice crackers.

✦ Hard-boiled egg.

✦ GF soup and/or GF crackers.

✦ GF crackers and cheese or cheese spread.

✦ Puddings (see page 184) or try any GF pudding.

✦ Yogurt.

Note: See pages 230-237 for GF snack products.

Healthy Meal Planning Tips

Here are some specific ideas how to incorporate more nutritious items into the gluten-free diet.

Breakfast Boosters		
If you eat this	**Add this**	**Or try this instead**
Cream of white rice cereal	Nuts, seeds, ground flax, dried fruits, or fresh fruit	Cream of brown rice, cream of buckwheat, amaranth, rolled oats (pure, uncontaminated gluten-free), quinoa flakes, or teff
Puffed rice or corn cereal	Fresh fruit	GF granola with nuts, seeds, ground flax, dried fruits
GF white rice bread or bagel	Nut butter, cheese, poached egg, or omelet with chopped vegetables	GF enriched bread or bagel; or make your own bread and substitute brown rice, ground flax, or bean flours for some of the white rice, cornstarch, tapioca starch or potato starch
Fruit beverage or fruit drink	Fresh or frozen fruit or fruit juice plus yogurt or skim milk powder and ground flax to make a fruit smoothie	Calcium-fortified juice or 100-percent fruit juice
GF waffle or pancakes with syrup	Cottage cheese or yogurt and fruit	Substitute brown rice, buckwheat, bean flour, ground flax, mesquite flour, oat flour (pure, uncontaminated, gluten-free), quinoa or teff flour for some of the white rice flour; or try GF fiber-rich frozen waffles

If you eat this	Add this	Or try this instead
Crêpes made with white rice flour and topped with syrup	A filling made with blended ricotta cheese, lemon or orange zest, and small amount of sweetener; a topping of berries, peaches, or other fruit, and maple syrup	Substitute almond or bean flour for some of the white rice flour
Fried egg and bacon	Low-fat mozzarella or feta cheese, veggies, and GF smoked salmon, turkey, or ham to make an omelet	Omega-3 rich egg; use a non-stick pan; try Canadian bacon or low-fat GF turkey or chicken sausage

Power Lunches and Dinners

If you eat this	Add this	Or try this instead
Chicken rice soup	Fresh or frozen vegetables	Soups made with lentils, dried beans or peas, vegetables (squash, pumpkin, tomato)
White rice pizza crust, salami and cheese	Vegetables such as peppers, onions, zucchini and tomatoes	Add some amaranth or brown rice flour to your dough; use low-fat cheese
White rice pasta with butter or margarine	Low-fat cheese and vegetables	Enriched gluten-free pasta, brown rice, or lentil pasta; use less butter or margarine
White rice bread sandwich, butter or margarine, mayonnaise and luncheon meat	Sprouts, lettuce, tomatoes, avocado, shredded carrots	GF enriched bread or bagel; low-fat mayonnaise, salsa, or mustard; salmon, tuna, low-fat GF deli meats such as chicken, turkey, pastrami or ham
White rice and meat, fish or chicken	Fresh or frozen vegetables	Brown rice or a combination of brown, wild, and white rice; quinoa, buckwheat, millet or teff
Baked or mashed potato with butter or margarine	Cheese and chopped veggies such as broccoli in the baked potato; milk and grated low-fat cheese in the mashed potato	Use yogurt or low-fat sour cream instead of butter or margarine; try a sweet potato for more vitamin A
Iceberg lettuce salad, GF croûtons, cucumbers, and celery with salad dressing	Tomatoes, peppers, cauliflower, broccoli, mushrooms, shredded carrots, chickpeas, sunflower seeds	Romaine or spinach with strawberries or mandarin oranges, toasted slivered almonds, and/or sesame seeds with a fruit dressing or low-fat salad dressing

Smart Snacks		
If you eat this	**Add this**	**Or try this instead**
GF pretzels	Unsalted nuts	Trail mix with GF granola, dried fruits, nuts and seeds
Rice cakes or rice crackers	Cheese (cubes or string), hummus, nut butter with banana or apple slices	GF snack bar made with seeds, dried fruits and healthy GF grains (amaranth, flax, quinoa); GF high-fiber snack crackers made with nuts and/or seeds
Fried corn chips	Salsa and shredded cheese	Baked corn chips with low-fat cheese and sour cream; popcorn
Celery sticks	Peanut butter, cheese spread or low-fat cream cheese with raisins	Carrot or turnip sticks, peppers, cherry tomatoes, broccoli or cauliflower
GF cookie	Fresh fruit and a glass of milk or enriched GF dairy substitute	Add brown rice, flax or quinoa to the recipe; choose ready-made cookies that are lower in sugar and fat or made with non-hydrogenated oils
GF brownie	Mug of warm, steamed milk or enriched GF dairy substitute	GF crispy rice square (still not so nutritious, but often less fat)
GF muffin with white rice flour	Chopped nuts, mashed banana, dried fruits (raisins, cranberries, apricots, dates), ground flax	Pumpkin, pineapple, carrot or banana muffins made with some brown rice flour, almond flour or bean flour
Full-fat fruit-flavored yogurt	Fresh fruit and nuts	Plain low-fat yogurt with chopped fruits, nuts and small amount of sweetener

Reprinted and adapted with permission from: **Rate Your Plate**, *Living Without* magazine, Fall 2003, pg. 26. www.livingwithout.com

Article by Julie Rothschild Levi and chart prepared by Shelley Case, RD.

Sample Seven-Day Gluten-Free Menu

Here is a sample menu to inspire you to eat safely, healthfully, and deliciously. Of course, different people have different tastes and nutritional needs, so adapt accordingly. Many of the meals and snacks work well when "on the go" (OTG). Stock up on these foods and cook extras for leftovers.

Monday:

Breakfast – Smoothie with fruit, yogurt and flax; gluten-free snack bar (OTG)

Lunch – Spinach salad with sunflower seeds, chickpeas, feta cheese, strawberries; gluten-free rice crackers

Hint: Make a homemade salad dressing to keep in the fridge at home and work.

Snack – Fresh pear and raw almonds (OTG)

Dinner – Gluten-free pasta with seafood or meat sauce and/or grated cheese, grilled veggies

Treat – Pudding* and gluten-free cookie

Tuesday:

Breakfast – Gluten-free bagel with nut butter, sliced bananas and yogurt (OTG)

Lunch – Baked white or sweet potato stuffed with broccoli and cheese and/or gluten-free deli meat; fresh fruit

Hint: Potato may be prepared the night before and reheated prior to eating. Cook extras for other dishes throughout the week.

Snack – Gluten-free granola with milk

Dinner – Turkey chili, gluten-free cornbread or corn chips, veggie sticks

Treat – Berries topped with real whipped cream (optional)

Wednesday:

Breakfast – Omelet with veggies and cheese, leftover fried potatoes, 1/2 grapefruit

Lunch – Tuna fish on mixed greens with seasonal fruit, gluten-free puréed vegetable soup (eg. carrot, squash, potato) with grated Parmesan cheese

Hint: Make soup monthly and freeze small batches for quick and healthy lunches.

Snack – Gluten-free snack bar and yogurt (OTG)

Dinner – Beef or chicken kabobs, millet or buckwheat pilaf with nuts and dried fruit, steamed asparagus

Treat – Piece of a dark chocolate bar

Thursday:

Breakfast – Gluten-free waffle with pure maple syrup, cottage cheese and peaches

Lunch – Gluten-free pasta salad with veggies and leftover chicken or beef, fresh fruit

Snack – Trail mix of gluten-free cereal, nuts and dried fruit; hot chocolate or decaf latte (OTG)

Dinner – Poached salmon, brown and/or wild rice, garlic green beans

Treat – Ice cream* or sorbet with fresh fruit

*Choose from dairy products or enriched, non-dairy, gluten-free substitutes (made from soy, rice or almond).

Friday:

Breakfast – Plain yogurt with fruit and unsweetened coconut, gluten-free toast with nut butter, calcium-fortified orange juice

Lunch – Gluten-free bagel with turkey, lettuce, tomato (option: sprouts, avocado); baby carrots, fresh fruit (OTG)

Snack – String cheese* and gluten-free crackers (OTG)

Dinner – Lamb stew with lentils, mixed greens salad

Hint: Use gluten-free starch, potato flakes, or diced potatoes to thicken.

Treat – Baked apple

Saturday:

Breakfast – Gluten-free cereal with nuts and/or seeds and milk;* fresh fruit or leftover baked apple

Hint: For a hot and healthy start, try cooked amaranth or quinoa, cream of buckwheat or cream of brown rice.

Lunch – Gluten-free grilled cheese* sandwich, gluten-free soup, veggie sticks

Hint: Use homemade stock or use gluten-free bouillon cubes as a safe and tasty base.

Snack – Gluten-free rice cakes with hummus (OTG)

Dinner – Hamburger patty or grilled chicken breast, corn on the cob, gluten-free coleslaw, watermelon

Treat – Vanilla ice cream* with warmed gluten-free brownie or cookie

Sunday:

Breakfast – Gluten-free blueberry pancakes, gluten-free breakfast sausage, glass of milk* or calcium-fortified juice

Lunch – Stir-fry with meat, seafood or tofu, Chinese veggies and brown rice topped with sesame seeds

Hint: Use gluten-free soy sauce. If dining out, bring your own soy sauce and ask the chef to use that in the preparation.

Snack – celery with nut butter and raisins (OTG)

Dinner – Gluten-free pizza, veggies and dip

Hint: Leftover pizza makes a great grab-and-go snack – even when cold.

Treat – Popcorn (OTG)

Other ethnic alternatives:

Fish or vegetable sushi with gluten-free soy sauce
Meat or veggie fajitas (made with gluten-free corn tortillas)
Seafood paella
Wild mushroom risotto or polenta
Veggie, fish, or meat curry over basmati rice
Pad thai and fresh spring rolls made with rice paper

*Choose from dairy products or enriched, non-dairy, gluten-free substitutes (made from soy, rice, or almond).

Reprinted with permission from: *Gluten-Free Guidance* by Shelley Case, **RD** and Cindy Kaplan. *Today's Dietitian*©, March 2003, page 49. Great Valley Publishing, Co.   www.todaysdietitian.com

Gluten-Free Cooking

Gluten-Free Baking

Gluten is the protein found in wheat flour that provides the structure for baked goods. In order to make tasty and satisfying gluten-free baked products it is essential to learn how to use different types and combinations of flours, starches and other ingredients, as well as specific baking techniques in order to compensate for the lack of gluten. This will take time and a lot of patience, perseverance and a sense of humor! But don't be discouraged, there are many excellent gluten-free cookbooks, newsletters and cooking classes/schools that provide detailed information about gluten-free baking and wonderful recipes (see pages 349-352). It is best to start with recipes that are easy to prepare such as pancakes, muffins and cookies. Once you master these, move on to more challenging recipes for breads, rolls, cakes and other items. But before you begin baking, read about the unique taste and texture properties of each flour and starch that are highlighted below. Also, a list of substitutions and general baking hints are found on pages 154-157.

Gluten-Free Flours and Starches

All flours and starches should be stored in airtight containers and labeled with their name and date. Some can be kept in a cool, dry, dark place, however, if you live in hot and/or humid climates, it is better to store them in the refrigerator or freezer. Also, regardless of the environment you live in, the following are best stored in the refrigerator or freezer for optimum freshness: amaranth flour, brown rice flour, corn bran, ground flax, millet flour, nut flours (almond, chestnut and hazelnut), potato flour, rice bran, rice polish and soy flour.

Almond Flour is made from blanched ground almonds which are high in fiber, protein and fat. Available in packages or grind your own in a small coffee grinder using blanched slivered almonds. Adds a rich texture and nutty flavor to baked products. Can also be used as a coating for chicken or fish.

Almond Meal is made from whole ground almonds with the skin on. It has a coarser texture and contains more fiber than almond flour.

Amaranth Flour is ground from the entire tiny, grain-like amaranth seed which is high in fiber, protein, calcium, iron and other nutrients. It has a nutty, slightly sweet toasted flavor and is best combined with other gluten-free flours. Very good in dark-colored baked products (e.g., chocolate cake, brownies, dark breads and muffins) and items with spices (e.g., pumpkin bread or muffins, spice cake). Also works well when combined with almond flour in light-colored, mild-flavored baked goods. Can also be used for thickening gravy.

Amaranth Starch is made from part of the amaranth seed and can be used as a thickener in puddings, sauces, gravy and soups.

Arrowroot Starch (Arrowroot Starch Flour) is ground from the root of a tropical plant. A neutral-flavored, white-colored finely powdered starch, it can be blended with different flours to make baked products. Also an excellent thickener for fruit sauces and other sauces. Can be used for breading as it produces a golden brown crust. Arrowroot can be exchanged for cornstarch.

Bean Flours* can be made from various ground dried beans such as black, cranberry (romano), fava, garbanzo (chickpea), navy, pinto, soy and white. In order to reduce as much of the flatulent effects of the beans as possible, some companies specially treat (precook or micronize) the beans before milling. Bean flours are high in fiber, protein, calcium, iron and B vitamins, especially folate. By combining bean flours with other flours to totally or partially replace white rice flour, the nutritional quality and texture of baked products can be greatly improved. Works well when combined with sorghum flour in intensely flavored recipes such as gingerbread and chocolate cake. Introduce bean flours gradually into the diet and choose those that have been "treated" for better tolerance.

* Reference: Bette Hagman. *Alas! Not All Bean Flours Are The Same*. Gluten Intolerance Group Newsletter, April 2001

Buckwheat Flour is ground from unroasted buckwheat groats (hulled buckwheat kernels). The dark flour has a strong, distinctive flavor as it contains a higher percentage of finely milled particles of the black buckwheat hull and is higher in fiber and nutrients. The light flour has a milder, mellow flavor as it contains fewer or no buckwheat hulls and is consequently lower in fiber and some nutrients. Either flour is best used in small amounts to add flavor to bland flours in breads, muffins, and pancakes. Make sure to purchase 100% pure buckwheat flour as some companies sell a combination of buckwheat flour and wheat flour in one package.

Chestnut Flour is made from ground chestnuts which are higher in starch and lower in protein and fat compared to other nut flours. This light beige silky-textured flour adds a nutty flavor to baked products. Best combined with other flours.

Corn Bran is very high in insoluble fiber. Light in color, with a mild flavor, it can be added in small amounts to baked products such as muffins, breads and loaves.

Corn Flour, milled from finely ground dried corn kernels, is very light in texture and gives a mild, nutty flavor to baked goods. It is best used in combination with other flours.

Cornmeal is made from dried kernels of yellow, white or blue corn, however, it is not as finely ground as corn flour. It can be used as a breading or in corn bread, corn muffins and polenta.

Cornstarch is made from the endosperm of corn that is highly refined, resulting in little nutritive value. This heavy white, flavorless powder is blended with various flours and/or other starches and used to lighten baked goods. Also an excellent thickener.

Flax Seed Meal (Ground Flax) is produced from ground flaxseed which is high in fiber, omega-3 fatty acids, protein, B vitamins, calcium and other minerals. This dark brown meal adds a nutty flavor, crunchy texture and improves the nutritional profile of baked products. Due to its high fat content, baked products made with flax brown quickly so the temperature and baking time may need to be reduced. It can be purchased already ground in vacuum-sealed packages on store shelves or in plastic bags in the refrigerated section. The flax seeds can also be ground in a coffee grinder and used as needed.

Garbanzo Bean Flour is ground from garbanzo beans (also known as chickpea, besan, gram or channa). This popular tan-colored bean flour is best combined with other flours. See Bean Flours for more information.

Garfava™ Flour, developed by Authentic Foods, is the trademark name for a blend of garbanzo bean and fava bean flours that are specially processed. Creates baked goods with excellent volume and a good moisture content. See Bean Flours for more information.

Garbanzo and Fava Bean Flour is also available from other companies that may or may not be specially processed. See Bean Flours for more information.

Hazelnut Flour is made from ground hazelnuts (also known as filberts). High in protein, fiber and other nutrients which can improve the nutritional quality of baked goods, it adds a rich texture and nutty flavor.

Mesquite Flour comes from the ground bean pods of the mesquite tree. Available as a light tan coarse meal or fine flour that is very high in fiber. Has a cinnamon-mocha aroma and slightly sweet chocolate, molasses-like flavor with a hint of caramel. Best combined with other flours to make pancakes, muffins, breads, cakes and cookies.

Millet Flour, ground from the tiny millet seed, is light yellow in color and has a slightly sweet corn-like, nutty flavor. High in protein and B vitamins as well as a source of fiber and minerals, it is best combined with other flours, comprising no more than 20-25% of the total flour blend.

Montina™ Flour is ground from the seeds of Indian ricegrass that is very high in fiber, iron and protein. A light brown, gray-colored flour with a sweet, nutty, almost "wheat-like" flavor, it can replace up to 25% of one of the primary flours in baked products.

Nut Flours are made from ground almonds, chestnuts or hazelnuts. Keep refrigerated or frozen in airtight containers for optimum freshness. See individual nut flours for more information.

Oat Flour (Pure, uncontaminated, gluten-free) is milled from whole grain oat groats (Cream Hill Estates uses the entire groat which includes the bran). It is a source of protein, iron, B vitamins and fiber. This flour has a sweet, nutty flavor; can use 50-75% in the total flour mixture of baked goods.

Potato Flour is not the same as potato starch and they cannot be substituted for one another. The flour is made from whole potatoes, including the skin, resulting in a heavier product with a light tan color and slight potato flavor. Due to its heavy texture, it is best used in small amounts and combined with other flours. Adds crispness and density to baked products.

Potato Starch is made only from the starch portion of the potato. This bland-flavored, fine white powder works well in many baked products when used at approximately 30-40% of the total flour mixture. Sift or whisk potato starch before measuring as it lumps easily.

Quinoa Flour is ground from the quinoa seed which is high in protein, iron and other nutrients and is also a source of fiber. This tan-colored flour has a slight nutty but strong flavor which can overpower baked goods, it is therefore best to limit to 25% of the total flour mixture. Works well in highly spiced or flavored baked products.

Rice Bran is the outer layer of the brown rice kernel and is high in fiber. It can be added in small amounts to baked goods to add a nutty flavor and improve the nutrient and fiber content.

Rice Cereal (Cream of Brown Rice or Brown Rice Cream) is made from whole-grain brown rice that is coarsely ground and can be cooked in 3-4 minutes as a hot cereal.

Rice Cereal (Cream of White Rice or White Rice Cream) is made from coarsely ground white rice and can be cooked in 3-4 minutes as a hot cereal.

Rice Flour (Brown) is made from whole-grain brown rice that is very finely ground. This slightly tan-colored flour is higher in fiber and other nutrients than white rice flour. If brown rice or white rice flour is used by itself in baked products, they tend to be gritty, crumbly and dry out quickly, therefore it is best combined with other flours and starches. Adds a nutty flavor to baked goods.

Rice Flour (Sweet), also known as sticky, sushi or glutinous rice flour, is different from white rice flour although they look alike. Made from ground sticky short-grain white rice that is higher in starch than brown or white rice, it makes an excellent thickener for sauces, gravy and puddings as it keeps liquids from separating when they are chilled or frozen. Can be used in small amounts in flour blends for baked products.

Rice Flour (White) is made from ground white rice (contains no bran or polish) thus is lower in fiber and nutrients than brown rice flour. This starchy white flour has a bland flavor and is best combined with other flours in baked products.

Rice Polish is made from part of the rice bran and rice germ (the layer underneath the rice bran). Lighter in color than pure rice bran, it is a good source of fiber and can be substituted for rice bran in other recipes.

Sorghum Flour is ground from new food-grade sorghum varieties (also known as milo). This light tan-colored flour has a slightly nutty, earthy flavor. Combine with other flours, especially bean flour, to produce a wide variety of excellent baked products.

Soy Flour, available as whole or defatted, is made from ground dried soybeans. This yellow, slightly nutty and "beany" tasting flour is best combined with other flours, especially rice, in baked products containing fruits, nuts, spices or chocolate. Very high in protein, fiber, B vitamins, iron and calcium.

Tapioca Flour (Tapioca Starch), also known as tapioca starch flour, is made from the root of the tropical cassava plant and is very low in nutrients. A pure white powder, it can be used to make up to 25-50% of the total flour blend. Used to lighten baked goods and create a chewy texture in breads. Also used as a thickener for soups, sauces, gravy and stir fries, and as a breading, as it browns quickly and produces a crispy coating.

Teff Flour is made from the ground whole grain tiny teff seeds from a grass native to Ethiopia. This nutty, molasses-like brown flour can comprise 25-50% of the total flour blend. It works well in dark baked breads, muffins, cakes and cookies (e.g., chocolate cake, brownies, pumpernickel bread, gingerbread) and can also be added to pancakes and puddings. This very nutritious flour is high in protein, fiber and minerals such as iron and calcium. Make sure to purchase 100% teff flour as teff flour may sometimes be combined with wheat flour.

Whole-Bean Flour, from ground cranberry (romano) beans, is high in fiber, protein, vitamins and minerals. It can be used in a variety of baked goods when combined with other flours as it is a dark, stronger-tasting flour. See Bean Flours for more information.

For more information and recipes using some of these flours and starches see pages 111-121, 158-201. A listing of companies that carry these flours can be found on pages 252-255.

Substitutions for Wheat Flour in Baking

A combination of gluten-free flours and starches makes a better product than single flours. A variety of gluten-free all-purpose baking flour mixes can be substituted for wheat flour and are available from many gluten-free companies (see pages 249-252). Also, the following are examples of gluten-free flour mixes that can be made at home and used in many different recipes.

CAROL FENSTER'S GLUTEN-FREE SORGHUM FLOUR BLEND

1 1/2 cups sorghum flour
1 1/2 cups potato starch OR cornstarch
1 cup tapioca flour
1/2 cup almond flour OR bean flour OR chestnut flour OR corn flour

✦ Mix ingredients and store in plastic self-seal bags or containers in the refrigerator. Before using in a recipe, take out the amount needed and allow to warm to room temperature before using.

✦ Makes 4 1/2 cups.

Reprinted with permission from: *Gluten-Free 101: Easy Basic Dishes without Wheat* by **Carol Fenster, PhD**, Savory Palate, Inc., 2006. www.glutenfree101.com

GLUTEN-FREE FLOUR MIXTURE BY CONNIE SARROS

2 1/2 cups white rice flour
1 cup potato starch
1 cup tapioca flour
1/4 cup cornstarch
1/4 cup bean flour
2 tbsp. xanthan gum

✦ Sift all of the ingredients together and store in plastic self-seal bags or containers and refrigerate until ready to use. If not used within 1 week, freeze the mixture. Before using in a recipe, take out the amount needed and leave at room temperature for 15 minutes before using.

✦ Makes 5 cups.

Reprinted with permission from: *Wheat-free Gluten-free Reduced Calorie Cookbook* by **Connie Sarros**, McGraw-Hill, 2003. www.gfbooks.homestead.com

GENERIC GLUTEN-FREE FLOUR MIXTURE

4 cups white rice flour
1 1/3 cup potato starch
1 cup tapioca flour

✦ Sift ingredients together and store in plastic self-seal bags or containers. Refrigerate for longer storage periods.

✦ Makes 6 1/3 cups.

Substitutions for Wheat Flour as a Thickener

Gluten-free flours, starches and other ingredients can be used as thickening agents in sauces, soups, stews, gravy, puddings and other food items. Each has its own unique properties, therefore some are more suitable than others for thickening. Starches should be mixed in cold water before using, added during the last 5 minutes of cooking and not overcooked. Flours should also be mixed in cold liquid before using. Gelatin needs to be softened in cold water, heated until the liquid is clear and then added to the food item to be thickened. Cooked starches are more clear and shiny, whereas cooked flours are more cloudy and opaque in appearance.

Substitutions for 1 tbsp. Wheat Flour

Starches	
Amaranth Starch	1 1/2 tsp.
Arrowroot Starch	1 1/2 tsp.
Cornstarch	1 1/2 tsp.
Flours	
Bean (e.g., garbanzo/chickpea)	1 tbsp.
Brown Rice Flour	1 tbsp.
Sweet Rice Flour	1 tbsp.
Tapioca Flour	1 tbsp.
White Rice Flour	1 tbsp.
Others	
Gelatin Powder (unflavored)	1 1/2 tsp.
Quick-Cooking Tapioca	2 tsp.

Food Item	Suitable Thickeners
Cream Soups	Amaranth starch, bean flour, rice flour (brown, sweet, white), tapioca flour
Fruit Sauces	Arrowroot starch, cornstarch, sweet rice flour
Fruit Pies and Cobblers	Cornstarch, quick-cooking tapioca
Gravy	Amaranth Flour, rice flour (brown, sweet, white), tapioca flour
Puddings	Amaranth starch, cornstarch, gelatin, sweet rice flour
Savory Sauces	Amaranth starch, arrowroot starch, bean flour, cornstarch, sweet rice flour
Stews	Bean flour, rice flour (brown, sweet, white), tapioca flour
Stir-Fry Dishes	Arrowroot starch, cornstarch, tapioca flour

General Baking Hints

Baking Tips

Store gluten-free flours and starches in plastic airtight containers with wide and tightly fitting lids. For optimum freshness keep in the refrigerator or freezer. Allow the cold flour or starch to return to room temperature before using.

✦ Label containers with the name of the item and date purchased.

✦ Measure flours and starches carefully. Inaccurate measurements can greatly affect the quality of gluten-free recipes because each flour and starch has very unique properties.

✦ Loosely spoon the flour or starch into the measuring cup, leveling the top with the flat side of a knife. Never pack down the flour.

✦ Use shiny, light-colored metal pans (gray not black) as products bake and brown more evenly in them than in dark pans which can leave edges crisp and over-browned.

✦ When using glass baking pans and non-stick metal baking pans (gray not black), reduce oven temperature by 25°F.

✦ Most gluten-free breads are better when baked at lower temperatures for longer periods of time. After the first 10-15 minutes of baking, tent the bread with foil to prevent over-browning.

✦ Baking is also affected by temperature and altitude. Slightly reduce the amount of liquid in the recipe if baking at a higher altitude or on a very humid day. For baking at very low altitudes, slightly increase the amount of liquid.

✦ Gluten-free bread dough tends to be softer, stickier and more batter-like. If it is too heavy and dry, the bread tends to be too crumbly.

✦ When making a gluten-free chocolate cake or brownies, grease the pan and then "flour" the pan with cocoa.

Texture Tips

✦ A combination of gluten-free flours and starches makes a better product than single flours.

✦ Gluten-free baked products often require more leavening than products made with wheat flour due to the lack of gluten which is necessary to form an elastic dough and enables the product to rise.

✦ It is important to use xanthan gum or guar gum in baked products in order to prevent crumbling. Add the gum to the dry ingredients as it does not mix with water. For every cup of gluten-free flour, use 1 teaspoon of gum for breads and ½ - ¾ teaspoon for other baked goods.

✦ Unflavored powdered gelatin also works as a binding agent and can prevent crumbling. If substituting gelatin for xanthan or guar gum, use twice as much gelatin. Soften the gelatin in half the water called for in the recipe before adding.

✦ Substituting buttermilk for the milk or water in recipes results in a lighter, more finely textured product. Carbonated beverages (not diet soft drinks) in place of water or milk can also result in a lighter-textured product (e.g., pancakes, cakes).

✦ Let gluten-free dough sit at least 30 minutes at room temperature to soften. This results in a better-textured product.

Flavor Tips

✦ To improve the flavor of gluten-free baked products use more herbs, spices and flavorings (approximately $1/3$ - $1/2$ more than normal).

✦ Adding chocolate chips, nuts, fruits (e.g., applesauce, bananas) dried fruits (e.g., apricots, cranberries, raisins) can also improve the flavor.

✦ Honey or molasses can provide more flavor than white sugar. You need to reduce the amount of liquid in the recipe if making this substitution. If a recipe calls for 1 cup of sugar, use $3/4$ cup honey or molasses.

✦ Most gluten-free breads taste better toasted or warm.

Storage Tips

✦ Baked products made with gluten-free flours have no preservatives, become stale quickly and are quite perishable. Wrap them tightly in plastic wrap and store in airtight plastic containers or self-seal plastic bags. If the product will not be eaten within one or two days, freeze to ensure minimum loss of moisture and flavor. For breads, it is best to thoroughly cool, slice and separate each slice with wax paper before bagging and freezing.

✦ Placing baked products such as muffins in plastic bags when still warm can preserve moisture.

✦ Thaw frozen baked goods at room temperature instead of microwaving at full power; microwaving causes them to become rubbery and tough.

Thanks to the following gluten-free culinary experts for some of the background information on gluten-free flours and starches, substitutions and many of the above baking tips:

Carol Fenster, PhD, President and Founder of Savory Palate, Inc., gluten-free publishing and consulting firm. Author of:
1,000 Gluten-Free Recipes
100 Best Gluten-Free Recipes
Gluten-Free 101: Easy Basic Dishes without Wheat
Wheat-Free Recipes and Menus: Delicious, Healthful Eating for People with Food Sensitivities
Cooking Free: 220 Flavorful Recipes for People with Food Allergies and Multiple Food Sensitivities
www.savorypalate.com

Connie Sarros, Author of gluten-free cookbooks and other resources:
Wheat-Free Gluten-Free Recipes for Special Diets
Wheat-Free Gluten-Free Cookbook for Kids and Busy Adults
Wheat-Free Gluten-Free Dessert Cookbook
Wheat-Free Gluten-Free Reduced Calorie Cookbook
Newly Diagnosed Survival Kit
All You Wanted to Know About Gluten-Free Cooking DVD
www.gfbooks.homestead.com

Donna Washburn, P.H.Ec. and **Heather Butt, P.H.Ec.**, partners in Quality Professional Services, specializing in recipe development and bread machine baking. Authors of:
Complete Gluten-Free Cookbook
125 Best Gluten-Free Recipes
The Best Gluten-Free Family Cookbook
www.bestbreadrecipes.com

SORGHUM BREAD

Yield: 1 Loaf/12 Slices

Bette Hagman, a.k.a. the "Gluten-Free Gourmet," is an expert in the area of gluten-free baking. She has been developing recipes combining the new food-grade sorghum varieties with other gluten-free flours.

1 cup	sorghum flour
2/3 cup	tapioca flour
2/3 cup	cornstarch
1 1/2 tsp.	xanthan gum
1/3 cup	non-fat dry milk powder OR nondairy substitute*
1/2 tsp.	salt
1 tsp.	unflavored gelatin
1 tsp.	GF baking powder
3 tbsp.	sugar
2 1/4 tsp.	dry yeast granules
2	eggs
1/2 tsp.	dough enhancer OR vinegar
3 tbsp.	vegetable oil
1 cup	lukewarm water (more or less)

✦ Grease a 4 1/2 x 8 1/2-inch loaf pan and dust with rice flour.

✦ Combine the dry ingredients in a medium bowl.

✦ In the mixing bowl of a heavy-duty mixer, whisk together the eggs, dough enhancer and oil. Add most of the water, holding back about 3 tbsp. to add as needed. Turn the mixer to low and add the flour mixture a little at a time. The batter should be the consistency of cake batter. Add the remaining water a little at a time to achieve this texture. Turn the mixer to high and beat for 3 1/2 minutes. Spoon the batter into the prepared pan, cover and let rise in a warm place; about 35 minutes for rapid rising yeast; 60 or so minutes for regular yeast, or until dough reaches the top of the pan.

✦ Bake for 50-55 minutes in a preheated 400°F oven, covering after 10 minutes with aluminum foil.

✦ Turn out immediately to cool. For a softer crust rub immediately with butter or margarine. Cool before slicing.

* *Bette wrote, "I used the adult drink powder Ensure as my nondairy substitute and it turned out very well. The extra flavor and vanilla in the powder made the best-tasting bread."*

This recipe was developed by **Bette Hagman** for **Twin Valley Mills**, and is reprinted with their permission. Twin Valley Mills, LLC., RR #1, Box 45, Ruskin NE, USA 68974;
Phone 402-279-3965;
www.twinvalleymills.com

Nutritional Analysis
1 serving = 1 slice

Calories (kcal)	152
Carbohydrates (g)	26
Dietary Fiber (g)	1
Fat (g)	5
Protein (g)	4
Iron (mg)	0.8
Calcium (mg)	56
Sodium (mg)	170

BASIC RYE BREAD

Reprinted with permission from: *Delicious Gluten-Free Wheat-Free Breads: Easy to make breads everyone will love to eat for the bread machine or oven* – by **LynnRae Ries** and **Bruce Gross**, What No Wheat Publishing, 2003, www.whatnowheat.com

Yield: **15 Slices** (1/2" thick)	

Caraway seeds add classic rye bread flavor to this versatile bread.

Note: This recipe provides options for both bread machine and mixer.

3	eggs
1/4 cup	vegetable oil
2 tbsp.	molasses
1 tsp.	vinegar
1 cup	water
3/4 cup	white rice flour
3/4 cup	brown rice flour
1/4 cup	sweet rice flour
1/2 cup	potato starch
1/2 cup	tapioca starch
1/4 cup	millet, amaranth OR sorghum flour
OR	use 3 cups of your favorite GF flour mix instead of the above flours
1 tsp.	salt
1/4 cup	light brown sugar
1 tbsp.	xanthan gum
1/2 cup	non-fat dry milk powder
1 tsp.	dough enhancer (optional)
2 1/2 tsp.	bread machine yeast
2 tbsp.	caraway seeds, if desired

✦ **Bread Machine:**

− Place ingredients into the bread machine according to the manual. Program the machine to knead (mix) the ingredients, rise once, then change to bake for 60-70 minutes. Rising time should be 50 minutes, or until the dough doubles in size. When done, remove the bread from the machine and place on a wire rack to cool. Remember to remove the bread machine paddles if they are stuck in the bread.

✦ **Mixer:**

− In a medium-sized bowl, mix all the liquid ingredients together and set aside.

− Place all the dry ingredients into mixer bowl and blend flours together on slow speed.

− Slowly add the liquid ingredients to the dry while the mixer is on low.

− Beat on high for 3-4 minutes. Mixture should look silky. If the dough is too dry, add liquid 1 tablespoon at a time.

✦ Place the dough into a 9 x 5-inch loaf pan that has been greased and dusted with rice flour. Bake in a preheated 350°F oven for 60-70 minutes. Start checking for the bread being done at 55 minutes. When done, remove from bread pan and place on cooling rack. Do not cut or package until the bread cools, approximately 2-3 hours.

Nutritional Analysis
(amaranth flour)
1 serving = 1 slice (1/2" thick)

Calories (kcal)	182
Carbohydrates (g)	31
Dietary Fiber (g)	2
Fat (g)	5
Protein (g)	4
Iron (mg)	0.9
Calcium (mg)	53
Sodium (mg)	210

(millet flour)
1 serving = 1 slice (1/2" thick)

Calories	183
Carbohydrates (g)	31
Dietary Fiber (g)	1
Fat (g)	5
Protein (g)	4
Iron (mg)	0.9
Calcium (mg)	50
Sodium (mg)	210

Brown Rice Bread

with variations for using Teff, Amaranth, Quinoa and Buckwheat

Yield: 1 Loaf/12 Slices	

So far, this is the best gluten-free bread we have tried. Recipe adapted from Barbara Emch's, a fellow celiac.

3	large eggs (egg-free: see substitution below*)
1/4 cup	vegetable oil
1 tsp.	lemon juice
2 cups	tapioca starch flour
2 cups	fine brown rice flour
2/3 cup	instant non-fat dry milk powder (for dairy-free: see substitution below **)
2 tsp.	xanthan gum
1 tsp.	salt
1 1/2 tbsp.	active dry yeast
4 tbsp.	sugar
1 1/4 cups	warm water (105°-115°F)

✦ Bring all refrigerated ingredients to room temperature. Grease a 5 x 9-inch loaf pan.

✦ In the bowl of a stand mixer, combine eggs, oil and lemon juice.

✦ In a medium bowl, combine tapioca starch flour, brown rice flour, dry milk powder, xanthan gum, salt, yeast and sugar. Add about 1 cup of the water to the egg mixture, then slowly add dry ingredients a little at a time until completely incorporated. If mixture is too dry, add remaining water (see humidity note). Mix batter on high speed for 3 1/2 minutes, then pour into prepared pan.

✦ Cover bread with foil and place in a cold oven. Set a pan of hot water on a lower shelf underneath the bread. Leave for 10 minutes with oven door closed. (This will cause the bread to rise quickly.) Remove bread from oven (do not uncover) and place in a warm place in the kitchen. Preheat oven to 400°F. Bread will continue to rise as oven preheats.

✦ Uncover bread and bake for 10 minutes to brown the top. Cover bread with foil and continue to bake bread for 30 minutes. Turn bread out onto a cooling rack. When completely cooled, wrap tightly to maintain freshness for as long as possible.

Notes: ✦ **Humidity:** If humidity is too high, reduce the amount of water in the recipe to avoid over-rising. Many gluten-free bakers experience the frustrating situation in which a beautiful loaf of bread deflates once removed from the oven. You will need to experiment a little to get just the right amount of water in your bread, depending on the humidity in the air. If in doubt, use less water than the recipe calls for.

✦ **Rapid Rise Yeast:** You may use rapid rise yeast or regular yeast. If using rapid rise yeast, eliminate the cold oven/pan of hot water rise method and instead follow yeast package directions for rise time.

* **Egg-Free Substitution, Flax Seed:** This seed has many health benefits such as high-quality protein, fiber, B and C vitamins, iron and zinc, anti-cancer properties, omega-3 fatty acids, and many other benefits. To use as an egg substitute: grind 3 tablespoons flaxseed and add 1/2 cup + 1 tablespoon boiling water, let sit for 15 minutes, then whisk with a fork – this mixture will replace 3 eggs in a recipe. A clean coffee grinder works well to grind the small flaxseed.

** **Dairy-Free Substitution, Ground Almonds:** Use 2/3 cup ground almonds to replace 2/3 cup dry milk powder.

BROWN RICE BREAD

(continued)

Variations:

Teff Bread, Quinoa Bread, Amaranth Bread, or Buckwheat Bread

Substitute the following combination of flours for the 2 cups brown rice flour and 2 cups tapioca flour in the original recipe.

1 1/2 cups	tapioca starch flour
1 1/2 cups	brown rice flour
1 cup	teff flour, quinoa flour, amaranth flour, OR light buckwheat flour

Light buckwheat flour is preferred to dark buckwheat flour. The dark flour gives a purple cast to the bread.

Reprinted with permission from: *Cooking Gluten-Free! A Food Lover's Collection of Chef and Family Recipes without Gluten or Wheat* by **Karen Robertson**, Celiac Publishing, 2002.

Nutritional Analysis
1 serving = 1 slice

	Original	Amaranth	Buckwheat	Quinoa	Teff	Dairy-Free & Egg-Free	Dairy Free	Egg Free
Calories	253	255	242	248	252	263	267	248
Carbohydrates (g)	47	45	42	44	45	47	46	48
Dietary Fiber (g)	2	3	3	2	2	3	3	3
Fat (g)	7	7	7	7	7	9	9	7
Protein (g)	6	7	6	6	6	4	5	5
Iron (mg)	1.0	1.8	1.2	1.8	1.6	1.1	1.2	1.0
Calcium (mg)	66	83	66	71	86	24	24	67
Sodium (mg)	257	258	256	258	258	217	234	240

Montina™ Bread

Yield: **1 Loaf/12 Slices**

The sweet, nutty flavor of Montina™ flour gives this bread a traditional "wheat-like" flavor.

Tip: For best results ... thin slices work well and toasting brings out additional flavor!

3 cups	Montina™ All-Purpose Baking Flour Blend*
1/4 cup	sugar
3 1/2 tsp.	xanthan gum
1 1/2 tsp.	salt
2/3 cup	non-fat dry milk powder
1 cup	water
1/4 cup	butter-flavored shortening
2 tsp.	sugar
1/2 cup	warm water (110°F)
4 1/2 tsp.	yeast granules
1 tsp.	apple cider vinegar **
3	eggs

✦ Combine Montina™, 1/4 cup sugar, xanthan gum, salt, dry milk powder in the bowl of a heavy mixer.

✦ In small saucepan, combine 1 cup water and shortening. Warm just until shortening is melted.

✦ Dissolve 2 tsp. sugar in 1/2 cup warm water and mix in the yeast. Let proof until bubbly.

✦ Turn the mixer on low, allowing all the dry ingredients to blend.

✦ Slowly add the warm water, shortening and vinegar. Blend thoroughly and then add the eggs.

✦ Add the yeast mixture to the bowl and beat on highest speed for 2 minutes.

✦ Cover the mixing bowl with plastic wrap and a towel and put in a warm place. Let the dough rise until doubled, approximately 1-1 1/2 hours.

✦ Return the bowl to the mixer and beat on high for 3 minutes.

✦ Spoon the dough into a greased 5 x 9-inch loaf pan, level dough as best you can, cover with plastic wrap and let rise until slightly above the top of the pan.

✦ Bake in a preheated 400°F oven for 10 minutes. At this point, place foil over the bread and bake 50 minutes longer.

✦ When baking is finished, remove bread from pan and cool on a wire rack.

Reprinted courtesy of: **Amazing Grains Grower Cooperative**, 405 Main St. S.W., Ronan MT, USA 59684; Phone 877-278-6585 or 406-676-3536; www.amazinggrains.com

* **Montina™ All-Purpose Baking Flour Blend** is a mixture of Montina Pure (100% Indian ricegrass), white rice flour and tapioca starch and is available from Amazing Grains Grower Cooperative.

** **Author's Note:** Other vinegars can be substituted for apple cider vinegar, except malt vinegar (which is not gluten-free).

Nutritional Analysis
1 serving = 1 slice

Calories (kcal)	232
Carbohydrates (g)	39
Dietary Fiber (g)	3
Fat (g)	6
Protein (g)	6
Iron (mg)	3.5
Calcium (mg)	63
Sodium (mg)	365

CAROL FENSTER'S PIZZA

Serves 6 (1 slice each)

This flour mixture produces a super pizza crust. Add the zesty sauce, grated mozzarella and your favorite toppings for a great lunch, dinner or snack.

Reprinted with permission from: *Gluten-Free 101: Easy Basic Dishes without Wheat* by **Carol Fenster, PhD.**, Savory Palate Inc. 2006; www.glutenfree101.com

Nutritional Analysis
(Brown Rice Flour)
1 serving = 1 slice

Calories (kcal)	147
Carbohydrates (g)	31
Dietary Fiber (g)	3
Fat (g)	2
Protein (g)	4
Iron (mg)	1.3
Calcium (mg)	54
Sodium (mg)	697

(Garbanzo/Fava Bean Flour)
1 serving = 1 slice

Calories (kcal)	130
Carbohydrates (g)	26
Dietary Fiber (g)	5
Fat (g)	2
Protein (g)	6
Iron (mg)	1.7
Calcium (mg)	66
Sodium (mg)	729

Sauce:

1 can	(8 oz.) tomato sauce
1/2 tsp.	dried oregano
1/2 tsp.	dried basil
1/2 tsp.	dried rosemary
1/2 tsp.	fennel seeds
1/4 tsp.	garlic powder OR 1 minced garlic clove
2 tsp.	sugar
1/2 tsp.	salt

Crust:

1 tbsp.	dry yeast
3/4 cup	warm milk (110°F) – cow, rice, OR soy milk
1/2 tsp.	sugar
2/3 cup	garbanzo/fava bean flour OR brown rice flour
1/2 cup	tapioca flour
2 tsp.	xanthan gum
1/2 tsp.	salt
1 tsp.	gelatin powder
1 tsp.	Italian seasoning
1 tsp.	olive oil
1 tsp.	cider vinegar

Sauce:

✦ Combine all sauce ingredients in a small saucepan and simmer for 15 minutes. (Makes about 1 cup, enough for a 12-inch pizza.)

Crust:

✦ Dissolve yeast and sugar in warm milk for five minutes. In a food processor, blend all crust ingredients, including yeast mixture, until a ball forms. Dough will be soft.

✦ Place dough on a greased 12-inch non-stick pizza pan. Liberally sprinkle rice flour over dough; then press dough into pan with your hands, continuing to sprinkle dough with flour to prevent sticking. Make edges thicker to contain toppings.

✦ Bake pizza crust in a preheated 400°F oven for 10 minutes. Remove from oven.

✦ Add sauce and toppings to crust. Bake another 20-25 minutes, or until top is nicely browned.

Injera (Ethiopian Flat Bread)

Yield: **1 Loaf/24 Slices**

This flat, thin porous bread is a traditional Ethiopian finger food. Injera is served with "wot," a sauce or stew made with chicken, beef or lamb or spicy ground lentils and peas.

Note: Authentic Injera is made from pure teff flour; however, many North American restaurants often use a combination of teff flour and wheat flour or barley flour.

2 tbsp.	yeast (2 packages)
6$\frac{1}{2}$ cups	warm water
1$\frac{1}{2}$ lbs.	teff flour (about 4$\frac{1}{2}$ cups)

✦ Dissolve the yeast in $\frac{1}{2}$ cup water.

✦ Combine the teff flour, yeast and 6$\frac{1}{4}$ cups water in a large bowl. Mix well. Ensure that no clumps are left at the bottom or side of the bowl.

✦ Cover the dough with plastic wrap and let it ferment for 2 to 3 days at room temperature. (Those with sensitive stomachs, may consider making the Injera the same day rather than waiting for 2-3 days. It will have a slightly "sweet" taste but that is considered normal.)

✦ Drain off the water that has risen to the top of the dough.

✦ Gradually add fresh warm water to the dough, just enough to make a thin smooth batter (like pancake batter); mix well. Cover the batter and let it stand until it rises, approximately 10 to 25 minutes.

✦ Heat a 10-inch skillet or frying pan until a drop of water bounces on the pan's surface.

✦ Scoop about $\frac{1}{3}$ cup of the batter and pour it into the pan quickly. Swirl the pan so that the entire bottom is evenly coated. Cover the pan quickly and let the Injera cook for 1-2 minutes. (Injera does not easily stick or burn.) Remove the cover and wait for a few seconds. It is cooked through when bubbles or "eyes" appear all over the top. If your first try is undercooked, cook the next one a little longer or use a smaller amount ($\frac{1}{4}$ cup) of batter. Do not turn the Injera over in the pan. Use a spatula to remove the cooked Injera and place it on a clean towel.

✦ Let the Injera cool and then stack them on a serving tray. Do not stack hot as they will stick together.

✦ Continue making the Injera until the batter is finished.

✦ Injera should be soft and pliable so that it can be rolled or folded like a crêpe or tortilla. Properly cooked, Injera will be thinner than a pancake but thicker than a crêpe.

Recipe courtesy of **Girma and Ethiopia Sahlu**, Regina SK, Canada

Nutritional Analysis
1 serving = 1 slice

Calories (kcal)	105
Carbohydrates (g)	21
Dietary Fiber (g)	2
Fat (g)	1
Protein (g)	4
Iron (mg)	2
Calcium (mg)	54
Sodium (mg)	7

APPLE DATE BREAD

Yield: **15 Slices** (¹/₂" thick)

Apple juice, applesauce and dates make this bread moist and flavorful.

Note: This recipe provides options for both bread machine and mixer.

Reprinted with permission from: *Delicious Gluten-Free Wheat Free Breads: Easy to bake breads everyone will love to eat for the bread machine or oven* by **LynnRae Ries** and **Bruce Gross**, What No Wheat Publishing, 2003; www.whatnowheat.com

Nutritional Analysis

1 serving = 1 slice (¹/₂" thick)

Calories (kcal)	187
Carbohydrates (g)	39
Dietary Fiber (g)	2
Fat (g)	2
Protein (g)	4
Iron (mg)	0.7
Calcium (mg)	51
Sodium (mg)	208

3	eggs
¹/₂ cup	chunky apple sauce
³/₄ cup	apple juice or water
1 tsp.	apple cider vinegar
1 tsp.	vanilla extract
1 tbsp.	vegetable oil
2 cups	white rice flour
¹/₂ cup	tapioca starch flour
¹/₂ cup	cornstarch

OR use 3 cups of your own favorite GF flour mix instead of the above flours

¹/₂ cup	non-fat dry milk
1 tsp.	salt
1 tbsp.	sugar
2 tsp.	cinnamon
1 tbsp.	xanthan gum
2¹/₄ tsp.	yeast
³/₄ cup	finely chopped GF pitted dates
1 tsp.	orange zest

✦ **Bread Machine:**

– Place ingredients into the bread machine according to the manual directions.

– Program the machine to knead (mix) the ingredients, add the dates and orange zest at the "add in time," allow the bread to rise once, then change to bake for 60-70 minutes. Rising time should be 50 minutes, or until the dough doubles in size.

– When done, remove the bread from the machine and place on a wire rack to cool. Remember to remove the bread machine paddles if they are stuck in the bread.

✦ **Mixer:**

– In a medium-sized bowl, mix all the liquid ingredients together and set aside.

– Place all the dry ingredients, including the yeast, into the mixer bowl and blend flours together on slow speed.

– Slowly add the liquid ingredients to the dry while the mixer is on low.

– Beat on high for 3-4 minutes. Mixture should look silky. If the dough is too dry, add liquid 1 tablespoon at a time.

✦ Add the dates and orange zest after the dough has been thoroughly mixed.

✦ Place the dough into a 9 x 5-inch loaf pan that has been greased and dusted with rice flour. Bake in a preheated 350°F oven for 60-70 minutes. Start checking for the bread being done at 55 minutes. When done, remove bread from pan and place on cooling rack. Do not cut or package until the bread cools, approximately 2-3 hours.

Banana Seed Bread

Yield: 1 Loaf/12 Slices

The combination of sorghum and bean flour really enhances the banana flavor of this loaf. Serve it for dessert or with a slice of old Cheddar for lunch or a snack.

1 cup	whole bean flour
1 cup	sorghum flour
1/4 cup	tapioca starch
1/4 cup	packed brown sugar
2 1/2 tsp.	xanthan gum
1 tbsp.	bread machine yeast OR instant yeast
1 1/4 tsp.	salt
1/2 cup	sunflower seeds*
3/4 cup	water
1 cup	mashed banana
1 tsp.	vinegar
1/4 cup	vegetable oil
2	eggs

✦ In a large bowl or plastic bag, combine whole bean flour, sorghum flour, tapioca starch, brown sugar, xanthan gum, yeast, salt and sunflower seeds. Mix well and set aside.

✦ Pour water, banana, vinegar and oil into the bread machine baking pan. Add eggs.

✦ Select the Rapid 2-Hour Basic Cycle. Allow the liquids to mix until combined. Gradually add the dry ingredients as the bread machine is mixing. Scrape with a rubber spatula while adding the dry ingredients. Try to incorporate all the dry ingredients within 1 to 2 minutes. When mixing and kneading are complete, leaving the bread pan in the bread machine, remove the kneading blade. Allow the bread machine to complete the cycle.

* Use raw, unroasted, unsalted sunflower seeds. For a nuttier flavor, toast the sunflower seeds.

Variation:
Pumpkin seeds or chopped pecans can replace the sunflower seeds.

Reprinted with permission from:
125 Best Gluten-Free Recipes
by **Donna Washburn** and
Heather Butt, Robert Rose Inc.
Publisher, 2003;
www.bestbreadrecipes.com

Nutritional Analysis
1 serving = 1 slice

Calories (kcal)	222
Carbohydrates (g)	30
Dietary Fiber (g)	4
Fat (g)	10
Protein (g)	7
Iron (mg)	2.0
Calcium (mg)	29
Sodium (mg)	282

MONTINA™ VEGETABLE SKILLET BREAD

	Serves: **8**

This bread is a good accompaniment to almost any type of meal or as a wonderful savory snack.

Note: A well-seasoned iron skillet or any heavy pan or baking dish will work. Salt can be eliminated. Any type of milk works well. Sautéed vegetables can be prepared ahead and refrigerated or frozen. Other vegetables such as yellow squash, zucchini or apple may be substituted or added. Do not overfill the pan since bread rises during baking.

This recipe was developed by **Michael and Bev Callihan** of Bozeman, MT for *Amazing Grains* and is used here with permission from: **Amazing Grains Grower Cooperative**, 405 Main Street S.W., Ronan MT, USA 59864; Phone 877-278-6585 or 406-676-3536; www.amazinggrains.com

Nutritional Analysis
per serving

Calories (kcal)	254
Carbohydrates (g)	35
Dietary Fiber (g)	3
Fat (g)	10
Protein (g)	9
Iron (mg)	2.7
Calcium (mg)	194
Sodium (mg)	554

1 ¼ cup	Montina™ Pure Baking Supplement*
1 cup	cornmeal, plain
4 tsp.	baking powder
1 tsp.	salt
1	medium onion, chopped
1	medium red pepper, chopped
1	medium green pepper, chopped
2	large ribs celery, chopped
3	small hot peppers, finely chopped (optional)
4 tbsp.	safflower oil
2	eggs, lightly beaten
1 cup	low-fat buttermilk

✦ Mix dry ingredients in a large bowl.

✦ Sauté vegetables in a 10-inch ovenproof skillet in 2 tbsp. oil for 5 minutes or until just softened.

✦ Add to dry ingredients and stir to coat.

✦ Add 1-2 tbsp. oil to skillet and heat in a preheated 400°F oven for 5 minutes.

✦ Combine eggs and milk and add to flour vegetable mixture. Allow to sit for 5 minutes. If needed, add more milk to make a very moist batter.

✦ Pour the batter into the hot skillet.

✦ Reduce oven temperature to 350°F and bake bread for about 40 minutes, or until lightly browned and firm.

✦ Slice and serve warm.

* **Montina™ Pure Baking Supplement** is 100% Indian ricegrass and is available from Amazing Grains Grower Cooperative.

MIGHTY TASTY MUFFINS

Yield: 12 Muffins	

The special flours and cereals used in these muffins complement the flavors of the brown sugar and spice mixtures.

2 tbsp.	Bob's Red Mill™ Mighty Tasty GF Hot Cereal *
2/3 cup	low-fat (1%) milk
1 tbsp.	apple cider vinegar **
1	large egg
1/3 cup	molasses
1 tsp.	vanilla
3/4 cup	Bob's Red Mill™ GF Garbanzo and Fava Flour
1/2 cup	potato starch
1/4 cup	tapioca flour
1/3 cup	brown sugar, packed
1 tsp.	GF baking powder
1/2 tsp.	baking soda
1 tsp.	xanthan gum
1/4 tsp.	nutmeg
1/2 tsp.	cinnamon
1/4 tsp.	ground ginger
1/4 tsp.	allspice
1/2 tsp.	salt

✦ In a large bowl, combine the first 6 ingredients. Let sit for 15 minutes, while the cereal softens.

✦ In a separate bowl, combine the remaining ingredients.

✦ Add the dry ingredients to the liquid ingredients and stir until just moistened.

✦ Spoon the batter into greased muffin tins. Fill tins 2/3 full.

✦ Bake in a preheated 350°F oven for approximately 20 minutes, or until the tops of the muffins are firm.

* Brown rice, corn, "sweet" white sorghum, buckwheat

** **Author's Note:** Distilled white vinegar is also gluten-free and can be substituted for apple cider vinegar.

Reprinted with permission from: **Bob's Red Mill Natural Foods, Inc.**, 5209 S.E. International Way, Milwaukie OR, USA 97222; Phone 800-553-2258 or 503-654-3215; www.bobsredmill.com Recipe adapted by **Carol Fenster, PhD**, author of gluten-free cookbooks and President of Savory Palate Inc. www.savorypalate.com

Nutritional Analysis
1 serving = 1 muffin

Calories (kcal)	123
Carbohydrates (g)	27
Dietary Fiber (g)	2
Fat (g)	1
Protein (g)	3
Iron (mg)	1.1
Calcium (mg)	72
Sodium (mg)	213

BLUEBERRY SORGHUM MUFFINS

Yield: **12 medium muffins**

Sorghum flour, cornstarch and soy flour make an interesting gluten-free combination for these muffins.

1 1/2 cups	sorghum/cornstarch mix*
1/4 cup	soy flour
1/4 cup	sugar
2 1/2 tsp.	GF baking powder
3/4 tsp.	salt
1 tsp.	xanthan gum
2	eggs
1 cup	low fat (1%) milk OR soy milk
1/3 cup	vegetable oil
1 tsp.	vanilla extract
1 cup	blueberries (rinsed and drained)

✦ In a large bowl, combine the dry ingredients and whisk together.

✦ Beat eggs lightly; add milk, oil and vanilla; beat until well mixed.

✦ Add wet ingredients to dry ingredients and beat until smooth. You can beat as long as needed, dough will not get "tough" like muffins made with wheat flour.

✦ Add blueberries and fold in gently.

✦ Spoon the batter into paper-cup-lined muffin tins. Fill cups 2/3 full.

✦ Bake in a preheated 350°F oven for 19 minutes, or until a toothpick comes out clean.

*	**Sorghum Cornstarch Mix:**
3 cups	sorghum flour
1 cup	cornstarch

Recipe courtesy of **Amy Perry** and **Meredith Wiking** of **Nebraska Grain Sorghum Board**, 301 Centennial Mall South, P. O. Box 94982, Lincoln NE, USA 68509;
Phone 402-471-4276;
www.sorghum.state.ne.us

Nutritional Analysis
1 serving = 1 muffin

Calories (kcal)	166
Carbohydrates (g)	21
Dietary Fiber (g)	2
Fat (g)	8
Protein (g)	4
Iron (mg)	0.9
Calcium (mg)	87
Sodium (mg)	262

CARROT PUMPKIN MUFFINS

1³/₄ cups	sugar
3	egg whites
1	whole egg
¹/₂ cup	vegetable oil
1 cup	unsweetened applesauce
1 cup	puréed pumpkin
1 tbsp.	vanilla
1¹/₃ cups	cooked puréed carrots
3 cups	flour mix*
1 tsp.	salt
1 tbsp.	baking soda
2 tsp.	GF baking powder
2 tsp.	xanthan gum
1 tbsp.	ground cinnamon

Yield: 30 Muffins

This recipe is moist and delicious. Using applesauce and pumpkin reduces the fat and sugar content as compared to traditional carrot muffins or cake.

✦ In a large bowl, combine sugar, eggs and oil, cream until light and fluffy. Add applesauce, pumpkin, vanilla and carrots.

✦ Sift dry ingredients together and slowly fold into batter.

✦ Spoon batter into paper-cup-lined small muffin tins, filling cups ²/₃ full, or into cake pans (one, 9 x 13-inch or two, 9-inch round).

✦ Bake in a preheated 350°F oven for 15-20 minutes (muffins) or 25-40 minutes for cake, depending on the size of the cake pans.

✦ Cool for 10 minutes. Remove cake from the pan and peel off the paper.

Tip: Use muffin liners instead of greasing pans (also helps maintain moisture for storing muffins). Use parchment paper (available from kitchen stores and some grocery stores) as the lining on the bottom of cake pans to avoid greasing pans (remove as much fat as possible).

* **Flour Mix:**

3 parts	rice flour
1¹/₂ parts	potato starch
1 part	tapioca starch

Variation:
To make **Carrot Cake**, eliminate the pumpkin and use all applesauce (total of 2 cups applesauce).

Recipe courtesy of **Laurel Hutton**, **Laurel's Sweet Treats, Inc.**, 16004 SW Tualatin – Sherwood Road, #123, Sherwood OR, USA 97140;
Phone 866-225-3432 or 503-625-3432;
www.glutenfreemixes.com

Nutritional Analysis
1 serving = 1 muffin

Calories (kcal)	148
Carbohydrates (g)	27
Dietary Fiber (g)	1
Fat (g)	5
Protein (g)	1
Iron (mg)	0.3
Calcium (mg)	26
Sodium (mg)	252

TEFF BANANA PANCAKES

Yield: 25 small pancakes

This basic pancake recipe is easy to make and is delicious with a variety of sweeteners and juices. Feel free to substitute maple syrup for honey, and juice for soy milk. Ground flax seeds easily take the place of eggs in these delicious pancakes made with naturally sweet teff and bananas. The batter is light and looks like pudding.

2 tbsp.	flax seeds
2	bananas, ripe
1 1/2 cups	vanilla soy milk
1 tbsp.	vanilla
1 tbsp.	honey
1 1/2 tsp.	vegetable oil
1 1/2 cups	teff flour
1 tbsp.	baking powder
1/4 tsp.	sea salt
1/2 tsp.	cinnamon

✦ Grind flax seeds in a blender until powdery. Add banana, vanilla soy milk, vanilla, honey and 1/2 tsp. oil. Blend well.

✦ In a large mixing bowl, combine teff flour, baking powder, sea salt and cinnamon. Stir in banana soy milk mixture.

✦ Place the griddle or skillet over medium heat. After a minute or two, brush on 1 tsp. of oil. Using a tablespoon, scoop up the batter and pour it on the hot griddle, 1 heaping tablespoon for each pancake.

✦ Cook pancakes for 3-4 minutes on the first side, or until you see tiny holes on the top of the pancakes. Flip them over and cook for another minute or two.

✦ Serve pancakes plain or dipped into yogurt.

Reprinted with permission from: **The Teff Company**, P.O. Box A, Caldwell ID, USA 83606; www.teffco.com; Phone 888-822-2221 and **Leslie Cerier**, 58 Schoolhouse Road, Amherst MA, USA 01002; www.lesliecerier.com

Nutritional Analysis
1 serving = 1 pancake

Calories (kcal)	54
Carbohydrates (g)	9
Dietary Fiber (g)	1
Fat (g)	1
Protein (g)	2
Iron (mg)	0.7
Calcium (mg)	64
Sodium (mg)	79

Hearty Mesquite Montina™ Pancakes

Yield: 8 - 4" Pancakes	

High-fiber mesquite and Montina™ add texture; banana and cinnamon add rich flavor – these are great breakfast pancakes

¹/₃ cup	mesquite flour
¹/₃ cup	Montina™ Pure Baking Supplement*
¹/₄ cup	GF Flour Blend **
2 tsp.	sugar
2 tsp.	baking powder
¹/₂ tsp.	baking soda
¹/₄ tsp.	cinnamon
¹/₄ tsp.	salt
1	large egg
1	medium ripe banana, mashed
1 cup	milk (cow, rice or soy)
1 tbsp.	canola oil
	additional oil for frying

✦ Blend all ingredients in a blender or whisk vigorously in a bowl. For lighter pancakes, sift the dry ingredients before blending.

✦ Let batter sit while preheating skillet or griddle to medium-high.

✦ Lightly oil hot skillet or griddle.

✦ Cook 1 "test" pancake using a scant ¹/₄ cup of batter. Adjust batter if necessary by adding more milk, a tablespoon at a time, if necessary. Cook until tops are bubbly (3-5 minutes). Turn and cook until golden brown (2-3 minutes).

* **Montina™ Pure Baking Supplement** is 100% Indian ricegrass flour sold under the trade name Montina by Amazing Grains Grower Cooperative.

** A variety of flours and starches can be used to make a GF Flour Blend (see page 154) or use an All-Purpose GF Flour Mix from gluten-free companies (see pages 249-252).

Adapted from and reprinted with permission from: *Gluten-Free 101: Easy Basic Dishes without Wheat* by **Carol Fenster, PhD.**, Savory Palate Inc. 2006. www.glutenfree101.com

Nutritional Analysis
1 serving = 2 pancakes

Calories (kcal)	229
Carbohydrates (g)	38
Dietary Fiber (g)	5
Fat (g)	6
Protein (g)	8
Iron (mg)	1.9
Calcium (mg)	233
Sodium (mg)	569

SHELLEY CASE'S HIGH-FIBER HOT CEREAL

Yield: **1 Cup**

This quick, heart-healthy breakfast is packed with fiber and omega-3 fatty acids. Add a spoonful of brown sugar, chopped nuts and/or dried apricots or raisins for more flavor and extra nutrients.

Tip: Mix dry flax and the hot cereal in self-seal plastic bags and take it when travelling. The cereal can be cooked in the microwave in your hotel room. Another option is to order juice and/or coffee/ tea and/or an egg at the restaurant and ask the server to heat the cereal and water in a bowl in their microwave. Most restaurants are very accommodating if you order some items off the menu.

3 tbsp.   Flax Seed Meal (Ground Flax)*
3 tbsp.   Cream of Brown Rice Hot Cereal
1 1/3 cup   water
            dash of vanilla

✦ Combine the first 3 ingredients in a medium to large glass bowl.

✦ Cook on high in a microwave for 3-4 minutes, or until thick and creamy.

✦ Stir in vanilla.

✦ Serve with brown sugar, nuts and/or dried fruits.

* As flax is very high in fiber, it is important to gradually introduce it in small portions until tolerated. Start with 5 tbsp. hot cereal and 1-3 tsp. of ground flax initially and then gradually work up to 3 tbsp. flax and 3 tbsp. hot cereal. See page 105 for fiber tips.

Variations:
Substitute Creamy Buckwheat Hot Cereal or Bob's Red Mill Mighty Tasty Gluten-Free Hot Cereal™ for the Brown Rice Hot Cereal.

Nutritional Analysis
1 serving = 1 cup

	Brown Rice	Buckwheat	Bob's Mighty Tasty
Calories (kcal)	225	217	225
Carbohydrates (g)	30	29	29
Dietary Fiber (g)	7	8	9
Fat (g)	10	10	10
Protein (g)	6	8	7
Iron (mg)	1.2	1.2	1.2
Calcium (mg)	60	60	60
Sodium (mg)	16	13	16

CRUNCHY GRANOLA

Yield: **11 Cups**

This high-fiber granola is loaded with nutrients. Great for breakfast, as a snack, or it can be used to make granola bars or as a topping for yogurt, ice cream or frozen yogurt, or a fruit crisp (apple, blueberry, peach). Various substitutions can be used for the nuts and dried fruits.

1/2 cup	shredded coconut
1/2 cup	sunflower seeds
1/4 cup	sesame seeds
1 cup	chopped nuts
1/2 cup	chopped GF dates
1/2 cup	chopped dried apricots
1/2 cup	raisins
	hot water
4 cups	GF corn flakes
3 cups	GF crisp rice cereal
3 tbsp.	flax seed meal (ground flax)
1/4 cup	oil
1/2 cup	honey
1 tbsp.	apple juice
1 tsp.	vanilla
1/2 tsp.	nutmeg
1/2 tsp.	cinnamon

✦ Combine the coconut, sunflower and sesame seeds and nuts in a shallow pan and toast under the broiler for a few minutes (watch carefully to prevent burning). Remove from the oven, stir and return to the oven to finish toasting. Remove from the oven and cool.

✦ Soak the dried fruit in hot water to clean and soften for 10 minutes. Drain. Chop the fruit into bite-sized pieces.

✦ Combine the cereals, flax, coconut, nuts and seeds.

✦ Mix the oil, honey, juice, vanilla, nutmeg and cinnamon together.

✦ Place the cereal/nut mixture in a large roasting or broiler pan; pour the oil/honey mixture over and mix well.

✦ Bake in a preheated 300°F oven for 1 hour, stirring every 10-15 minutes. Add the dried fruits and return to the oven for the last 15 minutes.

✦ Remove the granola from the oven and let it cool. Stir a few times as it cools.

✦ Store in an air-tight container in a cool place (refrigerator or freezer).

Recipe courtesy of **Laurel Hutton**, **Laurel's Sweet Treats, Inc.**, 16004 SW Tualatin – Sherwood Road, #123, Sherwood OR, USA 97140;
Phone 866-225-3432 or 503-625-3432
www.glutenfreemixes.com

Nutritional Analysis
1 serving = 1/2 cup

Calories (kcal)	190
Carbohydrates (g)	25
Dietary Fiber (g)	2
Fat (g)	10
Protein (g)	3
Iron (mg)	2.8
Calcium (mg)	35
Sodium (mg)	83

AMARANTH GRAIN-FREE GRANOLA

Yield: 7-8 cups

Eat this chunky granola out of hand as a snack, top it with fruit juice or milk for a quick healthy breakfast or sprinkle it over yogurt or ice cream for dessert

1 1/2 cups	amaranth flour
1 cup	chopped walnuts OR other nuts
1/2 cup	potato starch
1/2 cup	peanuts
1/2 cup	sunflower OR sesame seeds
1/2 cup	unsweetened coconut
1 1/2 tsp.	cinnamon
3/4 cup	mashed bananas OR puréed fruit
1/4 cup	maple syrup OR honey
1 tbsp.	lemon juice
1/4 cup	vegetable oil
1 1/2 tsp.	pure vanilla extract
2/3 cup	raisins

✦ Combine the flour, walnuts, potato starch, peanuts, sunflower seeds, coconut and cinnamon in a large bowl.

✦ Mix the bananas or fruit purée, maple syrup, lemon juice, oil and vanilla in a small bowl. If the honey is very thick, heat the mixture briefly to liquefy.

✦ Pour the liquid mixture over the dry mixture. Stir well to coat dry ingredients. If the mixture seems too dry, add a few tablespoons of water.

✦ Spread the granola on a lightly oiled jelly-roll pan. Bake in a preheated 300°F oven for 45-60 minutes, stirring every 15 minutes. Remove the granola from the oven and let it cool. Stir in the raisins.

Recipe courtesy of **Nu-World Amaranth, Nu-World Foods**, PO Box 2202, Naperville IL, USA 60567; Phone 630-369-6819; www.nuworldfoods.com

Nutritional Analysis
1 serving = 1/2 cup

Calories (kcal)	248
Carbohydrates (g)	27
Dietary Fiber (g)	4
Fat (g)	14
Protein (g)	6
Iron (mg)	2.0
Calcium (mg)	42
Sodium (mg)	6

FIG BARS

Yield: **16 Fig Bars**

A healthy high-fiber treat for snacks or in the lunch bag.

1 1/2 cups	(9 oz.) dried figs
1/4 cup	(4 oz.) finely ground pecans OR other nuts
1 cup	brown rice flour
1 cup	packed brown sugar
1/2 cup	tapioca flour
1/4 cup	rice bran
2 tsp.	baking powder
1 1/2 tsp.	xanthan gum
1/4 tsp.	salt
1/2 cup	margarine OR butter, softened
1	large egg

✦ Place the figs in a saucepan. Add enough water to almost cover the figs, about 1 cup. Bring to a boil. Remove from heat. Allow figs to cool in the saucepan with water.

✦ Meanwhile, in a mixing bowl, combine pecans, brown rice flour, brown sugar, tapioca flour, rice bran, baking powder, xanthan gum and salt.

✦ With a mixer on low, cut the margarine into the flour; mix until crumbly. Add the egg and mix well. Add 2 tbsp. of the reserved fig juice and mix well. Set aside.

✦ Put cooled figs in a food processor or blender and chop until the consistency is like thick preserves. Add 1 tbsp. reserved fig juice at a time, as needed, to get to spreading consistency, but no more than 4 tbsp. Set aside.

✦ In a well-greased 8 x 8-inch square baking pan, spread one half of the dough evenly. Spread the fig paste, carefully, over the dough. Spread or pat the remaining dough carefully over the figs.

✦ Bake in a preheated 375°F oven for 45-50 minutes, or until a toothpick inserted near the center comes out clean and the top is lightly browned. Remove from the oven. Cool for at least 10 minutes before slicing.

✦ Slice into 2 x 2-inch bars. Remove from the pan and allow to cool completely.

✦ The bars will keep, refrigerated, for up to a week.

Reprinted with permission from: *Incredible Edible Gluten-Free Foods For Kids* by **Sheri L. Sanderson**, Woodbine House, 2002; www.woodbinehouse.com

Nutritional Analysis
1 serving = 1 bar

Calories (kcal)	245
Carbohydrates (g)	36
Dietary Fiber (g)	3
Fat (g)	12
Protein (g)	3
Iron (mg)	1.3
Calcium (mg)	77
Sodium (mg)	175

CARROT APPLE ENERGY BARS

Yield: **18 Bars**

For a quick, easy, on-the-move breakfast or snack, choose these moist nutritious bars.

1 1/4 cups	sorghum flour
1/2 cup	amaranth flour
1/3 cup	rice bran
1/4 cup	ground flaxseed
1/4 cup	non-fat (skim) milk powder
1 1/2 tsp.	xanthan gum
1 tbsp.	GF baking powder
1/4 tsp.	salt
2 tsp.	ground cinnamon
2	eggs
1 cup	unsweetened applesauce
1/3 cup	packed brown sugar
1 1/2 cups	grated carrots
3/4 cup	dried fruit mix (see tips, at left)
1/2 cup	chopped walnuts

✦ Line a 13 x 9-inch baking pan with foil and grease lightly.

✦ In a large bowl or plastic bag, combine sorghum flour, amaranth flour, rice bran, ground flaxseed, milk powder, xanthan gum, baking powder, salt and cinnamon. Mix well and set aside.

✦ In a separate bowl, using an electric mixer, beat eggs, applesauce and brown sugar until combined.

✦ Add flour mixture and mix just until combined. Stir in carrots, dried fruit and nuts. Spoon the batter into the prepared pan; spread to edges with a moist rubber spatula and allow to stand for 30 minutes.

✦ Bake in a preheated 325°F oven for 30-35 minutes, or until a cake tester inserted in the center comes out clean.

✦ Let cool in pan on a cooling rack and cut into bars.

✦ Store in an airtight container at room temperature for up to 1 week or individually wrapped and frozen for up to 1 month.

Tips: ✦ For the dried fruit mix, we used 1/4 cup dried cranberries, 1/4 cup raisins, 2 tbsp. chopped dried mangoes, 1 tbsp. dried blueberries and 1 tbsp. chopped dried apricots.

✦ For a lactose-free bar, omit the milk powder.

✦ Try substituting grated zucchini for all or half of the carrots.

✦ Substitute cardamom for the cinnamon.

Reprinted with permission from: *The Best Gluten-Free Family Cookbook* by **Donna Washburn** and **Heather Butt**, Robert Rose Inc. Publisher, 2005; www.bestbreadrecipes.com

Nutritional Analysis
1 serving = 1 bar (3"x2")

Calories (kcal)	144
Carbohydrates (g)	24
Dietary Fiber (g)	3
Fat (g)	4
Protein (g)	5
Iron (mg)	1.7
Calcium (mg)	99
Sodium (mg)	139

ALMOND DELIGHTS

Yield: **24 Cookies**

Apricots and almonds are a luscious combination.

1¼ cups	slivered, blanched almonds
³/₄ cup	sugar
3	egg whites, unbeaten
¹/₄ cup	finely-chopped dried apricots

✦ In a blender, grind almonds as fine as possible.

✦ Mix nuts, sugar and egg whites in a saucepan.

✦ Cook over medium heat, stirring constantly, for 8-10 minutes, or until a path stays clean when a spoon is drawn through.

✦ Remove the pan from the heat; stir in apricots.

✦ Drop the batter by heaping teaspoonfuls onto a greased cookie sheet.

✦ Let cookies "rest" for ¹/₂ hour, then bake in a preheated 300°F oven for 12-15 minutes, or till delicately golden on exterior but soft inside.

✦ Remove from cookie sheets immediately.

Reprinted with permission from: *Wheat-Free, Gluten-Free Recipes for Special Diets* by **Connie Sarros**, 2003; www.gfbooks.homestead.com

Nutritional Analysis
1 serving = 1 cookie

Calories (kcal)	73
Carbohydrates (g)	9
Dietary Fiber (g)	1
Fat (g)	4
Protein (g)	2
Iron (mg)	0.3
Calcium (mg)	19
Sodium (mg	8

SORGHUM PEANUT BUTTER COOKIES

Yield: **72 Cookies**

Peanut butter and brown sugar are a dynamite flavor combo, and sorghum and garbanzo flours add interesting texture to a favorite cookie recipe.

1 1/2 cups	creamy peanut butter
1 cup	shortening OR margarine
2 1/3 cups	firmly packed brown sugar
6 tbsp.	low-fat (1%) milk
2 tsp.	vanilla
2	eggs
3 cups	sorghum flour
1/2 cup	garbanzo bean (chickpea) flour
1/2 cup	sweet rice flour
4 tsp.	xanthan gum
1 tsp.	salt
1 1/2 tsp.	baking soda

✦ Combine the peanut butter, shortening, brown sugar, milk and vanilla in a large bowl. With an electric mixer, beat on medium speed until well blended.

✦ Add the eggs. Beat just until blended.

✦ Combine the flours, salt and baking soda. Add to creamed mixture at low speed. Mix just until blended.

✦ Using a mini ice cream scoop, drop dough portions 2 inches apart on baking sheets lined with parchment paper. Flatten slightly in a crisscross pattern with the tines of a fork.

✦ Bake in a preheated 375°F oven for 8-10 minutes, or until set and just beginning to brown.

✦ Cool for 2 minutes on the baking sheets. Remove the cookies from the pan and cool completely.

Recipe courtesy of **Barbara Kliment, Executive Director** of **Nebraska Grain Sorghum Board**, 301 Centennial Mall South, P. O. Box 94982, Lincoln NE, USA 68509;
Phone 402-471-4276;
www.sorghum.state.ne.us

Nutritional Analysis
1 serving = 1 cookie

Calories (kcal)	113
Carbohydrates (g)	14
Dietary Fiber (g)	1
Fat (g)	6
Protein (g)	2
Iron (mg)	0.6
Calcium (mg)	11
Sodium (mg)	71

RUM AND QUINOA CRUNCH COOKIES

3/4 cup	butter OR margarine
1 cup	sugar
2	eggs, beaten
2 tsp.	rum extract
2 cups	NorQuin quinoa flour
1/4 cup	white rice flour
1 1/2 tsp.	baking powder
1/3 cup	toasted quinoa grain

Yield: **50 Cookies**

Quinoa has more high-quality protein than any other grain. These crisp cookies can be flavored to suit your taste.

✦ In a large bowl, cream butter; add sugar; cream together thoroughly.

✦ Add beaten eggs and rum extract.

✦ Mix dry ingredients together and add to wet ingredients. Mix well.

✦ Chill the dough for several hours or overnight.

✦ Roll out a small amount of dough at a time on a lightly floured surface (use rice flour). Cut the dough into desired shapes and place on greased cookie sheets OR shape the dough into balls OR drop by teaspoonfuls onto a cookie sheet. Flatten with a rice-floured glass to 1/4" thickness.

✦ Bake in a preheated 350°F oven for 10-15 minutes.

Variation:

2 tsp. lemon extract or 2 tsp. almond extract may be substituted for the rum extract.

Recipe is courtesy of: **El Peto Products Ltd.**, 65 Saltsman Dr, Cambridge ON, Canada N3H 4R7; Phone 800-387-4064 or 519-650-4614; www.elpeto.com and **Northern Quinoa Corporation**, Box 519, Kamsack SK, Canada S0A 1S0; Phone 866-368-9304 or 306-542-3949; www.quinoa.com

Nutritional Analysis
1 serving = 1 cookie

Calories (kcal)	67
Carbohydrates (g)	9
Dietary Fiber (g)	0.4
Fat (g)	3
Protein (g)	1
Iron (mg)	0.6
Calcium (mg)	13
Sodium (mg)	35

CRANBERRY PISTACHIO BISCOTTI

Yield: **64 Cookies**

These have the appearance and texture of traditional twice-baked biscotti, but are much easier and faster to make. We like to dip them in a sweet Italian dessert wine or in coffee.

Tips: ✦ Biscotti will be medium-firm and crunchy; for softer biscotti, bake for only 10 minutes in Step 5; for very firm biscotti, bake for 20 minutes.

✦ Store in an airtight container at room temperature for up to 3 weeks, or freeze for up to 2 months.

✦ If you prefer, you can use a 13 x 9-inch baking pan instead of the two 8-inch pans.

✦ Try orange-flavored cranberries and substitute orange zest for the lemon zest.

✦ Substitute pecans or hazelnuts for the pistachios.

Reprinted with permission from:
The Best Gluten-Free Family Cookbook by **Donna Washburn** and **Heather Butt**, Robert Rose Inc. 2005;
www.bestbreadrecipes.com

Nutritional Analysis
1 serving = 1 cookie

Calories (kcal)	62
Carbohydrates (g)	10
Dietary Fiber (g)	1
Fat (g)	2
Protein (g)	2
Iron (mg)	0.5
Calcium (mg)	15
Sodium (mg)	17

1 1/2 cups	amaranth flour
1/2 cup	soy flour
1/3 cup	potato starch
1/4 cup	tapioca starch
1 1/2 tsp.	xanthan gum
1 tsp.	GF baking powder
pinch	salt
4	eggs
1 1/4 cups	sugar
1 tbsp.	grated lemon zest
1 tsp.	vanilla
1 1/2 cups	coarsely chopped pistachios
1 cup	dried cranberries

✦ Line two 8-inch square baking pans with foil and grease lightly. For the second baking, use ungreased baking sheets.

✦ In a large bowl or plastic bag, combine amaranth flour, soy flour, potato starch, tapioca starch, xanthan gum, baking powder and salt. Mix well and set aside.

✦ In a separate bowl, using an electric mixer, beat eggs, sugar, lemon zest and vanilla until combined.

✦ Slowly beat dry ingredients into the egg mixture and mix just until combined. Stir in pistachios and cranberries. Spoon into the prepared pans. Using a moistened rubber spatula, spread the batter to the edges and smooth the tops.

✦ Bake in a preheated 325°F oven for 30-35 minutes, or until firm or tops are just turning golden. Let cool in the pans for 5 minutes.

✦ Remove Biscotti from the pans, remove foil and let cool on a cutting board for 5 minutes.

✦ Cut Biscotti into quarters, then cut each quarter into 8 slices. Arrange slices upright (cut sides exposed) at least 1/2 inch apart on baking sheets. Bake for an additional 15 minutes, until dry and crisp. Transfer to a cooling rack immediately.

Flax Pumpkin Squares

Yield: **9 Servings**

Cinnamon, nutmeg and cloves add the perfect flavor note to this pumpkin dessert.

Crust:

3/4 cup	GF cornflakes (crushed)
1/4 cup	flaxseed (ground)
1/4 cup	butter, melted
1 tbsp.	sugar
1/4 tsp.	cinnamon
1/4 tsp.	nutmeg

Filling:

8 oz.	cream cheese (at room temperature)
1/4 cup	sugar
1	egg
2/3 cup	canned pumpkin
1/4 tsp.	cinnamon
1/4 cup	ground flaxseed
1/4 tsp.	ground cloves
1/4 tsp.	salt

✦ In a small bowl, combine cornflakes, flaxseed, butter, sugar, cinnamon and nutmeg. Mix thoroughly and press into a foil-lined, 8-inch square pan.

✦ In a large mixing bowl, beat cream cheese until fluffy.

✦ Beat in sugar and then egg.

✦ Beat in pumpkin, cinnamon, flaxseed, cloves and salt.

✦ Spoon the batter over the prepared crust. Level out the top of the cake.

✦ Bake in a preheated 325°F oven for 40 minutes. Remove from the oven and cool on a wire rack for 1 hour.

✦ Refrigerate until completely cooled. Remove and cut into squares. Top with whipped cream if desired.

Reprinted with permission from: *The Essential Flax* by **Saskatchewan Flax Development Commission**, 2005, A5A 116 - 103rd St. East, Saskatoon SK, Canada S7N 1Y7; Phone 306-664-1901; www.saskflax.com

Nutritional Analysis
1 serving = 3"x3" piece

Calories (kcal)	272
Carbohydrates (g)	20
Dietary Fiber (g)	5
Fat (g)	20
Protein (g)	6
Iron (mg)	2.8
Calcium (mg)	63
Sodium (mg)	242

CHOCOLATE MESQUITE BROWNIES

Yield: 12

Brown sugar brownies – irresistible!

1/2 cup	mesquite meal (flour)
1/2 cup	unsweetened cocoa
1 cup	brown rice flour
1 cup	brown sugar
2 tbsp.	tapioca starch
1 tsp.	baking powder
1 tsp.	baking soda
2 tsp.	cornstarch
1/2 tsp.	sea salt
1	large egg
1 cup	water
1/2 cup	vegetable oil
1 tsp.	vanilla extract

✦ In a large bowl, combine all of the dry ingredients.

✦ Add the wet ingredients and mix until smooth.

✦ Pour the batter evenly into a greased 9 x 12-inch baking pan.

✦ Bake in a preheated 350°F oven for 25-35 minutes, depending on the depth of the pan, altitude and your patience.

Tips: ✦ For a more chocolatey brownie, add 1/2 cup chocolate chips to batter.

✦ For mocha brownies, substitute strong coffee or espresso for the cup of water.

Recipe courtesy of: **San Pedro Mesquite Company**, P.O. Box 338, Bowie AZ, USA 85605

Nutritional Analysis
1 serving = 1 slice

Calories (kcal)	241
Carbohydrates (g)	37
Dietary Fiber (g)	4
Fat (g)	11
Protein (g)	3
Iron (mg)	1.4
Calcium (mg)	53
Sodium (mg)	258

Creamy "I can't believe it's not rice!" Pudding

| Yield: **5 Servings** |

A traditional dessert favorite, this "rice pudding" version uses buckwheat groats instead of rice. Serve warm or cold, garnished with whipped cream and chopped nuts and/or fresh fruit. A splash of maple syrup is also a delicious option.

4 cups	water
1/4 tsp.	salt
2 tbsp.	butter OR margarine (optional)
2 cups	whole white buckwheat groats (Wolff's or Pocono)
2 eggs	
1 cup	low-fat (1%) milk
1/3 cup	honey (preferably clover OR other mild honey)
1 tsp.	vanilla extract
1/2 tsp.	ground cinnamon
1/2 tsp.	grated lemon peel
dash	fresh nutmeg
1 tbsp.	dark rum (optional)
1 cup	grated apple, cored but not peeled
1/4 cup	raisins
1/2 cup	sour cream
	whipped cream and chopped nuts OR fresh fruit, for garnish

Note: Groats are hulled crushed kernels of grain that are often cooked as rice is cooked. Buckwheat groats (kasha) are the most common, but oat and barley groats are also available.

✦ In a medium saucepan, heat water, salt and butter. Quickly stir in buckwheat groats. Reduce heat to low and cover pan tightly. Simmer for 15 minutes, until groats are tender and the liquid is absorbed.

✦ Beat together the eggs, milk and honey until well-blended. Add the vanilla, cinnamon, lemon peel, nutmeg and rum.

✦ In a large bowl, combine groats, apple, raisins and milk/egg mixture.

✦ Spread the pudding evenly in a buttered 8-inch square pan.

✦ Bake at 350°F for 25-30 minutes, stirring every 5 minutes.

✦ Remove the pudding from the oven. Let it cool for 15 minutes, then stir in the sour cream.

✦ Garnish individual servings as you prefer.

Recipe courtesy of: **The Birkett Mills**, 163 Main St, Penn Yan NY, USA 14527;
Phone 315-536-3311;
www.thebirkettmills.com

Nutritional Analysis
1 serving

Calories (kcal)	440
Carbohydrates (g)	82
Dietary Fiber (g)	8
Fat (g)	9
Protein (g)	13
Iron (mg)	2.4
Calcium (mg)	122
Sodium (mg)	195

WILD RICE FRUIT DESSERT

Yield: 10 Servings	

This version of the ever-popular "Ambrosia" has the added texture of wild rice. The whole family will love this one.

1 cup	wild rice (4 cups cooked)
14 oz.	can pineapple chunks, drained
10 oz.	can mandarin oranges, drained
14 oz.	can fruit cocktail, drained
1/2 cup	chopped walnuts
3 cups	miniature marshmallows
3 oz.	cherry gelatin powder
1 cup	whipping cream

✦ Wash wild rice in a wire strainer and run cold water over it.

✦ Combine 4 cups of water and 1 cup of wild rice in a large heavy saucepan. Bring to a boil; cover and simmer over low heat for approximately 45 minutes, until the rice kernels have burst their shells and fluffed out. Drain off any excess water. Stir with a fork; cover and let stand for 15 minutes.

✦ Place the wild rice in a large bowl and let cool.

✦ Drain the juice from the canned fruits.

✦ Add the fruit, rice, nuts and marshmallows to the cooled, wild rice.

✦ Mix in the dry gelatin powder.

✦ Whip the cream until stiff and fold into the fruit mixture.

✦ Refrigerate for at least 1 hour.

✦ Garnish with fresh fruit before serving.

Recipe courtesy of: **Riese's Canadian Lake Wild Rice**, La Ronge SK, Canada S0J 1L0; Phone 306-425-2314; www.wildlakerice.com

Nutritional Analysis
1 serving

Calories (kcal)	329
Carbohydrates (g)	50
Dietary Fiber (g)	2
Fat (g)	13
Protein (g)	6
Iron (mg)	0.9
Calcium (mg)	26
Sodium (mg)	64

Moroccan Salad

Serves: 10	

This salad has been a catering favorite of mine and my clients for many years. When I first started making it, I used rice. Now I use other grains like quinoa and millet, and I have even used a variety of rice. The blending of sweet and savory in this salad makes it exotic.

3 cups	cooked quinoa – can use rice, millet or a combination of millet and quinoa
1/2	EACH, red, yellow and orange pepper, 1/4 inch diced
1	medium red onion, 1/4 inch diced
1/2 cup	chopped GF pitted dates
1/2 cup	diced dried apricots
1/2 cup	dried cherries OR cranberries
	grated zest and juice of 1 orange and 1 lemon
2-3 tbsp.	extra-virgin olive oil
1/8 tsp.	turmeric
	salt and freshly ground black pepper to taste
1/3 cup	toasted, slivered almonds
2 tbsp.	sunflower seeds
2 tbsp.	chopped parsley OR cilantro

✦ Wash the quinoa, changing the water at least 5 times. Rub the grains with your hands and then let the grains settle to the bottom of the bowl each time before pouring off the water and then adding more fresh cold water.

✦ Bring a pot of lightly salted water to a boil.

✦ Add the quinoa and cook for 10 minutes.

✦ Drain the quinoa into a sieve. Rinse under cold water.

✦ Set the sieve over a saucepan of boiling water. Do not allow the water to touch the quinoa. Cover with a kitchen towel and lid. Steam the quinoa until it is fluffy and dry, about 10 minutes. Check the water level in the pan, adding more if necessary.

To Make the Salad:

✦ Toss everything together, except the almonds, sunflower seeds and the parsley.

✦ Taste for seasoning.

✦ Just before serving, stir in the almonds, then sprinkle the sunflower seeds and the parsley over the salad. Serve.

Recipe courtesy of: **Rebecca Reilly**, Culinary Expert and Author of *Gluten-Free Baking: More Than 125 Recipes for Delectable Sweet and Savory Baked Goods, Including Cakes, Pies, Quick Breads, Muffins, Cookies, and Other Delights.*

Nutritional Analysis
1 serving

Calories (kcal)	219
Carbohydrates (g)	32
Dietary Fiber (g)	5
Fat (g)	8
Protein (g)	6
Iron (mg)	0.9
Calcium (mg)	41
Sodium (mg)	123

QUINOA SALAD

Yield: 6 Servings

The delicate flavor of quinoa is similar to couscous. Cooked quinoa can be used as a pasta substitute in cold pasta salads.

Lemon Garlic Dressing:

4	garlic cloves, minced
1/4 cup	red wine vinegar
1/4 cup	canola oil
1/4 cup	water
1	lemon, juiced
	salt and pepper to taste
4 cups	cooked NorQuin quinoa
1 cup	grated carrots
1/2 cup	sliced green onions
1/2 cup	chopped celery
1/4 cup	sunflower seeds
1/4 cup	slivered almonds
3 tbsp.	sesame seeds
1/2 cup	sliced mushrooms

✦ In a small bowl, combine all of the dressing ingredients and let stand for at least 10 minutes.

✦ Prepare the salad ingredients and combine in a large bowl.

✦ Toss the salad with the dressing and serve.

Recipe courtesy of **Northern Quinoa Corporation**, Box 519, Kamsack SK, Canada S0A 1S0; Phone 866-368-9304 or 306-542-3949; www.quinoa.com

Nutritional Analysis
1 serving = 1 cup

Calories (kcal)	358
Carbohydrates (g)	30
Dietary Fiber (g)	8
Fat (g)	22
Protein (g)	12
Iron (mg)	1.6
Calcium (mg)	100
Sodium (mg)	220

THAI HOT-AND-SOUR SAUCE

Yield: **1¹/₃ Cups**	

This delectable, spicy sauce is fabulous on tossed green salads, sliced tomatoes, steamed cabbage wedges, stir-fried vegetables and rice, and rice noodles with steamed veggies. You're bound to think of many other uses as well.

¹/₃ cup	sesame tahini, other seed butter OR almond butter
¹/₃ cup	fresh lime juice
3 tbsp.	water
2 tbsp.	balsamic vinegar
2 tbsp.	dark sesame oil OR extra-virgin olive oil
2 tbsp.	sugar
2 tsp.	dried basil
1 tsp.	dried spearmint
1 tsp.	ground ginger
1 tsp.	crushed garlic
¹/₄ tsp.	crushed hot red pepper flakes

✦ Combine all of the ingredients in a small bowl and whisk until thick and smooth.

Reprinted with permission from: **Food Allergy Survival Guide – Surviving and Thriving with Food Allergies and Sensitivities** by **Vesanto Melina, MS, RD**, **Jo Stepaniak, MSEd** and **Dina Aronson, MS, RD**, Healthy Living Publications, 2004

Nutritional Analysis
1 serving = ¹/₃ cup

Calories (kcal)	218
Carbohydrates (g)	15
Dietary Fiber (g)	2
Fat (g)	18
Protein (g)	4
Iron (mg)	1.4
Calcium (mg)	52
Sodium (mg)	11

TEFF POLENTA

Serves: 4

Flavored with sweet juicy tomatoes, fresh basil, garlic, and decorated with bright green peppers, here is an irresistible summer repast. Serve garnished with grated Fontina, Parmesan, Manchego, or sliced rounds of chèvre.

Note: Like the traditional Italian polenta made with cornmeal, this polenta can be served as a first course or a side dish, or sliced and toasted or grilled.

2 cups	water
2 tbsp.	extra-virgin olive oil
8 cloves	garlic, thickly sliced
1 cup	coarsely chopped onions
1 cup	coarsely chopped green pepper
2/3 cup	teff grain
1/2 tsp.	sea salt
2 cups	coarsely chopped plum tomatoes
1 cup	coarsely chopped fresh basil

✦ Boil the water in a tea kettle.

✦ Place the oil in a 10-inch skillet and warm over medium heat. Add the garlic and onions and sauté, stirring occasionally, for 5 minutes, or until fragrant. Add peppers and sauté for 2 minutes, or until bright green. Stir in the teff.

✦ Turn off the heat to prevent splattering and add the boiling water and salt. Turn the heat on and let the polenta simmer for 2 minutes. Add the tomatoes and basil.

✦ Cover and simmer for 10-15 minutes, stirring occasionally, until the water is absorbed. There may be some extra liquid from the tomatoes, but as long as the teff is not crunchy, the polenta is done.

✦ Taste and adjust the seasonings, if desired.

✦ Transfer the polenta to an un-oiled 9-inch pie plate. Let it cool for about 30 minutes. Slice and serve.

Reprinted with permission from: **The Teff Company**, P.O. Box A, Caldwell ID, USA 83606; www.teffco.com; Phone 888-822-2221 and **Leslie Cerier**, 58 Schoolhouse Road, Amherst MA, USA 01002; www.lesliecerier.com

Nutritional Analysis
1 serving = 1 slice

Calories (kcal)	223
Carbohydrates (g)	33
Dietary Fiber (g)	5
Fat (g)	8
Protein (g)	6
Iron (mg)	2.9
Calcium (mg)	107
Sodium (mg)	306

Quinoa and Wild Rice Pilaf

Yield: 6¹/₂ Cups	

Mushrooms and bacon give this pilaf a rich satisfying flavor.

1 cup	wild rice
1 cup	quinoa seed
¹/₃ cup	chopped GF bacon
1 tbsp.	margarine OR vegetable oil
¹/₂ cup	celery
1	onion, chopped
1 cup	sliced mushrooms

✦ Wash the wild rice in a wire strainer and run cold water over it.

✦ In a large heavy saucepan, cook the wild rice in 4 cups of boiling water. Bring to a boil, cover and simmer over low heat for about 1 hour, until all the water has been absorbed.

✦ During the last 15 minutes, add quinoa and, if the rice is almost dry, 1 additional cup of boiling water.

✦ While the rice is cooking, fry the bacon in a pan. When crisp, remove and drain.

✦ Melt the margarine in a skillet and add the celery, onion and mushrooms; sauté for about 5 minutes.

✦ In a casserole, combine the vegetables and bacon with the rice and quinoa mixture.

✦ Microwave on high for 10 minutes or bake in a preheated 350°F oven for 30 minutes.

Recipe courtesy of **Northern Quinoa Corporation**, Box 519, Kamsack SK, Canada S0A 1S0; Phone 866-368-9304 or 306-542-3949; www.quinoa.com

Nutritional Analysis
1 serving = ¹/₂ cup

Calories (kcal)	121
Carbohydrates (g	21
Dietary Fiber (g)	2
Fat (g)	2
Protein (g)	5
Iron (mg)	1.7
Calcium (mg)	14
Sodium (mg)	111

MOROCCAN MILLET

<table>
<tr><td>2 tbsp.</td><td>coconut OR olive oil OR organic canola OR safflower oil</td></tr>
<tr><td>1</td><td>EACH, large red and green bell pepper, sliced into strips</td></tr>
<tr><td>1</td><td>large onion, sliced into half-moons</td></tr>
<tr><td>2 tbsp.</td><td>crushed garlic</td></tr>
<tr><td>2 tsp.</td><td>paprika</td></tr>
<tr><td>1/2 tsp.</td><td>salt</td></tr>
<tr><td>1 tsp.</td><td>ground cumin</td></tr>
<tr><td>1/2 tsp.</td><td>ground cinnamon</td></tr>
<tr><td>1/4 tsp.</td><td>ground turmeric</td></tr>
<tr><td>1/4 tsp.</td><td>ground ginger</td></tr>
<tr><td>1/8 tsp.</td><td>ground cayenne</td></tr>
<tr><td>1 1/2 cups</td><td>millet</td></tr>
<tr><td>3 cups</td><td>GF vegetable stock*</td></tr>
<tr><td>1 3/4 cups</td><td>drained cooked chickpeas OR a 15 oz. can</td></tr>
<tr><td>1/4 cup</td><td>raisins OR chopped GF dates</td></tr>
<tr><td>1/4 cup</td><td>sunflower seeds, pumpkin seeds OR pine nuts (optional)</td></tr>
<tr><td></td><td>salt and pepper to taste</td></tr>
</table>

Yield: 6 Servings

This pilaf is great as a one-dish meal or served with a fresh green salad. Peppers, especially red peppers, are among our best sources of vitamin C and the protective group of phytochemicals known as carotenoids. Millet and chickpeas are good sources of the yellow vitamins riboflavin and folate.

✦ Place 1 tbsp. of the oil in a large roasting pan. Add the peppers, onion, garlic, paprika and salt. Toss until everything is evenly coated with the oil and well combined.

✦ Place in a preheated 450°F oven to roast for 20 minutes, stirring 2 or 3 times during the cooking cycle.

✦ Remove the vegetables from the oven and allow them to cool until safe to handle; then chop them coarsely.

✦ Meanwhile, heat the remaining tablespoon of oil in a large saucepan. Add the cumin, cinnamon, turmeric, ginger and cayenne. Stir over medium-high heat until the spices are uniform in color and well combined, about 30 seconds.

✦ Add the millet and stir quickly to coat, about 1 minute.

✦ Immediately pour in the vegetable stock and bring to a boil. Reduce the heat, cover and cook the millet until all the liquid is absorbed, about 20 minutes.

✦ Place the millet in a large bowl and fluff with a fork.

✦ Add the roasted vegetables, chickpeas, raisins and optional seeds. Season with salt and pepper to taste. Toss gently and serve.

* **Author Note:** Choose a lower-sodium gluten-free vegetable stock or broth.

Reprinted with permission from: *Food Allergy Survival Guide – Surviving and Thriving with Food Allergies and Sensitivities* by **Vesanto Melina, MS, RD**, **Jo Stepaniak, MSEd** and **Dina Aronson, MS, RD**, Healthy Living Publications, 2004.

Nutritional Analysis
1 serving

Calories (kcal)	369
Carbohydrates (g)	63
Dietary Fiber (g)	10
Fat (g)	8
Protein (g)	12
Iron (mg)	3.8
Calcium (mg)	57
Sodium (mg)	1763

HEARTY VEGETARIAN KASHA CASSEROLE

Yield: 6 Servings	

Hearty legumes and kasha are complemented by succulent leeks and piquant cayenne in this savory and substantial casserole.

Note: Kasha is the Russian name for savory or sweet dishes of boiled, baked or roasted buckwheat groats or whole-grain buckwheat. It is sometimes used for cooked millet and oats.

Reprinted with permission from: ***Buckwheat Recipes*** by **Canadian Special Crops Association**, 1215 - 220 Portage Ave., Winnipeg MB, Canada R3C 0A5; Phone 204-925-3780; www.specialcrops.mb.ca www.specialcrops.mb.ca/CSCA_B W_Recipes.pdf

28 oz. can	tomatoes
3 cups	diced cabbage
2	leeks, thinly sliced
1/3 cup	dried peas OR small white beans
1/2 cup	coarse kasha
5 cups	vegetable broth OR water
1/2 cup	brown rice
1/2 tsp.	salt
1/2 tsp.	cayenne pepper
1 tsp.	dried basil or 1 tbsp. chopped fresh
1/4 cup	chopped fresh parsley

✦ Combine the tomatoes, cabbage, leeks, peas, kasha and vegetable broth in a crock-pot or large Dutch oven.

✦ Simmer, covered, for an hour. Add the brown rice, salt, cayenne and basil. Add more liquid if needed.

✦ Cook for an additional 20-30 minutes. Add the parsley just before serving.

Nutritional Analysis
1 serving

Calories (kcal)	210
Carbohydrates (g)	43
Dietary Fiber (g)	8
Fat (g)	1
Protein (g)	10
Iron (mg)	3
Calcium (mg)	102
Sodium (mg)	3002

WILD RICE & VEGETABLE CASSEROLE

Yield: **8 Servings**

Creamy wild rice has a nutty flavor that is wonderful with the robust flavor of broccoli, and also with the more delicate flavors of cauliflower and asparagus.

¹/₂ cup	wild rice (2 cups cooked)
	pepper and sage to taste
10 oz.	can GF cream soup
1 bunch	broccoli, cauliflower OR asparagus, cut into florets or bite-sized pieces
1 cup	grated Cheddar cheese

✦ Wash the wild rice in a wire strainer and run cold water over it.

✦ Combine 2 cups of water and ¹/₂ cup of wild rice in a heavy saucepan. Bring to a boil, cover and simmer over low heat for approximately 45 minutes, until the rice kernels have burst their shells and fluffed out. Drain off excess water. Stir the rice with a fork; cover and let stand for 15 minutes.

✦ Put the cooked rice, seasoned with a little pepper and sage, into a greased 1¹/₂-2 quart casserole.

✦ Cover with the undiluted cream soup.

✦ Steam the vegetables for 5 minutes, then place over the soup.

✦ Sprinkle with the cheese.

✦ Bake in a preheated 350°F oven for about 20 minutes.

Recipe courtesy of **Riese's Canadian Lake Wild Rice**, La Ronge SK, Canada S0J 1L0; Phone 306-425-2314; www.wildlakerice.com

Nutritional Analysis
1 serving

Calories (kcal)	131
Carbohydrates (g)	14
Dietary Fiber (g)	3
Fat (g)	6
Protein (g)	8
Iron (mg)	1.1
Calcium (mg)	144
Sodium (mg)	155

Black Bean Chili

Yield: **6-8 Servings** (8 cups)

The goodness of chili in a flash. The range of ingredients provides a powerful phyto-chemical mix. This vegetarian chili is packed with a rainbow of carotenoids and allium family members and their perks, topped off with a hit of both soluble and insoluble fiber.

2 tsp.	extra-virgin olive oil
1 cup	chopped onions
3	large cloves garlic, finely chopped
1	green bell pepper, diced
1 cup	1/2 inch cubes zucchini (1 medium)
1 tsp.	finely chopped jalapeño pepper
2x19 oz. cans	black beans, rinsed and drained
28 oz. can	whole tomatoes, coarsely chopped, with juice
1 cup	frozen corn kernels
1 tbsp.	chili powder
1 tsp.	ground cumin
1 tsp.	dried oregano
	salt to taste
3 tbsp.	chopped fresh coriander, for garnish
	shredded light Cheddar cheese, for garnish (optional)

✦ Heat the oil in a large, heavy pot over medium heat.

✦ Add the onions and garlic; sauté for 5 minutes.

✦ Add the green pepper, zucchini and jalapeño pepper; sauté another 3 minutes.

✦ Add the black beans, tomatoes with juice, corn, chili powder, cumin and oregano.

✦ Reduce heat to medium-low and simmer, uncovered and stirring occasionally, for 30 minutes.

✦ Season with salt to taste.

✦ Garnish with coriander and Cheddar, if using, before serving.

Author's Note:
For a hearty Turkey, Chicken or Beef Black Bean Chili, sauté 1 lb. of ground meat in a heavy skillet. Drain off all fat; place the cooked meat in a colander and rinse with very hot or boiling water. Add to sautéed onions and garlic.

Reprinted with permission from:
The Enlightened Eaters™ Whole Foods Guide – Harvest the Power of Phyto Foods by **Rosie Schwartz**, Penguin Group, 2003

Nutritional Analysis
1 serving = 1 cup

Calories (kcal)	143
Carbohydrates (g)	31
Dietary Fiber (g)	9
Fat (g)	2
Protein (g)	8
Iron (mg)	3.1
Calcium (mg)	92
Sodium (mg)	581

LENTIL LEAF ROLLS

Yield: **10 Servings**

These rice and lentil-filled "cabbage rolls" are beautifully flavored with dill.

³/₄ cup	short-grain rice
³/₄ cup	water
¹/₂ tsp.	salt
1 tbsp.	canola oil
¹/₂ cup	finely chopped onion
2 tbsp.	chopped fresh dill
1 tsp.	salt
¹/₈ tsp.	pepper
1¹/₂ cups	lentils, cooked
30	lettuce, Swiss chard, beet, spinach OR cabbage leaves*
1	GF vegetable bouillon cube
¹/₂ cup	boiling water
¹/₂ cup	cream milk (10% MF)

✦ Combine the rice, water and salt in a small saucepan. Bring to a boil, stir once and reduce the heat to simmer. Cover; cook for 12 minutes, until the water is absorbed.

✦ In a small skillet, over medium heat, heat the oil and sauté the onions for 4 minutes, until they start to turn brown.

✦ Combine the onions with dill, salt, pepper, lentils and rice.

✦ Prepare the leaves by washing them and cutting larger leaves into smaller pieces (approximately 3-4" squares).

✦ Blanch the leaves by putting them into a large bowl; pour boiling water over leaves; blanch for 30 seconds*.

✦ Drain the leaves, rinse in cold water and drain again.

✦ At the base of each leaf, put 1¹/₂ tbsp. rice and lentil filling.

✦ Roll up leaves while tucking in sides.

✦ Place the rolls, seam down, in a lightly oiled 2-quart casserole.

✦ Dissolve the bouillon cube in boiling water. Pour over the rolls.

✦ Pour cream milk over the rolls.

✦ Cover with a few remaining leaves.

✦ Cover with a lid or foil. Bake in a preheated 325°F oven for 1¹/₂ hours.

✦ Check the rolls after 1 hour. If they need more liquid, add a little cream milk.

* Cabbage leaves may need to be steamed longer to make them more pliable.

Adapted from and reprinted with permission from: **Saskatchewan Pulse Growers**, 104 - 411 Downey Road, Saskatoon SK, Canada S7N 4L8; Phone 306-668-5556; www.saskpulse.com

Nutritional Analysis
1 serving

Calories (kcal)	123
Carbohydrates (g)	20
Dietary Fiber (g)	4
Fat (g)	3
Protein (g)	5
Iron (mg)	1.9
Calcium (mg)	54
Sodium (mg)	454

Lentil Pizza Squares

Yield: **12 Servings**

Serve these pizza squares with a green salad for a casual main course or as a substantial snack.

1/4 cup	canola oil
3/4 cup	chopped onion
1 cup	sliced mushrooms
1	garlic clove, minced
4	eggs
1 1/2 cups	lentil purée*
1 1/2 cups	low-fat sour cream
7 1/2 oz.	can tomato sauce
3/4 cup	cornmeal
1 tsp.	crumbled dried basil
1 tsp.	crumbled dried oregano
1/2 tsp.	salt
1 1/2 cups	grated low-fat Cheddar cheese
1 1/2 cups	grated low-fat mozzarella cheese
1/2 cup	sliced pepperoni OR salami **
1/2 cup	diced sweet green pepper

✦ In a skillet, heat the oil and add the onion, mushrooms and garlic. Sauté until the onion is translucent. Remove from the heat and let cool.

✦ In a large mixing bowl, beat the eggs. Blend in lentil purée, sour cream, tomato sauce, cornmeal, basil, oregano, salt and the mushroom mixture. Stir in the cheeses.

✦ Spoon the batter into a 9 x 13-inch baking dish sprayed with nonstick vegetable spray.

✦ Garnish with the pepperoni and green peppers.

✦ Bake in a preheated 350°F oven for 40-45 minutes, or until firm to the touch. Let stand 10 minutes before cutting. Cut into 12 squares.

* **Lentil Purée:**

3/4 cup	lentils
2 cups	water

✦ To prepare Lentil Purée, rinse the lentils and drain.

✦ Cover with water and bring to a boil. Reduce heat and simmer for 45-50 minutes.

✦ Drain off any excess liquid and mash the lentils with a potato masher.

✦ Cool the purée before adding to recipe.

**Gluten-free brand required.

Adapted from and reprinted with permission from: *Discover the Pulse Potential* (1994), by the **Saskatchewan Pulse Growers**, 104 - 411 Downey Road, Saskatoon SK, Canada S7N 4L8; Phone 306-668-5556; www.saskpulse.com

Nutritional Analysis
1 serving = 1 square

Calories (kcal)	292
Carbohydrates (g)	20
Dietary Fiber (g)	4
Fat (g)	17
Protein (g)	16
Iron (mg)	2.2
Calcium (mg)	226
Sodium (mg)	542

TURKEY MEATBALLS WITH LEMON SAUCE

Yield: **4 Servings**

Kasha (roasted buckwheat groats) adds a distinctive nutty flavor to these tasty meatballs. This serves four as an hors d'oeuvre or serves two as a main dish with a marinated vegetable or tossed green salad.

1 cup	cooked kasha (any granulation)
1	egg, beaten
1 tsp.	grated lemon zest
1 1/2 lbs.	99% fat-free ground raw turkey
2 tbsp.	vegetable oil
1 cup	GF chicken OR turkey broth
1/4 cup	plain yogurt
1 tbsp.	cornstarch
1 tbsp.	lemon juice
1	small carrot, finely shredded
1	green onion, diced

✦ Prepare the kasha according to package directions, using chicken broth (gluten-free).

✦ Combine the kasha, egg, lemon zest and turkey in a mixing bowl; blend well.

✦ Shape the mixture into 12 balls.

✦ In a large skillet, heat the oil and brown the turkey balls on all sides. Add the broth; cover and simmer for 20 minutes. Use a slotted spoon to transfer the meatballs to a serving dish.

✦ In a small bowl, combine the yogurt, cornstarch and lemon juice.

✦ In the skillet, combine the yogurt mixture with the pan juices and cook until the sauce is thickened and bubbly. Add the carrot and onion. Cook for a few minutes and pour the sauce over the meatballs.

Author Note: The original recipe had 1 tsp. Worcestershire sauce, however, some brands of Worcestershire sauce contain malt vinegar (which is not gluten-free) and/or soy sauce (which often contains wheat).

Recipe adapted and reprinted with permission from **The Birkett Mills**, 163 Main St, Penn Yan NY, USA 14527;
Phone 315-536-3311;
www.thebirkettmills.com

Nutritional Analysis
1 serving

Calories (kcal)	326
Carbohydrates (g)	13
Dietary Fiber (g)	2
Fat (g)	11
Protein (g)	46
Iron (mg)	2.8
Calcium (mg)	45
Sodium (mg)	369

Oven-Fried Chicken

	Yield: **6 Servings**

Ground flax seed and GF crackers or corn flakes are used to add crunch to this crispy chicken dish.

1	egg, beaten
3 tbsp.	non-fat (skim) milk
1/2 cup	ground flax seed (flax seed meal)
1/2 cup	GF crackers OR GF corn flakes (finely crushed)
1/4 tsp.	black pepper
1 tbsp.	dried parsley flakes
1 tsp.	chili powder
1 tsp.	garlic powder
1 tsp.	salt
2-3 lbs.	chicken pieces
2 tbsp.	melted butter*

✦ In a small bowl, combine the egg and milk.

✦ In a shallow container, combine the ground flax, GF cracker or corn flake crumbs, pepper, parsley, chili powder, garlic and salt.

✦ Skin the chicken and rinse with warm water. Pat dry.

✦ Dip the chicken pieces into the egg mixture; coat with the crumb mixture.

✦ Place the chicken on a greased 10 x 15-inch baking pan so pieces do not touch.

✦ Drizzle the chicken pieces with melted butter.

✦ Bake in a preheated 350°F oven for 45 minutes, or until chicken is tender and no longer pink. Do not turn chicken pieces while baking.

* For a lower-fat version, omit the butter.

Adapted from and reprinted with permission from: *Flax: Family Favorites – Recipes and Healthful Tips* by **The Flax Council of Canada**, 465 – 167 Lombard Ave., Winnipeg MB, Canada R3B 0T6; Phone 204-982-2115; www.flaxcouncil.ca and **Saskatchewan Flax Development Commission**, A5A - 116 - 103rd St. E., Saskatoon SK, Canada S7N 1Y7; Phone 306-664-1901; www.saskflax.com

Nutritional Analysis
1 serving

Calories (kcal)	291
Carbohydrates (g)	10
Dietary Fiber (g)	3
Fat (g)	12
Protein (g)	34
Iron (mg)	3.1
Calcium (mg)	56
Sodium (mg)	564

CAJUN FLAX COATING

Yield: **12 tablespoons**

Suggested foods for coating: chicken, veal, beef, pork, catfish, turkey, redfish, shrimp.

2 tbsp.	paprika
1/2 cup	ground flaxseed
1 tbsp.	black pepper
1/2 tsp.	ground cumin
1/2 tsp.	cayenne pepper
1/2 tsp.	ground oregano
1/2 tsp.	ground thyme
1/2 tsp.	dried basil
	GF seasoning salt, to taste

✦ Combine all ingredients, adding seasoning salt to taste.

Note: Used as a seasoning, this coating doesn't require the use of seasoned flour or an egg wash.

Reprinted with permission from: *The Amaxing Flax Cookbook* by **Jane Reinhardt-Martin, RD, LD**, 2004; www.flaxrd.com

Nutritional Analysis
1 serving = 1 tbsp.

Calories (kcal)	32
Carbohydrates (g)	3
Dietary Fiber (g)	2
Fat (g)	2
Protein (g)	1
Iron (mg)	0.6
Calcium (mg)	20
Sodium (mg)	66

CAROL FENSTER'S SAVORY PIE CRUST

for your favorite pot pie

Yield: 1 Pie/6 Slices	

This savory crust uses Montina™ Pure (Indian rice grass) to add fiber and a hearty texture. The crust is surprisingly easy to handle and the dough can be made ahead and frozen for later use.

³/₄ cup	gluten-free flour blend of your choice OR Carol's GF Sorghum Flour Blend*
³/₄ cup	tapioca flour
¹/₂ cup	sweet rice flour
¹/₂ cup	Montina™ Pure Baking Supplement**
1 tbsp.	sugar
1 tsp.	EACH, xanthan gum and guar gum
1 tsp.	dried thyme leaves
¹/₂ tsp.	salt
¹/₂ cup	shortening***
2 tbsp.	butter OR margarine (non-diet)
¹/₄ cup	milk (cow, rice or soy)
1	egg, beaten for egg wash (optional)

✦ Place the dry ingredients, shortening and butter in a food processor. Mix well. Add milk and blend until dough forms a ball. If dough is too stiff, add water a tablespoon at a time until you can shape the dough into a ball.

✦ Flatten the dough to 1-inch disk, wrap tightly and refrigerate for 1 hour so the liquids are well-distributed throughout the dough.

✦ Massage the dough between your hands until warm and piable, making the crust easier to handle. Roll half of the dough (keep the remaining half wrapped tightly to avoid drying out) to a 10-inch circle between 2 pieces of heavy-duty plastic wrap dusted with rice flour. (Use damp paper towel between countertop and plastic wrap to anchor plastic wrap.) Be sure to move the rolling pin from the center of the dough to the outer edge, moving around the circle in a clockwise fashion to assure uniform thickness.

✦ Remove the top plastic wrap and invert the crust, centering it over the pie plate. Remove the remaining plastic wrap and press the crust into place. If the dough cracks or splits, simply press the edges together again.

✦ Pour your favorite pot pie filling into the crust (see Note on page 201).

✦ Roll the remaining dough to a 10-inch circle between floured plastic wrap. Invert and center on filled crust. Don't remove the top plastic wrap until the dough is centered. Shape a decorative ridge around the rim of the pie plate. Prick the crust several times with a fork to allow the steam to escape. Freeze for 15 minutes. Brush with beaten egg, if desired, for shinier crust. Place the pie on a non-stick baking sheet.

✦ Bake the pie in a preheated 375°F oven for 15 minutes on the lowest oven rack to brown the bottom crust. Move to the next highest oven rack and bake another 25-35 minutes OR until the crust is nicely browned. Cover loosely with foil if the edges brown too much.

✦ Cool for 10 minutes on a wire rack before serving.

Adapted from and reprinted with permission from: *Gluten-Free 101: Easy Basic Dishes without Wheat* by **Carol Fenster, PhD**, Savory Palate Inc. 2006. www.glutenfree101.com

Nutritional Analysis
1 serving = 1 slice

Calories (kcal)	359
Carbohydrates (g)	44
Dietary Fiber (g)	1
Fat (g)	22
Protein (g)	3
Iron (mg)	1.2
Calcium (mg)	28
Sodium (mg)	247

CAROL FENSTER'S SAVORY PIE CRUST

(continued)

* **Carol's Gluten-Free Sorghum Flour Blend**
(makes 4 1/2 cups)

1 1/2 cups	sorghum flour
1 1/2 cups	potato starch OR cornstarch
1 cup	tapioca flour
1/2 cup	corn flour OR bean flour OR almond flour OR chestnut flour

** **Montina™ Pure Baking Supplement** is 100% Indian ricegrass flour sold under the trade name Montina by Amazing Grains Grower Cooperative.

***Non-hydrogenated shortenings, made by Spectrum® or Smart Balance®, are available at health food stores.

Note: ✦ Filling options could include your favorite chicken, turkey or beef stew, or a hearty vegetable stew.

✦ If you prefer to make a **single-crust pot pie**, put your favorite filling into a greased casserole dish. Roll half of the dough to the appropriate size and lay it over the filling, shaping a decorative edge around the rim of the dish. Prick the top with a fork a few times to let steam escape. Brush the crust with beaten egg. Bake at 375°F for 25-35 minutes, or until the filling is hot and bubbly and the crust is golden brown. Freeze the remaining dough for another use.

✦ For a dessert pie crust, omit thyme leaves, add pie filling and proceed as on the previous page.

Eating Away From Home

Once you've mastered the basics of the gluten-free diet, it is possible to eat away from home, whether it be at a restaurant or in the home setting of a friend, acquaintance, or stranger. A positive attitude and a game plan are essential for a safe and successful experience. Some excellent resources on the subject of eating out and traveling, including books; dining cards in English and foreign languages; gluten-free travel clubs; websites and bed & breakfasts are found on pages 352, 353. Here are some helpful tips for eating out.

Restaurants

1. Selecting a place to eat

Successful dining out depends on a variety of factors, including the type of restaurant chosen.

- ◆ Be careful in restaurants where language may be a communication barrier. Food service and wait staff may not easily understand gluten-free restrictions. Foreign language restaurant cards listing allowed and not allowed ingredients and foods can be helpful (see page 353 for specific resources).

- ◆ Allow extra time to discuss specific needs for a gluten-free meal.

    - Fast food and quick service restaurants may have little time to thoroughly check ingredients and food preparation methods. Fortunately, some chains have an ingredient listing of their menu items which can be helpful in making safe food choices.

    - Fine dining restaurants offer a less hurried atmosphere and usually have more time to accommodate special needs. Call the restaurant the day before or earlier the same day and ask to speak to the chef to discuss meal options. Chefs are generally aware of gluten and can often substitute other ingredients and/or create an alternative dish.

2. Timing of Meals

- ◆ Avoid peak meal times. Dining early or late will allow more time and easier access to staff who can answer questions and usually accommodate special needs.

3. Explain Dietary Restrictions Briefly

- ◆ The terms "celiac disease" and "gluten-free" may be unfamiliar to those in the food service industry. However, many understand the concept of "food allergy." Briefly indicate that you have a serious food sensitivity and must avoid foods containing wheat, barley and rye in order to prevent getting sick. Ask the server and/or chef if they could help you with selection of safe menu items.

4. Ask Specific Questions

- ◆ It is essential to inquire about cooking methods, specific ingredients that are in the item and how it is served. Unfortunately, many servers are from a generation with little knowledge of cooking, where food comes from and food preparation methods, therefore it may be advisable to have the server or manager ask the chef very specific questions.

- ◆ Here are examples of foods and the potential problems involved with them:

    a) **Salads and Salad Dressings**

    - May contain croûtons; wheat-based Asian noodles; won tons; pasta or taco shells; or salad dressings containing unsafe ingredients (e.g., wheat flour or wheat starch, hydrolyzed wheat protein, soy sauce).

- Emphasize that no croûtons or other bread products be used. If no safe salad dressings are available, ask for oil and a lemon wedge or balsamic vinegar to be served on the side.

b) **Marinades**

- Teriyaki or soy sauce (made with wheat) or beer may be used to marinade meat, fish or poultry.

c) **Soups and Sauces**

- Soups and sauces are often made with commercial soup bases or soup cubes containing wheat flour, wheat starch or hydrolyzed wheat protein. Roux (pronounced 'roo') is a combination of butter and flour which is used to thicken sauces. Many restaurants also use commercial canned, frozen or dry sauce mixes that contain unsafe ingredients.

d) **Meat, Fish and Poultry**

- May be dusted (or 'dredged') with flour or bread crumbs before grilling or frying.

- Some hamburger patties may contain wheat flour, wheat starch or bread crumbs.

- Seasonings containing wheat flour or wheat starch may be added to meat, fish or poultry.

- If prime rib is too rare for the customer's taste, the chef may "cook" it in a pot of au jus until it reaches the desired doneness. Au jus may come from a can or mix containing unsafe ingredients.

- Self-basting turkeys and imitation bacon bits may contain hydrolyzed wheat protein.

- Imitation seafood may contain wheat starch.

e) **Fried Foods**

- The oil used to deep-fry foods may be used for both breaded and non-breaded items, in which case they should be avoided. In large restaurants and fast food establishments, French fries are often cooked in separate fryers where there is less chance of cross contamination.

f) **Hash Browns and Rice**

- Some frozen hash brown potatoes may contain wheat starch. Ask for ingredient information and whether any other ingredients have been added while cooking them (e.g., seasonings which may contain wheat flour, wheat starch or hydrolyzed wheat protein).

- Rice pilafs may have seasonings or added ingredients that may need to be avoided. Also, many restaurants use commercially packaged rice that is seasoned with unsafe ingredients (e.g., broth, soup bases, seasonings that contain wheat flour, wheat starch, hydrolyzed wheat protein). It is best to choose plain steamed rice cooked in water.

g) **Pasta**

- Some restaurants have gluten-free pasta, or check to see if you can bring your own pasta. Ask that fresh water be used, not the water that has been used to cook wheat pasta.

h) **Vegetables**

- Avoid battered vegetables or those prepared in sauces which are usually thickened with flour. Some vegetables may be sautéed or stir-fried with seasonings or soy sauce that contain wheat.

5. Food Preparation Equipment

✦ Request that your food be prepared on a clean grill or in a clean pan. If this is a problem, suggest cooking it on clean aluminum foil.

✦ Cooking methods such as steaming, poaching or baking are often safer choices.

6. Confirm Your Order Before Eating

✦ Is this the "special" meal I ordered?

✦ Were your instructions followed?

7. Thank the Chef and Food Server

Leave a generous tip for good service and patronize the establishment again.

Adapted from ***Restaurant Dining: Seven Tips for Staying Gluten-Free*** by the Gluten Intolerance Group, Seattle, WA.   www.gluten.net

Social Events

1. Call the hostess or catering staff before the event.

✦ If your hostess is not aware of your food restrictions, explain that you are on a special diet.

✦ When attending a banquet, contact the catering department and/or chef several days ahead of time to explain your dietary restrictions.

✦ Briefly explain your dietary restrictions and the need for plain foods. It is often possible for the planned menu items to be prepared without marinades, sauces or other unsafe ingredients (e.g., plain steak, chicken, fish, salad, vegetables, fruits) or a safe substitute may be available. Most people are more than willing to accommodate this special request if they know in advance, rather than scrambling at the last minute to make changes to the menu or food preparation methods or, worse yet, feeling awkward about not having something safe for you to eat. For those individuals who know you well, they may change the preparation method for the items or the menu choices altogether so that it is suitable for everyone. Many people find preparing a gluten-free meal an interesting challenge, while others may feel uneasy. If the hostess is concerned about what to serve, offer to bring something that is safe for you to eat.

✦ When invited to an event where you are unable to determine ahead of time what's on the menu, you may want to eat something before you leave home or take something with you to be on the safe side.

2. Always say thank you.

✦ A thank-you note, telephone call or email to the host or catering department for accommodating your special dietary needs is always greatly appreciated.

Gluten-Free Shopping

In the beginning, be prepared to spend a lot more time in the stores shopping for gluten-free foods. You need to read every label and begin to learn which ingredients are gluten-free and which contain gluten. Excellent resources to take with you are:

Canadian Celiac Association *Pocket Dictionary: Acceptability of Foods and Food Ingredients for the Gluten-Free Diet*

> Available in a pocket-sized book or a software version (Windows, Pocket PC's and Smart Phones) that provides a brief description of each item along with an assessment of its acceptability for the gluten-free diet.

Clan Thompson Food Lists

> 1. Available in a "Celiac SmartList" for Palm OS Handhelds, Pocket PC's, Windows, Mobile, Blackberry Smartphones or Macs that includes many foods from major brands found in the USA that are gluten-free.
>
> 2. Available in a "Celiac SmartList" for Palm OS Handhelds, Blackberry Smartphones, Windows or Macs that includes many foods from major brands found in Canada that are gluten-free.

Caution

Manufacturers often change ingredients in their products. Always check ingredient labels for changes and the inclusion of suspect ingredients. If in doubt, phone the manufacturers. Be very explicit in your request for information:

✦ Is there any wheat, rye, triticale, spelt, kamut, barley or regular oats or their derivatives in the product?

✦ Are the components of a particular ingredient also free of the offending grains?

– baking powder (may contain wheat starch).

– seasonings (may contain wheat starch, wheat flour or hydrolyzed wheat protein).

– modified food starches made from wheat.

– hydrolyzed plant or vegetable protein from wheat.

– soy sauce (often contains wheat).

– worcestershire sauce (some contain malt vinegar).

To order these resources see pages 347, 348.

Helpful Hints

Set up files in a 3-ring binder to organize all the product information you collect. Divide it into two sections:

✦ Regular Supermarket Foods

✦ Foods from Gluten-Free Companies

Take notes, including the date, when you call the manufacturers. Keep product lists from gluten-free companies and indicate whether or not you liked the product.

Gluten-Free Shopping List

The following is a sample list to get you started on your gluten-free diet.

Bread Products
__ GF bread, bagels, buns, pizza crusts
__ GF freezer waffles
__ GF muffins

Cereals
__ Amaranth, buckwheat, corn, millet, quinoa, rice, soy
__ GF corn flakes, GF crisp rice
__ Cream of buckwheat or rice (brown or white), cornmeal

Pasta
__ Corn, legume, potato, quinoa, rice, soy

Crackers/Rice Cakes
__ GF rice crisp/crunch crackers
__ GF plain or flavored rice cakes

Rice
__ Brown, wild, white

Gluten-Free Flours
__ Amaranth flour
__ Arrowroot or tapioca starch
__ Bean flours
__ Cornstarch
__ Cornmeal
__ Mesquite flour
__ Montina™ flour
__ Potato starch
__ Quinoa flour
__ Rice flour (white, brown)
__ Sorghum flour
__ Soy flour
__ Teff flour

Gluten-Free Ingredients & Baking Mixes
__ GF bread mix
__ GF pancake/waffle mix
__ GF muffin mix
__ GF baking powder
__ Baking soda
__ Xanthan gum or Guar gum

Legumes (dry or ready to eat)
__ Beans (e.g., garbanzo, kidney, white)
__ GF canned baked beans
__ Lentils, Split Peas

Grains, Other
__ Amaranth
__ Buckwheat groats
__ Flax seed or flax seed meal

__ Millet
__ Quinoa
__ Teff

Spices
__ Black pepper
__ Onion powder
__ Garlic powder, fresh garlic

Miscellaneous
__ Honey, molasses, sugar (brown, white)
__ Jam, jelly, marmalade
__ GF puddings
__ Gelatin (flavored)
__ Vanilla
__ Vinegar (except malt vinegar)

Sauces
__ Ketchup, plain mustard and relish
__ GF barbecue sauce
__ GF pizza and pasta sauces
__ GF salsa
__ GF soy sauce

GF Soups, (see pages 266-270)

Nuts & Seeds
__ Almonds, peanuts, pecans, walnuts
__ Pumpkin, sesame & sunflower seeds
__ Nut butters (almond, cashew, peanut)

Meat, Fish and Poultry
__ Fresh or frozen (plain)
__ GF deli meats

Dairy
__ Milk (whole, 2%, 1%, or skim)
__ Milk powder
__ Yogurt
__ Cheese
__ Eggs

Fruits
__ Fresh, canned or frozen (plain)
__ Dried fruits

Vegetables
__ Fresh, canned or frozen (plain)
__ Tomato paste
__ Tomatoes, canned

Fats and Oils
__ Butter or margarine
__ Vegetable oil (e.g., canola, olive)
__ GF salad dressings

CROSS-CONTAMINATION

In addition to always checking about ingredients in gluten-free foods, you must also be aware of the possibility of cross-contamination (a process by which a gluten-free product comes into contact with something that is not gluten-free).

Avoiding Cross-Contamination at Home

✦ Store all **gluten-free** products in separate labeled containers. Some families buy bright stickers and put them on everything that is and/or should remain gluten-free. In addition, you may want to keep all **gluten-free** foods in a separate place in the cupboard and refrigerator.

✦ Buy separate containers of items like peanut butter or jam and label "gluten-free" to prevent them from becoming cross-contaminated by other family members preparing gluten-containing products (e.g. toast, sandwiches).

✦ Buy squeeze bottles of condiments such as ketchup, mustard, relish and mayonnaise.

✦ Have a separate butter or margarine container and cutting board that are used for **gluten-free** foods only.

✦ Have your own toaster. If not, use a toaster oven, where the rack can be removed and washed if others have used it. Another option is to buy special toaster bags for gluten-free bread that can be placed in a regular toaster. These bags can be washed and re-used.

✦ Always make sure that the counter space you are using to prepare **gluten-free** foods is freshly washed to ensure it is free from crumbs or flour dust.

✦ Make sure pots, utensils, etc., that are also used for other foods are thoroughly scrubbed before using with **gluten-free** foods.

✦ Do not boil gluten-free pasta in the same water that previously had gluten-containing pasta. Also use a separate colander to drain gluten-free pasta, as it is difficult to remove traces of pasta from the colander.

✦ Have your own set of utensils and other items for gluten-free baking, e.g., wooden spoons, sifter.

Cross-Contamination Outside of the Home

✦ Avoid buying products from bulk bins. Gluten-free products can become contaminated by:
(1) scoops that have been used in another bin with gluten-containing products and
(2) being placed in a bin that previously had gluten-containing items that was not thoroughly cleaned.

✦ Be aware that French fries may have been cooked in the same oil where battered gluten-containing foods (e.g., fish, chicken fingers) have been fried.

✦ Request that the cook: (1) use clean utensils, (2) clean the grill or pan before preparing your food, and (3) keep your meal away from meals that contain gluten.

✦ Be careful at buffets as spoons may have been used for more than one dish.

✦ Check with airlines to see if a gluten-free meal can be ordered. However, always put "extra" snacks such as dried fruits, nuts and seeds, fresh fruit and/or mini rice cakes in your carry-on bag as the meal may not be appropriate or suitable. Also, you may encounter flight delays and need gluten-free snacks.

GLUTEN-FREE PRODUCTS

Gluten-free products listed on pages 210 to 278 were exhaustively researched from sources believed to be reliable at the time of printing and recorded from August-December 2009. The author assumes no liability for any errors, omissions or inaccuracies in this section.

Many of the products are made by companies who manufacture gluten-free products exclusively, usually in dedicated facilities. Other companies manufacture gluten-free and gluten-containing products in the same facility and/or may have separate areas of the plant or separate lines to produce gluten-free products. Most manufacturers have strict quality control policies/procedures and take extra precautions to prevent cross-contamination. A growing number of companies test their ingredients and/or products using the highly sensitive ELISA test. They may also request that ingredient suppliers provide documentation of any testing that has been done and gluten-free status of the ingredients. Some also have third party certification from organizations such as the Gluten-Free Certification Organization (GFCO). See page 342.

As mentioned on pages 60, 61 and 67, the lack of international consensus on the definition and regulation of the term gluten-free, as well as, limited scientific data on a safe threshold level of gluten for individuals with celiac disease, has created challenges for the food industry and consumers. This has resulted in a wide variety of statements, use of symbols on food product labels and answers from company consumer relations department. These are some of the type of statements that companies may give when asked if the product is gluten-free:

1. Ingredients that contain gluten are always listed on the ingredient label.

2. There are no gluten-containing ingredients in the product or they are made with non-gluten ingredients. The product is gluten-free.

3. There are no gluten-containing ingredients in the product or they are made with non-gluten ingredients. Products are tested using the ELISA test and/or products have been certified by the Gluten-Free Certification Organization (GFCO). The product is gluten-free.

4. There are no gluten-containing ingredients in the products or they are made with non-gluten ingredients, however: a) they are made on the same line as gluten-containing products, although the equipment is thoroughly cleaned and sanitized and/or b) they do not test for gluten or there may be a risk for cross-contamination, therefore, they may or may not make a gluten-free declaration.

5. May contain traces of wheat or gluten.

6. Made in the same facility where wheat is used or made on shared equipment with gluten-containing ingredients.

7. They will not make a statement about the gluten-free status of the product.

When a company will not guarantee that a product is gluten-free, both consumers and health professionals are often confused and left to make their own decisions on the safety of the product. Although there is no one perfect answer, it should be noted that the vast majority of food companies are very concerned about food safety. They have strict quality control procedures to prevent or reduce the risk of cross-contamination, as they do not want consumers to have serious health problems and/or result in a food recall that is not only costly but can damage the reputation of the company.

The following gluten-free product lists are not all-inclusive and the availability of some products will vary depending on where you live in Canada or the USA. Also, companies may discontinue products. Finally, manufacturers of regular commercial food products often change ingredients used in their products. Carefully reading the labels on a regular basis, and contacting the company (if in doubt), is of utmost importance to confirm that the products have remained gluten-free.

The tables on pages 210 to 278 were designed to assist you in purchasing gluten-free products. The package sizes of these products are listed in ounces with the equivalent weight in grams. Gluten-free products can be purchased from a variety of sources:

MANUFACTURERS OF GLUTEN-FREE PRODUCTS

A very large selection of products can be purchased from gluten-free specialty manufacturers and other companies who produce gluten-free products in addition to other items (see pages 279 to 320).

GLUTEN-FREE SPECIALTY STORES AND DISTRIBUTORS

Some stores and distributors specialize in selling gluten-free and/or allergen-free products exclusively (see pages 332 to 338).

HEALTH FOOD STORES

Often carry a wide selection of products.

Be aware of cross-contamination, especially for items in bulk bins or those bulk bagged in the store. Ask what procedures they use to reduce the risk of cross-contamination (e.g., cleaning the area and equipment used to portion and package bulk items; keeping gluten-free foods separate from gluten-containing foods.

GROCERY STORES

Most large chains carry a variety of gluten-free products throughout the store or have special designated areas for natural or health foods. Examples include baking mixes, cereals (cornmeal, hominy grits, cream of rice, gluten-free cold cereals), cookies, crackers, rice cakes, gluten-free flours (potato, rice, soy) and starches (corn, potato, rice, tapioca), mixes, pasta (corn, rice), snack bars and frozen entrees.

GLUTEN-FREE BAKERIES

There are a growing number of specialty bakeries that produce only gluten-free items. Several bakeries listed in this section produce gluten-free products in a shared facility (some in segregated areas) on dedicated equipment or equipment that has been thoroughly cleaned and sanitized to prevent cross-contamination (see pages 321 to 331).

REGULAR COMMERCIAL BAKERIES

Some bakeries make gluten-free products in addition to regular gluten-containing bakery items.

Be aware of the strong possibility of cross-contamination. Ask the bakery what procedures they use to reduce the risk of cross-contamination (e.g., cleaning of the area and equipment, baking gluten-free products in a separate area and in separate pans and/or on specific days when no gluten-containing items are produced).

CEREALS

✦ Most regular cereals (rice, corn) are **NOT** gluten-free as they usually contain barley malt (extract or flavoring), e.g., **Kellogg's Corn Flakes, Rice Krispies**.

✦ Some cereals labeled "**wheat free**" are **NOT** gluten-free: e.g., **Erewhon Crispy Brown Rice Cereal (Original and No Salt Added)** – contains organic barley malt.

✦ Products containing spelt or kamut are **NOT** gluten-free.

Company	Cereals	Grams	Ounces
AMY'S KITCHEN	Cream of Rice Organic Hot Cereal	255	9
ANCIENT HARVEST	Organic Quinoa Flakes	340 g, 4.54 kg	12 oz., 10 lbs.
ARROWHEAD MILLS	Corn Grits (white or yellow)	680	24
	Maple Buckwheat Flakes	341	12
	Sweetened Rice Flakes	341	12
	Rice and Shine Hot Cereal	680	24
BAKERY ON MAIN	**Gluten-Free Granola*** Apple Raisin Walnut, Cranberry, Orange Cashew, Extreme Fruit & Nut**, Nutty Maple Cranberry**, Rainforest	340	12
	Made from corn and rice flours, rice bran, nuts, seeds. *Dairy-Free. **Also in 22 oz.		
BARBARA'S BAKERY	Brown Rice Crisps	284	10
	Fruit Juice Sweetened Corn Flakes	255	9
	Puffins Honey Rice	340	12
BARKAT	Porridge Flakes (rice and millet)*	500	17.6
	Breakfast Pops*, Corn Flakes*, Corn Flakes, Chocolate Corn Flakes*, Chocolate Rice Crunchies*, Rice Crunchies*, Muesli*	250	8.8
	*Organic and Dairy-Free. Non-organic corn flakes are also Dairy-Free		
THE BIRKETT MILLS	Pocono Cream of Buckwheat Hot Cereal*	369	13
	*Also available in bulk.		
BOB'S RED MILL	Brown Rice Farina Hot Cereal	737	26
	Creamy Buckwheat Hot Cereal	510	18
	Gluten-Free Corn Grits/Polenta	680	24
	Gluten-Free Whole Grain Rolled Oats	907	32
	Mighty Tasty GF Hot Cereal*	680	24
	Millet Grits/Meal	454	16
	*Whole grain brown rice, corn, "sweet" white sorghum, buckwheat.		
CHOICES BEST RICE BAKERY	Granola*, Muesli**	454	16
	* Made with organic brown rice flakes and quinoa flakes, dried fruits, nuts and seeds. ** Made with organic brown rice flakes and quinoa flakes, dried fruit, nuts, seeds, millet, puffed millet and puffed rice.		
CREAM HILL ESTATES	Lara's Old Fashioned Rolled Oats*	500 g, 1 kg, bulk	1.1 and 2.2 lbs., bulk
	*Pure, uncontaminated oats		
CREAM OF THE CROP	Organic Buckwheat Hot Cereal	400	14.1

Company	Cereals		Grams	Ounces
EL PETO	**Cream of Rice***	Apple Cinnamon, Brown, White	500 g, 1 kg, 2.5 kg	17.5 oz., 2.2 lbs., 5.5 lbs.
	Corn Balls, Cocoa Balls		250	8.8
	Corn Flakes	Sweetened, Unsweetened	250	8.8
	*Also available in bulk.			
ENJOY LIFE	**Crunch Granola***	Cinnamon, Cranapple, Very Berry	363	12.8
	Perky's	Crunchy Flax, Crunchy Rice	340	12
	* Fortified with thiamin, niacin, folate, iron, magnesium, zinc, Vitamin B_6, Pantothenic Acid.			
ENVIROKIDZ	**Organic Cereals**	Gorilla Munch*	28.5, 37, 284, 650	1, 1.3, 10, 23
		Koala Crisp	324, 725	11.5, 26
		Leaping Lemurs Peanut Butter & Chocolate	284	10
		Peanut Butter Panda Puffs	300, 700	10.6, 25
	*Available in single serving packages (bag or cup).			
EREWHON	Aztec Crunchy Corn & Amaranth (organic)		284	10
	Brown Rice Cream (organic)		454	16
	Cocoa Crispy Rice		340	12
	Corn Flakes (organic)		312	11
	Crispy Brown Rice (gluten-free label) (organic)		284	10
	Crispy Brown Rice with Mixed Berries (gluten-free label)		284	10
	Rice Twice		284	10
	Strawberry Crisp		326	11.5
AVENA (FARMPURE FOODS) [ONLY OATS™]	**Oat Flakes***	Quick, Regular	650 g	23 oz.
			2 kg	4 lb. 6 oz.
			10, 20 kg	22 & 44 lb.
	Breakfast Blends*	Apple Cinnamon, Maple Roasted Flax	650 g, 2 kg	23 oz., 4 lbs. 6 oz.
	*Pure, uncontaminated oats.			
GIFTS OF NATURE	Gluten-Free Rolled Oats*		1.23 kg	2.75 lbs.
	*Pure, uncontaminated oats.			
GLUTENFREEDA FOODS	**Gluten-Free Honey Granola*** 4 packages/box	Apple Almond, Cranberry Cashew, Raisin Almond	298	10.5
	Instant Oatmeal*	Apple Cinnamon, Banana Maple, Maple Raisin, Natural	296	10.4
	*Made with certified gluten-free oats.			
GLUTEN-FREE OATS®	Old Fashion Rolled Oats*		566 g	20 oz.
			1.16 kg	2 lbs. 9 oz.
			11.35 kg	25 lbs.
	*Pure, uncontaminated oats.			
GLUTINO	**Cereal O's**	Apple & Cinnamon, Honey Nut	285	10.1
GOGO QUINOA	Amaranth Puffs		180	6.4
	Quinoa Puffs (Plain)		180	6.4
	Quinoa Puffs (Cocoa)		225	8
	Quinoa Flakes		500	17.6

Company	Cereals	Grams	Ounces
Health Valley	Blue Corn Flakes (organic)	312	11
	Corn Crunch Ems, Rice Crunch Ems	403	14.25
Holly's Oatmeal	**Gluten-Free Oatmeal Porridge Cereal*** Plain, Cranberry	454	16
	*Made with pure, uncontaminated gluten-free oats, quinoa flakes, amaranth, flax, whole grain brown rice, corn, sorghum, buckwheat.		
Kinnikinnick	Kinni-Crisp Rice Cereal*	375	13
	*Casein-Free.		
Lundberg	Hot 'n Creamy Purely Organic Rice Cereal	280 g, 11.35 kg	10 oz., 25 lbs.
Nature's Own Bakery	Granola	300	10.6
Nature's Path	Organic Crispy Rice	284	10
	Organic Crunchy Sunrise - Maple, Vanilla	300	10.6
	Organic Fruit Juice Sweetened Corn Flakes*	28.5, 300, 750	1, 10.6, 26.4
	Organic Honey'd Corn Flakes	300, 750	10.6, 26.4
	Organic Mesa Sunrise Multigrain**	300, 750	10.6, 26.4
	Organic Whole O's	325	11.5
	*Available in single serve bag. **Cornmeal, buckwheat, flax, amaranth.		
New Morning	Cocoa Crispy Rice Cereal	284	10
Nonuttin' Foods	**Granola*** Vanilla Caramel, Vanilla Cinnamon	250	8.8
	*Made with pure, uncontaminated oats.		
Nu-World Amaranth	Puffed Amaranth	198	7
	Puffed Amaranth Cereal (Berry Delicious, Cinnamon Delight)	198	7
Orgran	Multigrain O's with Quinoa	300	10.6
	Puffed Amaranth Cereal*	100	3.5
	*Dairy-Free.		
Udi's	**Granola*** Au Natural, Cranberry, Original, Vanilla	340	12
	*Made with certified gluten-free oats.		
Whole Foods GF Bakehouse	Fruit & Nut Granola*	454	16
	*Made with certified gluten-free oats. Dairy-Free.		

Baked Products

✦ Most gluten-free bread products are found in supermarket freezer sections or at some local bakeries.

✦ Some breads are vacuum-packed for a shelf life of 4 months to 1 year from the date of manufacture, e.g., **Ener-G Foods, PaneRiso/Kingsmill**.

✦ Ready-to-eat gluten-free bread products are convenient but are expensive. More economical options include:

    ✦ Use gluten-free mixes and bake your own, see pages 238-252.

    ✦ Make your own using various gluten-free flours, see page 154.

    ✦ A variety of bread, cookie, muffin and pastry recipes are found in the recipe section on pages 158-201.

    ✦ There are many gluten-free cookbooks and other cooking resources available (see pages 348-351).

BREADS

Company	Breads		Grams	Ounces
ANDREA'S FINE FOODS	CF French Loaf*, White Sandwich Loaf		736	26
	*Casein-Free.			
BARKAT	**Sliced Bread***	Brown, Multi-Grain, White, Whole-Meal	500	17.6
	Par-Baked	Country Loaf	250	8.8
		White Bread	550	19.4
		White Sliced	300	10.6
	*Dairy-Free. Par-Baked bread made in a factory which uses dairy and may contain traces of dairy.			
BI-AGLUT	**SfornaGusto**	Sliced Bread (Pan Carrè)	400	14.1
		Rustic-Style Bread (Pane Rustico)	400	14.1
CELIAC SPECIALTIES	Apple, Cheddar Herb, Cinnamon Raisin*, Flaxseed*, Mock Rye*, Multigrain*, Navy Bean*, Onion Poppy*, White*		672	24
	Garlic Bread		142	5
	*Casein-Free.			
CHOICES BEST RICE BAKERY	Brown Rice Bread*, Quinoa Multigrain*		454	16
	Cinnamon Raisin*, Multiseed*		530	18.7
	Cinnamon Raisin Soda*, Soda*		500	17.7
	Flaxseed*		525	18.6
	Foccacia*		195	6.9
	Jalapeño Cheddar Cornbread		200	7.1
	Sourdough*		540	19.1
	*Dairy-Free. All breads also available frozen.			
EL PETO	Brown Rice*, White Rice*		various weights	various weights
	Cheese		670	23.5
	Flax*, Gourmet, Italian Style, Millet*, Supreme Italian, Multi Grain*, Potato*, Raisin*, Tapioca*		650	22.5
	*Dairy-Free. All breads are egg-free. Breads are vacuum-packed for orders shipped outside of Ontario. Not shelf-stable.			
ENER-G FOODS	Brown Rice*, Hi-Fiber Rice*, Papa's, Raisin (no egg)*, Tapioca*, White Rice*, White Rice Flax*		454	16
	Corn*, Light Brown Rice*, Light Tapioca*, Light White Rice*, Light White Rice Flax*		228	8
	Four Flour		576	20.3
	Seattle Brown*		600	21.2
	Raisin*		672	23.7
	Rice Starch (low protein)*		490	17.3
	Breads are in shelf-stable vacuum packages and are enriched with thiamin, riboflavin, niacin, iron and folic acid. *Also available in 2-slice travel packages.			
ERAGRAIN	Enriched with Natural Whole Grains (Frozen Bread)*		795	1.75 lb.
	*Made with garbanzo flour, potato starch, tapioca starch and teff flour. Dairy-Free.			

Company	Breads		Grams	Ounces
Everybody Eats	Egg Challah*		509	18
	Multigrain High Fiber		N/A	N/A
	White Bread		566	20
	*Dairy-Free.			
Food For Life	Bhutanese Red Rice*, Brown Rice*, Fruit & Seed Medley*, Raisin Pecan*, Rice Almond*, Rice Pecan*, White Rice*		680	24
	Made with brown rice flour and rice bran. *Dairy-Free.			
French Meadow Bakery	Cinnamon Raisin*, Multigrain*		425	15
	Sandwich*		396	14
	*Casein-Free.			
Gillian's Foods	Cinnamon Raisin*, French*		350	12
	Crostini*		142	5
	Garlic*, No Rye Rye*, Sandwich*		510	18
	*Dairy-Free.			
Gluten-Free Bagel Company	Cinnamon Raisin*		695	24.4
	Crusty French*, Crusty Herb*, Marble Rye*, Pumpernickel*		525	18.6
	Primo White*		635	22.4
	Pita Bread* (4)		340	12.0
	*Dairy-Free.			
Gluten-Free Creations	Cheddar Cheese, Sandwich		792	28
	Herb*, White*		679	24
	Seeded Multigrain*, Whole Grain*		820	29
	*Dairy-Free. All breads enriched with thiamin, niacin, riboflavin, folic acid, iron and calcium.			
Glutino	**Original Corn Breads**	Cheese	620	21.9
		Corn	540	19
		Fiber	580	20.5
		Raisin	640	22.6
	Premium Corn Breads	Cinnamon Raisin*	640	22.6
		Corn*	540	19
		Fiber*	575	20.2
		Flax*	600	21.2
	Premium Brown Rice Bread Homestyle*		670	24
	Premium Brown Rice Bread*		670	24
	All products (except Premium Brown Rice Breads) are enriched with thiamin, riboflavin, niacin, iron, calcium and Vitamin B$_6$. Homestyle bread contains mesquite flour and inulin (prebiotic). Brown Rice bread contains inulin and sugar beet fiber. *Dairy-Free.			
Kinnikinnick	Brown Sandwich		585	21
	Cheese Tapioca Rice, Robin's Honey Brown Rice, Raisin Tapioca Rice, Sunflower Flax Rice		650	23
	Festive (seasonal), Italian White Tapioca Rice, Tapioca Rice		600	21.5
	Many Wonder Multigrain Rice		660	23.5
	White Sandwich		565	20
	All products are Casein-Free except Cheese Tapioca Rice Bread. Breads are enriched with thiamin, riboflavin, niacin, folic acid and iron.			

Company	Breads		Grams	Ounces
MARIPOSA BAKING COMPANY	Challah*, Cinnamon Raisin Bread*, Country French Loaf*, Multi-Grain Bread*, Sandwich Bread Loaf*, "Rye" Round		540	19
	*Casein-Free.			
NATURE'S OWN BAKERY	Breads	Golden Rice*, Sandwich*	750	26.5
	*Dairy-Free.			
O'DOUGHS	Breads*	Flax (Half Loaf)	350	12.3
		Flax (Full Loaf)	700	24.7
		White (Half Loaf)	350	12.3
		White (Full Loaf)	700	24.7
	*Dairy-Free.			
PANERISO/KINGSMILL	Rice Breads*	Brown, Flax Seed, Raisin & Cinnamon, Rye No Rye, White	500	17.6
	*Dairy-Free. Available as shelf-stable or frozen bread.			
PANNE RIZO	Brown Rice, Cinnamon Raisin, Dairy-Free Brown Rice*, Herbed Olive, Sesame White Rice		610	21.5
	Cheddar Scallion, Fruit & Nut		625	22
	Egg-Free		600	21.2
	Foccacia (Thyme Scallion)*		375	13.3
	*Dairy-Free.			
SCHÄR	Breads	Classic White	400	14.1
		Hearty Grain	400	14.1
		Hearty White*	400	14.1
		Multigrain**	400	14.1
	*Enriched with thiamin, riboflavin, niacin, iron and calcium. **Enriched with calcium and folic acid. Note: Classic White and Multigrain are shelf stable, vacuum-packed. Hearty Grain and Hearty White are frozen.			
STERK'S BAKERY	Breads	Italian Cinnamon, Italian, Italian Hi-Fiber, Italian Raisin, Italian Whole Brown, Sandwich*	600	21.2
	*Dairy-Free.			
UDI'S	White Sandwich, Whole Grain, Cinnamon Raisin		340	12
WHOLE FOODS GF BAKEHOUSE	Cinnamon Raisin, Honey Oat Bread*, Prairie, Sandwich, Sourdough, Sundried Tomato & Roasted Garlic		794	28
	Cornbread		510	18
	*Made with certified gluten-free oats and is Dairy-Free.			

YEAST-FREE BREADS

Company	Yeast-Free Breads	Grams	Ounces
EL PETO	Flax Seed, Hi-Fibre Brown Rice, Millet, Potato	650	22.5
	Yeast-Free breads are all Dairy-Free.		
ENER-G FOODS	YF Brown Rice Loaf*	540	19
	YF White Rice Loaf*	636	22.4
	*Available in 2-slice travel packages.		

Company	Yeast-Free Breads		Grams	Ounces
FOOD FOR LIFE	YF Rice Breads*	Brown	800	28.2
		Multigrain	725	25.6
	*All breads are Dairy-Free.			
GLUTEN-FREE CREATIONS	Yeast Free Bread*		454	16
	*Enriched with thiamin, riboflavin, niacin, folic acid and calcium.			
KINNIKINNICK	Candadi Yeast Free Multigrain Rice Bread*		650	23
	YF Tapioca Rice Bread*		600	21.5
	*Casein-Free and enriched with thiamin, riboflavin, niacin, folic acid and iron.			
NATURE'S OWN BAKERY	Rice Breads*	Brown, Multi Seed	800	28.2
		Fruit & Seed Medley, Potato, White	725	25.6
	*Corn, Dairy and Soy-Free.			

BAGELS, BAGUETTES, BUNS, MUFFINS, PIZZA CRUSTS, ROLLS

Company	Bagels, Baguettes, etc.		Grams	Ozs.	Number
ANDREA'S FINE FOODS	Buns	Hamburger	792	28	6
		Hot Dog	650	23	6
	Pizza Crust*	Individual (6")	100	3.5	1
		Large (12")	340	12	–
	Rolls	CF Dinner Rolls*	481	17	6
		White Dinner Rolls	425	15	6
	*Casein-Free.				
BARKAT	Baguettes	Home Fresh Par Baked	200	7	1
		Par Baked	200	7	1
	Rolls	Home Fresh Par Baked	300	10.5	6
		Par Baked	200	7	2
	Pizza Crusts*	Brown Rice, White Rice	150	5.3	1
	*Dairy-Free.				
BI-AGLUT	SfornaGusto	Baguette	360	12.7	2
		Mini Baguette	300	10.6	4
		Bread Rolls	280	1	4
		Buckwheat Rolls	200	9.8	4
CELIAC SPECIALTIES	Buns	Hamburger, Hot Dog, Sub	392	14	4
	Dinner Rolls		454	16	2
	English Muffins*		454	16	4
	Muffins (Pumpkin)*		454	16	2
	Pizza Crust – 10"		672	24	1
	Wraps		392	14	4
	*Casein-Free.				
CHEBE	Frozen Dough	Bread Sticks (Plain, Tomato Basil)*	340	12	12
		Rolls*, Sandwich Buns*	340	12	12
		"On-the-Go" Pizza Dough*	284	10	2
	*Free of yeast, soy, potato, rice. Made from cassava (manioc).				

Company	Bagels, Baguettes, etc.		Grams	Ozs.	Number
CHOICES BEST RICE BAKERY	Buns	Hamburger*, Multiseed Hamburger*	400	14	4
		Cheddar and Herb	110	3.9	1
		Flaxseed*	420	14.8	4
		Sourdough Hamburger*	425	15	4
		Hot Dog	NA	NA	2
	Pizza Crust*		280	9.9	2
	*Dairy-Free.				
DIETARY SPECIALTIES	English Muffins	Plain, Cinnamon Raisin	400	14.1	4
EL PETO	Hamburger Buns	Brown*, Italian with Sesame, Multi-Grain*, Potato*	500	17.5	8
	Hot Dog Buns	Italian with Sesame, Potato*	500	17.5	8
	Dinner Rolls	Brown*, Italian, Gourmet, Multi Grain*	500	17.5	8
	Gourmet Mini Sub Buns		480	16.9	4
	Rolls	Cheese, Fruit*, Raisin*	500	17.5	8
	Pizza Crusts*	Basil, Millet, Plain (pre-baked)	420	14.8	2
	Muffins**	Apple Spice, Banana, Blueberry, Carrot, Chocolate Chip, Cranberry, Lemon Poppyseed, Raisin Rice Bran, Tropical Delight	460	16.2	6
	Waffles	Belgian (Regular; Corn/milk-free)*	300	10.5	2
	*Dairy-Free. **Also make Sugar-Free muffins sweetened with fruit juice.				
ENER-G FOODS	Dinner Rolls	Tapioca Dinner*	280	9.9	6
	Hamburger Buns	Brown Rice*	292	10.3	4
		Seattle Brown*	460	16.2	4
		Tapioca*	220	7.8	4
		White Rice*	292	10.3	4
	Hot Dog Buns	Tapioca*	220	7.8	4
		Seattle Brown*	440	16.2	4
	English Muffins	Brown (with flax)*	488	17.2	4
		Plain	428	15	4
	Rice Pizza Shells (6") (low protein)*		252	8.9	3
	Rice Pizza Shells (10") (low protein)*		520	18.4	3
	Products are in shelf-stable, vacuum packages. *Enriched with thiamin, riboflavin, niacin, iron and folic acid.				
ENJOY LIFE	Bagels*	Classic Original, Cinnamon Raisin	454	16	6
	*Casein, Egg, Nut and Soy-Free. Enriched with thiamin, riboflavin, niacin, folate, calcium, magnesium, Vitamin B$_6$.				
EVERYBODY EATS	Bagels		906	32	8
	Baguettes		340	12	2
	Deli Rolls*		454	16	6
	Ficelle Dinner Rolls		340	12	12
	Pizza Shells		NA	NA	2
	*Dairy-Free.				
FOOD FOR LIFE	Tortillas*	Brown Rice	340	12	6
		Sprouted Corn	283	10	6
	*Dairy-Free.				

Company	Bagels, Baguettes, etc.		Grams	Ozs.	Number
Foods By George	**Muffins**	Blueberry, Corn	482	17	6
	English Muffins*	Cinnamon Currant, Plain, No-Rye Rye	397	14	4
	Pizza Crusts (6")*		255	9	3
	*Dairy-Free/Casein-Free.				
French Meadow Bakery	GF Italian Roll*		1 kg	35.2	8
	GF Par Baked Pizza Crust (7")*		272	9.6	2
	GF Par Baked Pizza Crust (10.5")*		220	7.8	6, 24**
	GF Tortillas*		255	9	6
	*Casein-Free. Frozen Pizza Crusts on foil pans. **Food service only.				
Gillian's Foods	**French Rolls***	Plain, Caramelized Onion, Cinnamon Raisin, Everything Dinner, Poppy Seed, Sesame Seed	624	22	6
	Pizza Crust*	7" Par Baked	454	16	2
	Pizza Dough	Frozen	454	16	1-2
	*Dairy-Free.				
Gluten-Free Bagel Company	**Bagels**	Cinnamon Raisin*, Plain*, Poppyseed*, Pumpernickel*, Sesame*	560	19.6	6
	Rolls	Dinner*	390	13.6	6
		French*	665	23.4	4
		Hamburger*	460	16.3	6
		Pita Bread	340	12	4
		Portuguese Cheese	220	7.8	3
		Portuguese Cheese (mini)	280	9.8	12
	Scones	Blueberry, Irish Soda Bread	170	6.0	3
	Soft Pretzels*		560	19.6	6
	*Dairy-Free.				
Gluten-Free Creations	**Bagels**	Berry*, Cinnamon Raisin*, Jalapeño Cheese, Plain*	454	16	4
		Everything*	340	12	4
	Pizza Crusts	Italian Herb*, Simply*, Whole Grain*	227	8	2
	*Dairy-Free. All items are enriched with thiamin, niacin, riboflavin, folic acid, iron and calcium.				
Gluten Free & Fabulous	Pizza Crust*		622	22	
	*Dairy-Free.				
Glutino	**Premium Bagels**	Cinnamon Raisin	700	24.7	5
		Plain, Poppyseed, Sesame	650	22.9	5
	Premium English Muffins		485	17	6
	Pizza Crusts (pre-baked)	Premium Corn*	375	13.2	4
	*Dairy-Free. Enriched with thiamin, riboflavin, niacin, iron, calcium and Vitamin B$_6$ except English Muffins.				

Company	Bagels, Baguettes, etc.		Grams	Ozs.	Number
KINNIKINNICK	Tapioca Rice English Muffins		375	13.5	4
	Tapioca Rice Hamburger Buns		400	14.5	4
	Tapioca Rice Hot Dog Buns		350	12.5	4
	Muffins	Blueberry, Carrot, Chocolate Chip	300	12.5	6
	Muffins (Jumbo)	Chocolate Lovers, Harvest Crunch, Lemon Poppy Seed	120	4.2	1
	Pizza Crust (7")	Personal Size	600	21	4
	Pizza Crust (10")	Family Size	660	23	3
	Tapioca Rice Bagels	Cinnamon Raisin, New York Style Plain, Sesame	400	13.5	4
	Tapioca Rice Multigrain Seed & Fibre Bun		400	14.5	4
	Tapioca Rice Tray Buns		350	12.5	6
	Waffles (Homestyle)	Original, Cinnamon & Brown Sugar	210	7	6
	All products are Casein-Free. All products except muffins and waffles are enriched with thiamin, riboflavin, niacin, folic acid and iron.				
LA TORTILLA FACTORY	**Smart & Delicious Gluten-Free Wraps** Ivory Teff		396	13.96	6
	Sonoma Gluten-Free Wraps* Ivory Teff		396	13.96	6
	*Organic, no preservatives (frozen).				
MARIPOSA BAKING COMPANY	**Bagels**	Plain*, Sesame*	855	30	5
	Crostini*		156	5.5	NA
	Baguette*		170	6	1
	Pizza Crust (10")*		342	12	1
	*Casein-Free.				
NATURE'S HILIGHTS	Brown Rice Pizza Crust (frozen, fully cooked, ready to heat)		284	10	2
NATURE'S OWN BAKERY	Golden Rice Buns		425	15	5
	Pizza Crusts (12")	Brown	400	14.1	1
NATURE'S PATH	**Toaster Waffles***	Buckwheat Wild Berry, Homestyle, Mesa Sunrise	210	7.5	6
	*Dairy-Free.				
NU-WORLD AMARANTH	**Flatbread/Pizza Crust** (pre-baked) – 6"				
		Amaranth Buckwheat	113	4	2
		Amaranth Garbanzo	113	4	2
		Amaranth Sorghum	113	4	2
O'DOUGHS	**Buns***	Apple Cranberry Breakfast, Flax, White	400	14.1	4
	Pizza Kit with Sauce	Flax, White	540	19	4
	*Dairy-Free.				

Company	Bagels, Baguettes, etc.		Grams	Ozs.	Number
PaneRiso/ Kingsmill	White Rice Pizza Crusts (pre-baked) (8")		150	5.3	1
	White Rice Pizza Crust (pre-baked) (12")		300	10.5	1
Panne Rizo	Dinner Rolls (Brown)		460	16.2	4
	Fruity Tea Buns		540	19.1	4
	Hamburger Buns Brown*, White		550	19.4	4
	Muffins	Banana Chocolate Chip*, Banana Pecan (sugar-free)*, Banana Strawberry*, Blueberry Lemon Poppy*, Carrot Walnut, Cranberry Orange*, Maple Pumpkin*, Raspberry White Chocolate	840	29.6	6
	Pizza Crusts (7")	Brown*, White	250	8.8	2
	*Dairy-Free.				
Rustic Crust	Pizza Crust (7")	Napoli Herb*	255	9	2
	*Dairy-Free.				
Schär	Baguettes*		350	12.3	2
	Ciabatta Parbaked Rolls*		200	7	4
	Classic White Rolls*		300	10.6	4
	Pizza Crusts*		300	10.6	2
	Sub Sandwich Rolls*		150	5.3	2
	*Vacuum-packed.				
Sterk's Bakery	**Bagels**	Plain*, Poppy Seed*, Sesame*	various weights		6
	Buns	Hamburger*, Hot Dog*, Italian, Italian Hi-Fiber	various weights		6
	Muffins	Apple Raisin*, Banana Blueberry*, Chocolate Blueberry*, Triple Berry*	various weights		6
	Pizza (12")	Italian, Yummy*	various weights		1
	*Dairy-Free.				
Udi's	**Bagels**	Cinnamon Raisin, Plain, Whole Grain	397	14	4
	Pizza Crust		227	8	2
Van's	**GF Toaster Waffles***	Apple Cinnamon, Blueberry, Buckwheat, Flax, Homestyle	255	9	6
	Toaster Mini Waffles (Wheat-Free) – Homestyle*		213	7.5	32
	Wheat-Free French Toast Sticks*		241	8.5	6
	Wheat-Free Homestyle Pancakes*		352	12.8	6
	Wheat-Free products are Gluten-Free. *Dairy-Free.				
Whole Foods GF Bakehouse	Almond Scones, Cranberry Orange Scones		340	12	4
	Cheddar Biscuits, Cream Biscuits		280	10	6
	Hamburger Buns		680	24	6
	Muffins	Blueberry, Cherry Almond Streusel, Lemon Poppyseed, Morning Glory*	397	14	4
	Pizza Crust		680	24	2
	*Dairy-Free.				

YEAST-FREE – BUNS AND ROLLS

Company	Buns and Rolls		Grams	Ozs.	Number
EL PETO	YF Hamburger Buns	Potato	650	22.9	8
	YF Hot Dog Buns	Potato	700	24.7	8
	YF Pizza Crust	Plain, Millet	420	14.8	2
	All products are Dairy-Free.				
ENER-G FOODS	YF Rice Pizza Shells (6")		354	12.5	3
	YF Rice Pizza Shells (10")		900	31.7	3

CAKES, LOAVES, PIES, MISCELLANEOUS

Company	Cakes, Loaves, Pies, Miscellaneous		Grams	Ozs.	Number
ANDREA'S FINE FOODS	Cakes	Banana**, Carrot, ChocoChunk**, Chocolate*, Lemon**, Red Velvet, Yellow*	595	21	–
		Fudged Ice Brownie	140, 540	5, 19	–
	Iced Cupcakes	Banana**, ChocoChunk**, Chocolate*, Lemon**, Yellow*	NA	NA	2
	Mini Loaf	Banana**, Chocolate Chunk**, Pumpkin**	170	6	–
	Muffins	Blueberry, Carrot Spice	140	5	2
	Rolls	Iced Cinnamon Rolls	284 g, 1.27 kg	10 oz., 40 oz.	2, 9
	*Also available in Casein-Free. **Casein-Free.				
BARKAT	Honey Cake*		250	8.8	–
	Rich Christmas Pudding*		454	16	–
	*Dairy-Free.				
BI-AGLUT	Chocolate Plumcake, Plumcake with Apricot		180	6.3	–
CELIAC SPECIALTIES	Angel Wings*		112	4	–
	Brownie Tray*		454	16	–
	Cakes	Angel Food*	425	15	–
		Pumpkin*	454	16	–
	Cupcakes	Chocolate*, Vanilla*	various weights		2
	Donuts	Cinnamon-Sugar, Coconut, Double Chocolate, Glazed, Plain, Powder Sugar	454	16	6
	Donut Holes*	Cinnamon Sugar, Glazed, Plain, Powder Sugar	192	7	12
	Pies (6")	Apple, Cherry, Blueberry	454	16	–
	Pie Crust (9")		280	10	–
	Strudel	Apple, Blueberry, Cherry	311	11	3
	*Casein-Free.				

Company	Cakes, Loaves, Pies, Miscellaneous		Grams	Ozs.	Number
CHOICES BEST RICE BAKERY	Brownies*	Bite Sizes	285	10.1	–
	Cake	Black Forest, Carrot, Sacher Torte	various weights		
		Chocolate, Vanilla (Dairy & Non-Dairy)	various weights		
	Cheesecake	Marble, Pistachio, Pumpkin, Sour Cherry	various weights		
	Cinnamon Buns (frozen)		NA	NA	4
	Pastry Shells	Pie (Frozen)*	200	7.1	2
		Tart (Frozen)*	NA	NA	12
	Pies	Apple*, Apple Cranberry*, Berry Rhubarb*, Peach Blackberry*, Pumpkin, Summer Berry	various weights		
	Pudding Cakes	Banana Bread*, Banana Vegan*, Blueberry Lemon*, Chocolate*, Chocolate Vegan*, Gingerbread Loaf*, Lemon Poppyseed*, Marble*, Pumpkin*	300	10.6	–
	Scones	Blueberry, Cranberry, Fruit & Nut	125	4.4	1
	Squares	Brownie*	200	7.1	NA
		Blueberry Almond, Cranberry Almond	210	7.4	3
		Granola Bars	95	3.4	2
		Lemon Square	430	15.2	NA
	Tarts	Butter	150	5.3	3
		Pecan	140	4.9	3
	Waffles	Frozen	360	12.7	4
	*Dairy-Free.				
DIETARY SPECIALTIES	Cheesecake		454	16	–
	Classic Pound Cake		369	13	–
	Pie Shells		400	14	2
EL PETO	Pies (8")	Apple*, Blueberry*, Cherry*, Peach Apricot*, Pumpkin*, Strawberry-Rhubarb*, Walnut	500	17.5	–
	Pie Dough*		400	14	–
	Tarts	Buttertart, Lemon*, Pecan, Raspberry*	NA	NA	6
	Tart Shells*	Sweetened, unsweetened	NA	NA	12
	*Dairy-Free.				

Company	Cakes, Loaves, Pies, Miscellaneous		Grams	Ozs.	Number
ENER-G FOODS	Brownies*		560	19.7	–
	Cinnamon Rolls		672	23.7	8
	Donut Holes*		235	8.3	20
	Plain Donuts*		200	7	6
	Pound Cake*		249	8.8	–
	*Enriched with thiamin, riboflavin, niacin, iron and folic acid.				
EVERYBODY EATS	Banana Bread		679	24	–
	Cinnamon Sticky Buns		792	28	16
	Cupcakes (yellow)	Chocolate or Vanilla Frosting	NA	NA	6
	Poundcake	Chocolate Swirl, Cinnamon Swirl, Plain	792	28	–
	Pie	Apple, Pumpkin	1.25 kg	44	–
	Rugelach	Apricot, Pineapple, Raspberry	454	16	–
FOODS BY GEORGE	Brownies*		397	14	6x8" tray
	Crumb Cake		567	20	6x8" tray
	Pecan Tart		113	4	1
	Pound Cake		454	16	7" loaf
	*Dairy-Free.				
FRENCH MEADOW BAKERY	GF Fudge Brownie*		80, 343	2.8, 12.1	1**, 9
	GF Fudge Brownie Bites (in tub)*		288	10.2	16
	GF Iced Cakes*	Chocolate, Yellow	225	9	1
	GF Iced Cupcakes*	Chocolate, Yellow	224	8	4
	GF Muffins*	Apple Cinnamon, Blueberry	59	2.1	1
	*Casein-Free. **Individually wrapped, single serve.				
GILLIAN'S FOODS	Brownies		509	18	–
	Pies (9")	Apple, Pumpkin	NA	NA	NA
	Pie Shell (9")		227	8	1
GLUTEN-FREE BAGEL COMPANY	Brownies*		340	12	4
	Bundt Cakes	Iced Chocolate*	3 small, 1 large		
		Orange Chiffon*	3 small, 1 large		
	*Dairy-Free.				
GLUTEN-FREE CREATIONS	Brownies	Rich	8x8" tray or 1 individual		
	Cakes	Chocolate, Yellow*	454	16	–
	Donuts	Cinnamon & Sugar*, Insane Chocolate, Plain Jane*, Simply Chocolate*, Superb Sprinkles	340	12	4
	Muffins	Chocolate Zucchini*, Cranberry Orange Pecan*, Lemon Poppyseed*	340	12	4
	*Dairy-Free. All items enriched with thiamin, niacin, riboflavin, folic acid, iron and calcium.				
GLUTINO	Carrot Cake		325	11.5	1 tray
	Cup Cakes	Chocolate, Marble, Vanilla	200	7.1	6
	Chocolate Fudge Cake		300	10.6	1 tray
GOOD EATZ	Brownies	Chocolate Chip, Walnut	113	4	–
	Cheesecake		240	8.5	–
	Mini Cakes	Carrot, Chocolate, Pecan Streusel, Spice, Vanilla	311	11	–

Company	Cakes, Loaves, Pies, Miscellaneous		Grams	Ozs.	Number
GOOD EATZ	Mini Loaves	Banana, Cran-Orange, Carrot Flax, Pumpkin	85	3	–
	Rice Crispie Treats	Cherry Vanilla, Chocolate Peanut Butter, Chocolate Peanut Butter Vegan, Plain, Plain Vegan	57	2	–
	Tarts	Apple Crumb, Cherry Crumb, Peach Crumb	various weights		
KINNIKINNICK	JB Brownie Squares		350	9	1
	Donuts	Cinnamon Sugar	270	9.5	6
		Chocolate Dipped, Maple Glazed, Vanilla Glazed	320	11.3	6
	Fruit Cake (seasonal item)		300	10.6	NA
	Tapioca Rice Cinnamon Buns		500	18	6
	All products are Casein-Free.				
MARIPOSA BAKING COMPANY	Breads/Loaves	Cranberry Orange Nut*, Pumpkin*	285	10	–
	Brownies	Mocha, Triple Chocolate, Walnut	65	2.25	–
		Brownie Bark	170	6	–
	Coconut Lemon Squares*		57	2	–
	Cakes	Apple Spice Peace*	220	7.75	–
		Sour Cream Coffeecake	205	7.25	–
	Muffins	Blueberry, Lemon Poppyseed, Morning*, Pumpkin*	115	4	–
	*Casein-Free.				
O'DOUGHS	Cakes*	Banana, Carrot, Chocolate,	400	14.1	
	*Dairy-Free.				
PAMELA'S PRODUCTS	Cakes (Frosted)	Coffee, Chocolate Fudge	various weights		6 svg.
	Cheesecakes	Agave Sweetened New York, Hazelnut, New York, White Chocolate Raspberry, Zesty Lemon	142, 564	5, 20	1, 6 svg.
PANNE RIZO	Applesauce Spice Bars		480	17	6
	Apple Crostada, Berry Crostada		350	12.4	1
	Brownies (Macadamia Nut)		360	12.7	4
	Berry Tarts, Buttertarts, Mincemeat Tarts		240	8.5	6
	Cinnamon Bun Swirls*		680	24	4
	Coconut Cherry Dream Bars		420	14.8	4
	Cakes	Carrot, Chocolate, Vanilla, Walnut	various weights		
	Gramma's Cinnamon Dots		200	7.1	5
	Pecan Toffee Squares		420	14.8	4
	Pies (6")	Apple Cinnamon*, Cherry*, Pumpkin, Peach Blackberry*, Strawberry Rhubarb*, Summer Berry*	various weights		
	*Dairy-Free.				

Company	Cakes, Loaves, Pies, Miscellaneous		Grams	Ozs.	Number
PATSYPIE	Double Chocolate Mini Brownies		300	10.5	–
	Morning Glory with Flax Mini Muffins		300	10.5	–
STERK'S BAKERY	**Cakes**	Chocolate Sponge*, Vanilla Sponge*	various weights		–
	*Dairy-Free.				
WHOLE FOODS GF BAKEHOUSE	Banana Bread		397	14	–
	Carrot Cake		510	18	–
	Cupcakes	Chocolate, Vanilla,	454	16	4
	Pies	Apple, Cherry*, Peach*, Southern Pecan*, Pumpkin*	454	16	–
	*seasonal				
	Pie Crust		513	18	–
UDI'S	Cinnamon Rolls		340	12	4
	Muffins	Blueberry, Double Chocolate, Lemon Struesel	340	12	4

COOKIES

✦ **NOT** all "**wheat-free**" cookies are gluten-free. Some may contain barley or regular oats.

Company	Cookies		Grams	Ounces
ALLERGYFREE FOODS	Oatmeal Raisin Bites*		454	16
	*Made with gluten-free oats. Casein, Soy, Egg and Nut-Free.			
ANDEAN DREAM	**Quinoa Cookies***	Chocolate Chip, Cocoa-Orange, Coconut, Orange Essence, Raisin & Spice	198	7
	*Casein, Nut and Soy-Free.			
ANDREA'S FINE FOODS	**Cookies**	Chocolate Chip, Oatmeal*, Pecan Shortbread, Sugar	140	5
	Cookie Dough	Chocolate Chip, Oatmeal*, Sugar	566	20
	*Casein-Free. Note: Oatmeal Cookies made with gluten-free oats.			
ARICO NATURAL FOODS	**Cookies*** (pouch)	Almond Cranberry, Chocolate Chunk, Double Chocolate, Lemon Ginger, Peanut Butter, Triple Berry	135	4.8
	*Made with organic brown rice flour. Casein-Free.			
AUNT GUSSIES	Chocolate Chip, Chocolate Spritz, Sugar-Free Chocolate Chip, Sugar-Free Vanilla Spritz		170	6
BARKAT	Chocolate Tea Cakes		168	5.9
	Coffee Biscuits*		200	7
	Cream Filled Wafers	Chocolate, Lemon, Vanilla	100	3.5
	Digestive Biscuits*		175	6.2
	*Dairy-Free.			

Company	Cookies		Grams	Ounces
BARKAT	Ginger Cookies		150	5.3
	GMAN Gingerbread Cookies		100	3.5
	Honey Cake*		250	8.8
	Shortcake Biscuits*		175	6.2
	*Dairy-Free.			
BI-AGLUT	**DolciSfizi**	Chocolate Filled Wafer	175	6.2
		Chocolate Coated Bars	25, 75	0.8, 2.6
	SfornaGusto Muffins (Merendine)	Plain	150	5.3
		Apricot Jam, Yoghurt with Raisin	180	6.4
		Cocoa with Milk Filling, Gianduia Filling	200	7
	SfornaGusto Cookies	Biscotti, CiocoStelle, Frollini (without sugar), Gocce, Ruote, Rustici	180	6.4
		Biscottino*	200	7
		Granular Biscotti	340	12
	*Dairy-Free.			
CELIAC SPECIALTIES	**Cookies**	Casein-Free Chocolate Chip*, Chocolate Chip, Sugar*	various	6
	Cookie Dough (Frozen)	Casein-Free Chocolate Chip*, Chocolate Chip, Sugar*	454	16
	*Casein-Free. Cookie dough makes 12 cookies.			
CHERRYBROOK KITCHEN	**Gluten-Free Dreams**	Mini Chocolate Chip, Mini Vanilla Graham	170	6
CHOICES BEST RICE BAKERY	**Cookies**	Bird's Nest*, Chocolate Chip*, Double Chocolate Fudge	200	7.1
		Butter Shortbread, Ginger*	150	5.3
		Mexican Wedding	160	5.6
		Raisin Sunflower*	220	7.8
	Biscotti	Cranberry Almond Spice	110	3.9
	Mediterranean Macaroons*		260	9.2
	*Dairy-Free.			
EL PETO	Almond Shortbread*, Carob Chip*, Chocolate Chip*, Chocolate Coconut Macaroons*, Coconut Macaroons*, Chocolate Hazelnut, Cinnamon Hazelnut*, Gingersnaps*, Raspberry Hazelnut*		200	7
	*Dairy-Free.			
ENER-G FOODS	Biscotti (Chocolate Chip)		208	7.3
	Biscotti (Plain)		280	9.9
	Chocolate, Cinnamon		250	8.8
	Chocolate Chip Potato*		272	9.6
	Sunflower		280	9.9
	*Also available in bulk.			

Company	Cookies		Grams	Ounces
ENER-G FOODS	Ginger*		224	7.9
	Vanilla, White Chocolate Chip		288	10.2
	*Also available in bulk.			
ENJOY LIFE	Chewy Chocolate Chip, Snickerdoodle		28*	1*
	Chewy Chocolate Chip, Double Chocolate Brownie, Gingerbread Spice, Happy Apple, Lively Lemon, No-Oats "Oatmeal", Snickerdoodle		170**	6**
	Casein, Egg, Nut and Soy-Free. *2 cookies/pack. **12 cookies/box.			
ENVIROKIDZ	Vanilla Animal Cookies		255	9
EVERYBODY EATS	Chocolate Chip Cookies		340	12
	Sugar Cookies		227	8
	Fudge Brownies*		566	20
	*Dairy-Free.			
FOODS BY GEORGE	Biscotti*		345	12.2
	*Dairy-Free.			
FRENCH MEADOW BAKERY	Chocolate Chip (individually wrapped)*		60	2.1
	Chocolate Chip Cookie Dough*		382	13.5
	*Casein-Free.			
GILLIAN'S FOODS	Chocolate Chip, M&M, Sugar		340	12
	*Also available as frozen cookie dough.			
GLUTEN-FREE CREATIONS	Cookies	Chocolate Chip, Oatmeal Raisin*	255	9
		Chocolate Delight*	679	24
		Pecan Wedding*	170	6
		Snickerdoodles	255	9
	Cookie Dough (frozen)	Chocolate Chip, Sugar	908 g	2 lbs.
	Note: Only available in-store. Makes 24-36 cookies.			
	*Dairy-Free. All items are enriched with thiamin, niacin, riboflavin, folic acid, iron and calcium. Note: Oatmeal Cookies made with pure, uncontaminated oats.			
GLUTEN FREE & FABULOUS	Brownie Bites		185	6.5
	Cookie Bites	Butterscotch, Chocolate Chip, Shortbread	185	6.5
	Chocolate Chip Cookie (Individually Wrapped)		85	3
GLUTEN-FREE BAGEL COMPANY	Brown Sugar Wafers, Chocolate Chip, Chocolate Chip Walnut, Cookie Jar Cut-outs, Decorated Cut-outs, Italian Ricotta Cheese, Orange, Peanut Butter, Pumpkin		340	12
	All are Dairy-Free except Italian Ricotta Cheese.			
GLUTENFREEDA FOODS	Real Cookies™	Chip Chip Hooray, Chocolate Minty Python, Peanut Envy, Peanut Paul and Mary,	454	16
		Sugar Kookies, Snicker Poodles	434	15.3
	Frozen, pre-formed cookie dough.			

Company	Cookies		Grams	Ounces
GLUTINO	Chocolate Chip		245	8.6
	Chocolate Vanilla Creme		300	10.6
	Vanilla Creme		300	10.6
	Wafer Cookies	Chocolate, Vanilla	130	4.6
		Lemon, Strawberry	200	7
GOOD EATZ	Chocolate Chip*, Ginger Molasses*, Peanut Butter, Peanut Butter Chocolate Chip, Snickerdoodle*, White Chocolate Chip Pecan		85, 284	3, 10
	*Dairy-Free.			
IAN'S NATURAL FOODS	**Cookie Buttons*** Chocolate Chip, Cinnamon		180	6.35
	*Single serve. 6 pouches/box.			
JENNIES	Almond Macaroons, Chocolate Macaroons, Coconut Macaroons		227	8
	Coconut Macaroons	Almond, Coconut, Dutch Chocolate,	57	2
	Unsweetened Macaroons	Carob, Chocolate, Coconut	127	4.5
KINNIKINNICK	Ginger Snap		170	6
	Kinni-Kritters Animal Cookies	Chocolate, Graham Style, Plain	200	7
	KinniTOOS Sandwich Cream Cookies Chocolate, Fudge, Vanilla		200	7
	Montana's Chocolate Chip		200	7
	S'Moreables (Graham Style Crackers)		200	7
	All products are Casein-Free			
LEDA NUTRITION	**Cookies***	Coconut, Gingernut	155	5.5
	Chocolate Coated Creme Filled Biscuits* Choculence, Minton		180	6.4
	*Dairy-Free.			
LE VENEZIANE	**Sorrisi di Mais Cookies***	Almond, Chocolate, Plain	200	7
	*Corn-based.			
MARIPOSA BAKING COMPANY	**Biscotti***	Almond, Cinnamon Toast, Ginger Spice	180	6.3
		Biscotti Crumbs	455	1 lb.
		Biscotti Ends & Pieces	228	8
	Chocolate Chip Cookies*		42	1.5
	*Casein-Free.			
NANA'S COOKIE COMPANY	**Nana's No Gluten Cookies**	Chocolate, Chocolate Crunch, Ginger, Lemon	100	3.5
	Nana's No Gluten Cookie Bars*	Berry Vanilla, Fudgy Wudgy, Nana Banana	175	6.2
	Nana's No Gluten Cookie Bites*	Fudge, Ginger Spice, Lemon Dreams	142	5
	*5/box.			

Company	Cookies		Grams	Ounces
NATURE'S OWN BAKERY	**Bites***	Double Chocolate Chip, Fruit & Seed	170	6
	Tropical Treats**	Regular, Lite	90 g, 2.8 kg	3.2 oz., 6.4 lbs.
	*Dairy-Free. **Available in single serve individually wrapped and box of 32. Dairy-Free.			
ORGRAN	**Biscotti***	Amaretti, Classic Choc	150	5.3
	Classic Choc Cookie* (single serve)		50	1.8
	Dinosaur Whole Fruit Cookies*	25% Whole Fruit (Currants), Wild Berry	175	6.2
	Outback	Chocolate, Vanilla	176	6.2
	Animal Cookies*	Mini Multipack (8/box)**	50	1.8
	Itsy Bitsy Bears*	(Vanilla cookies with chocolate bits)	175	6.2
	Wild Raspberry Flavored Fruit Biscuits*		175	6.2
	*Dairy-Free. **Mini Multipack contains vanilla and chocolate flavors.			
PAMELA'S PRODUCTS	**Biscotti**	Almond Anise, Chocolate Walnut, Lemon Almond	170	6
	Cookies (Organic)	Chocolate Chunk Pecan Shortbread*, Dark Chocolate-Chocolate Chunk, Espresso Chocolate Chunk*, Old Fashioned Raisin Walnut*, Peanut Butter Chocolate Chip, Spicy Ginger*	33, 150	1.2, 5.3
	Made with organic ingredients. 33 g (1.2 oz.) package contains 2 cookies.			
	Cookies (Traditional Shortbread)	Butter, Lemon, Pecan, Swirl	206	7.25
	Cookies (Traditional)	Chunky Chocolate Chip, Chocolate Chip Walnut, Ginger with Sliced Almonds*, Peanut Butter*	206	7.25
	Simple Bites (Mini Cookies)	Chocolate Chip, Extreme Chocolate, Ginger Mini Snapz*	200	7
	*Dairy-Free.			
PANERISO/ KINGSMILL	Chocolate Chip		110	4
	Cinnamon, Coconut, Orange		125	4.4
PANNE RIZO	**Biscotti**	Almond, Cranberry Pistachio (low fat), Mocha Almond (low fat), Star Anise Almond, Triple Chocolate	220	7.8
		Chocolate Swirled	225	7.9
	Cookies	Chocolate Dipped Macaroons* Ginger Chocolate, Tollhouse Regular, Tollhouse Dairy-Free/Low Sugar*, Frosted Raspberry Swirls, Gingerbread Hearts, Pecan Snowballs	various weights	
	Shortbread	Buttery, Pecan	240	8.5
		Sugar	265	9.3
	*Dairy-Free.			

Company	Cookies		Grams	Ounces
PatsyPie	Biscotti	Almond, Almond & Raisin, Chocolate Chip, Cranberry Orange	275	9.7
		Pecan	250	8.8
	Cookies	Chocolate Chip, Lemon, Peanut Butter, Raisin, Snappy Ginger	275	9.7
Schär	Chocolate Dipped Cookies		150	5.3
	Chocolate Hazelnut Bars		105	3.7
	Chocolate O's		165	5.8
	Lady Fingers		150	5.3
	Sandwich Creme Cookies	Chocolate, Vanilla	125	4.4
	Shortbread Cookies		200	7
	Wafers	Cocoa, Vanilla	125	4.4
		Hazelnut	51	1.8
Sterk's Bakery	Cherry Shortbread, Chocolate Chip, Coconut Macaroons, Shortbread		various weights	
Sunstart Bakery	Cookies	Chocolate Chip, Chocolate Wrapped Golden Crunch, Raspberry, Stem Ginger	150	5.3
	Bars	Caramel and Chocolate Dessert Delights, Rocky Road Bars	150	5.3
Whole Foods GF Bakehouse	Cookies	Almond*, Chocolate Chip, Molasses, Ginger*, Nutmeal Raisin, Peanut Butter	284	10
	Walnut Brownies		454	16
	*Dairy-Free.			

SNACK BARS

Company	Snack Bars		Grams	Ounces
Bakery on Main	Gluten-Free Granola Bars*	Cranberry Maple Walnut, Extreme Trail Mix, Peanut Butter Chocolate Chip	170	6
	*Dairy-Free. 5 bars/box.			
BumbleBar	Original		45	1.6
	Original With	Almond, Cashew, Hazelnuts, Mixed Nuts	45	1.6
	Awesome Apricot, Chewy Chocolate, Chunky Cherry, Tasty Tropical		40	1.4
	Chai with Almonds, Chocolate Crisp, Lushus Lemon		45	1.6
	All bars are Dairy-Free.			
Ener-G Foods	Chocolate Chip Snack Bars*		420	14.8
	*Package of 10.			
Enjoy Life	Snack Bars* (5/box)	Caramel Apple, Coco Loco, Very Berry, Sunbutter Crunch	140	5
	*Casein, Egg, Nut and Soy-Free. Fortified with thiamin, riboflavin, niacin, folate, Vitamin B_6.			

Company	Snack Bars		Grams	Ounces
EnviroKidz	Crispy Rice Bars (6/box)	Berry, Chocolate, Fruity Burst, Peanut Butter, Peanut Choco Drizzle	170	6
Glutino	Breakfast Bars (5/box)	Apple, Blueberry, Chocolate, Cranberry	200	7
	Organic Bars (5/box)	Chocolate Banana, Chocolate Peanut Butter, Wild Berry	140	5
Heaven Scent	Crispy Rice & Marshmallow Bars			
		Original, Chocolate Chip, Soy Protein	57	2
Jennies	Omega-3 Energy Bar*	Almond, Chocolate, Coconut	57	2
		*Made with coconut and seeds (flax, pumpkin, sunflower)		
Lärabar	Energy Bars*	Apple Pie, Pecan Pie, Tropical Fruit	45	1.6
		Cashew Cookie, Cherry Pie, Coconut Cream Pie, Peanut Butter Cookie, Peanut Butter & Jelly	48	1.7
		Banana Bread, Chocolate Coconut Chew, Cinnamon Roll, Cocoa Môle, Ginger Snap, Key Lime Pie, Lemon, Pistachio	51	1.8
		*Made with dried fruits, nuts, spices. Dairy-Free.		
	JamFrakas*	Apple Crispalicious, Banana Chocolate Blastocrisp, Chocolate Chip Cosmocrisp, Peanut Butter Bliss Crisp, Strawberry Crispiscrumptious	28	1
		*Made with dried fruits, nuts, honey and crisp rice. Dairy-Free		
	Jŏcolat*	Chocolate, Chocolate (Cherry, Coffee, German, Hazelnut, Mint)	48	1.7
		*Made with dates, nuts and cocoa. Dairy-Free.		
Leda Nutrition	Leda Bars*	Apple Cinnamon, Apricot, Banana	85	3
	Multipack Bars** (5/box)	Apple Cinnamon, Strawberry, Triple Berry	190	6.7
	Nurture Bars**	Apple & Pomegranate, Blueberry & Goji	38	1.3
		*Made with chickpea, corn, tapioca, rice and dried fruits. Dairy-Free. **Baked fruit-filled bars made with chickpea, tapioca and rice flours. Dairy-Free.		
Mrs. May's Naturals	Classic Crunch*	Almond, Cashew, Cran-Blueberry, Cran-Tropical, Pecan, Pom-Raspberry, Pumpkin, Strawberry Pineapple, Sunflower, Ultimate, Walnut, White Sesame	142	5
		Black Sesame, Coconut Almond, Walnut	156	5.5
	Trio Bars*	Blueberry, Cranberry, Strawberry, Tropical	34	1.2
	Ultimate Plus Bars*	Banana Blueberry, Black Sesame, Cranberry Crunch, Mango Strawberry	40	1.4
		*Snacks and snack bars made from nuts, seeds and/or dried fruits. Sweetened with rice malt (gluten-free).		

Company	Snack Bars		Grams	Ounces
Nonuttin' Foods	**Granola Bars***	Apple Cinnamon, Chocolate Chip, Double Chocolate Chunk, Raisin	30	1
	*Made with pure, uncontaminated oats. Free of dairy, peanuts, tree nuts, eggs.			
Omega Smart	**Nutritional Bars***	Apricot Almond, Banana Chocolate Chip, Carrot Cake, Chocolate Nut, Cinnamon Apple, Pomegranate Strawberry Colada, Pumpkin Spice, Raisin Spice	63	2.2
	*Dairy-Free.			
	Youth in a Bar**	Almond Macaroon, Dark Chocolate Cherry, Wild Blueberry	65	2.3
	**Made with flax, dried fruits and goat milk.			
Orgran	**Fruit Filled Bars***	Apricot, Blueberry	50	1.8
	*Dairy-Free.			
Perfect 10	**Bliss Bars***	Apricot Chocolate, Cranberry Chocolate, Lemon Chocolate	50	1.8
	*Made with dried fruits, nuts, seeds and dark chocolate chips. Dairy-Free.			
	Natural Energy Bars**	Apple Cinnamon, Apricot, Cherry, Cranberry, Lemon	50	1.8
	**Made with dried fruits, nuts and seeds. Dairy-Free.			
PureFit	**Nutrition Bars***	Almond Crunch, Berry Almond Crunch, Chocolate Brownie, Granola Crunch**, Peanut Butter Crunch	56.7	2
	*Soy-based with nuts. Dairy-Free. **Made with pure gluten-free oats. Dairy-Free.			
Think Products	**thinkThin Desserts**	Chocolate Covered Strawberries, Lemon Cream Pie, Tangerine Cremesicle	50	1.76
	thinkThin Bars	Brownie Crunch, Chocolate Fudge, Chocolate Mudslide, Chunky Peanut Butter, Creamy Peanut Butter, Dark Chocolate, White Chocolate Chip	60	2.1
	thinkThin Bites	Chocolate Toffee Nut, Cookies and Cream, White Chocolate Raspberry	39	1.37
Wellness Foods	**The Simply Bar***	Cocoa Coffee, Lemon Coconut	37	1.3
		Cinnamon, Cocoa CaCo Raspberry, Peanut Butter Chocolate	40	1.4
	Organic Protein Bar*		40	1.4
	Contains berries (blueberry, cranberry, Goji)			
	*High protein, low fat, dairy-free, vegan and kosher. Made with non-GMO soy crisp and agave nectar.			

CRACKERS AND RICE CAKES

✦ Most crackers contain wheat, rye, regular oats, and/or barley. Read labels carefully.

✦ The majority of large and mini rice cakes are gluten-free, however, some multigrain rice cakes may contain barley or wheat flour, regular oats, barley malt flavoring, barley malt extract or barley malt and are **NOT** gluten-free.

CRACKERS

Company	Crackers		Grams	Ounces
BARKAT	Crackers*, Matzo Crackers*		200	7.1
	Cracker Bread		275	9.7
	*Dairy-Free.			
BI-AGLUT	**Bread Sticks**	Grissini (plain), Pizza, Sesame	150	5.3
	Cracker*		150	5.3
	Crispbread (Fette Tostate)*, Crispbread (Fette Tostate Mediterranee)*		240	8.5
	Toasted Bread (Pane Biscottato)		300	10.6
	*Dairy-Free.			
BLUE DIAMOND	**Nut Thins**	Almond, Cheddar Cheese, Country Ranch, Hazelnut, Pecan, Smokehouse	120	4.25
CRUNCHMASTER	**Baked Rice Crackers**	Artisian Four Cheese, Toasted Sesame Rice*	100	3.5
	Baked Multi-Grain Crackers*		128	4.5
	Baked Multi-Seed Crackers	Original*, Roasted Garlic, Rosemary & Olive Oil, Sweet Onion	128	4.5
	*Dairy-Free.			
EDEN FOODS	Brown Rice Crackers		75	2.6
	Brown Rice Chips		50	1.7
	Nori Maki Rice Crackers		68	2.4
EDWARD & SON'S TRADING CO.	**Brown Rice Snaps** (organic)	Black Sesame*, Cheddar, Salsa*, Toasted Onion*, Unsalted Plain*, Vegetable*	100	3.5
	Brown Rice Snaps*	Onion Garlic, Tamari Seaweed, Tamari Sesame, Unsalted Sesame	100	3.5
	Exotic Rice Toast*	Jasmine Rice & Spring Onion, Purple Rice & Black Sesame, Thai Red Rice & Flax Seeds	65	2.25
	*Dairy-Free.			

Company	Crackers		Grams	Ounces
Ener-G Foods	Broken Melba Toast*		454	16
	Cinnamon Crackers		168	5.9
	Gourmet Crackers (low protein)		200	7
	Gourmet Onion Crackers		200	7
	Seattle Crackers		125	4.4
	All products are Dairy-Free. *Enriched with thiamin, riboflavin, niacin, iron and folic acid.			
Gluten Free & Fabulous	Sweet Savory Bites (cracker type snack with nuts & seeds)		185	6.5
Glutino	**Bread Sticks**	Sesame, Pizza Flavored	150	5.3
	Crackers ("Ritz" Style)		150	5.3
	Crackers	Cheddar, Multigrain, Vegetable	125	4.4
Hol•Grain	**Brown Rice Crackers**	Lightly Salted, Lightly Salted Onion & Garlic, Lightly Salted Sesame, Unsalted	127	4.5
Kitchen Table Bakers	**Parmesan Cheese Gourmet Wafer Crisps**	Aged Parmesan, Everything, Flax Seed, Garlic, Italian Herb, Jalapeño, Rosemary, Sesame	85	3
Mary's Gone Crackers	**Organic Crackers**	Original, Black Pepper, Caraway, Herb, Onion	184	6.5
Orgran	**Crispbreads***	Essential Fibre, Toasted Buckwheat, Toasted Corn, Multi-Grain with Quinoa	125	4.4
	CrispiBites*	Balsamic Herb, Original Sea Salt Corn, Onion & Chive	100	3.5
	Multi-Grain Deli Crackers*		100	3.5
	*Dairy-Free.			
Panne Rizo	Crostini Toasts*		115	4.1
	*Dairy-Free.			
San-J	**Brown Rice Crackers**	Black Sesame, Sesame	100	3.5
		Tamari	80	2.8
Schär	Cheese Bites		125	4.4
	Crispbread		125	4.4
	Italian Bread Sticks		150	5.3
	Snack Crackers		300	10.6
	Table Crackers		200	7

Corn & Rice Cakes – Large

Company	Corn & Rice Cakes – Large		Grams	Ounces
Lundberg	**Eco-Farmed Rice Cakes**	Apple Cinnamon, Buttery Caramel, Honey Nut	269	9.5
		Brown Rice, Brown Rice (Salt-Free), Wild Rice	241	8.5
		Sesame Tamari, Toasted Sesame	255	9.0

Company	Corn & Rice Cakes – Large		Grams	Ounces
LUNDBERG	Organic Brown Rice Cakes	Brown Rice, Brown Rice (Salt-Free), Mochi Sweet, Popcorn, Tamari Seaweed, Wild Rice	241	8.5
		Flax with Tamari	273	9.6
		Caramel Corn, Cinnamon Toast, Koku Seaweed, Sweet Green Tea with Lemon	269	9.5
		Sesame Tamari	255	9.0
PLUM-M-GOOD	Organic Rice Cakes	Brown Rice (Salted), Brown Rice (Unsalted), Brown Rice Sesame (Salted), Brown Rice Sesame (Unsalted), Multigrain (Salted),* Multigrain (Unsalted)*	185	6.5
	Regular Rice Cakes	Multigrain (salted), Plain (salted and unsalted), Sesame (salted)	185	6.5
	*Made with brown rice, buckwheat, millet.			
QUAKER (CANADA)	Butter Popcorn, Original		127	4.5
	Caramel Corn		186	6.6
	Caramel Chocolate Chip		199	7
	Savory Tomato and Basil		173	6.1
	White Cheddar		140	4.9
QUAKER (USA)	Apple Cinnamon, Caramel Corn		185	6.5
	Butter Pop Corn, Lightly Salted, Salt Free		127	4.5
	Chocolate Crunch		205	7.2
	White Cheddar		140	4.9
REAL FOODS	Corn Thins (Crispbreads)	Cracked Pepper & Lemon*, Flax & Soy*, Multigrain*, Original*, Sesame*	150	5.3
		Feta & Sundried Tomato, Sour Cream & Chives, Tasty Cheese	165	5.8
	Rice Thins	Whole Grain Brown Rice*	150	5.3
	*Dairy-Free.			

RICE CAKES – MINI

Company	Rice Cakes – Mini		Grams	Ounces
QUAKER (CANADA)	Crispy Mini Rice Chips*	Butter Pop Corn, Caramel Kettle Corn, Cheddar, Crunchy Dill, Ketchup, Salt & Vinegar, Sea Salt & Lime, Sour Cream & Chives	100	3.5
	Note: *BBQ contains barley malt flavor and is NOT gluten-free.			
QUAKER (USA)	Quakes Rice Snacks*	Apple Cinnamon, Cheddar Cheese, Caramel Corn, Chocolate, Honey Nut, Kettle Corn, Nacho Cheese, Ranch, Sour Cream and Onion	various sizes	various sizes
	Note: *BBQ contains barley malt flour and is NOT gluten-free			

SNACKS

Candy, Chips, Nuts, Seeds, Pretzels

✦ Read labels carefully. **Many snack foods contain wheat, regular oats or barley:** e.g., flavored tortilla chips, potato chips, soy nuts, licorice.

Company	Snacks		Grams	Ounces
ARICO	Cassava Chips*	Barbeque Bliss, Ginger on Fire, Original Sea Salt Mist	142	5
	*Dairy-Free.			
BARBARA'S BAKERY	Cheese Puffs	Original (Natural)	200	7
		Original Bakes	155	5.5
		White Cheddar Bakes	155	5.5
BARKAT	Pretzels*, Pretzel Sticks*, Sesame Pretzels*		75	2.7
	*Dairy-Free.			
CANDY TREE	Black Licorice	Bites, Laces, Rope, Vines	74	2.6
	Cherry Licorice	Bites, Laces, Vines	74	2.6
	Raspberry Licorice	Bites, Laces, Vines	74	2.6
	Strawberry Licorice	Bites, Laces, Vines	74	2.6
	Organic corn-based candy.			
CHEECHA	Gluten-Free Cheecha Potato Puffs	Luscious Lime, Mediterranean Ginger, Original Potato, Sea Salt & Spiced Pepper, Sea Salt & Vinegar	70	2.5
	Note: Also make regular "Cheecha Krackles" (various flavors) that contain wheat flour.			
ENER-G FOODS	Crisp Pretzels (low protein), Sesame Pretzel Rings		75	2.7
	Wylde Pretzels	Lightly Salted, Sesame	113, 227	4, 8
		Poppy Seed	113	4
ENJOY LIFE	No Nuts Trail Mix*	Beach Bash, Mountain Mambo	170	6
	*Dairy-Free.			
GLUTINO	Pretzels	Sticks, Twists	75, 227, 400	2.6, 8, 14.1
		Sesame Rings	227	8
		Unsalted Twists	227	8
GOGO QUINOA	Quinoa Crunchies*	Cinnamon, Original, Oregano	99	3.5
	*Organic rice and quinoa flours.			
LUNDBERG	Rice Chips	Fiesta Lime, Honey Dijon, Pico De Gallo, Nacho Cheese, Santa Fe BBQ, Sea Salt, Sesame & Seaweed, Wasabi	170	6
MARY'S GONE CRACKERS	Sticks & Twigs*	Curry, Chipotle Tomato, Sea Salt	227	8
	*Made with brown rice, flax, sesame, quinoa, amaranth, millet and chia seeds. Dairy-Free.			

Company	Snacks		Grams	Ounces
MOCHI	Bake & Serve Rice Puffs	Original, Cashew-Date, Chocolate Brownie, Raisin-Cinnamon, Sesame-Garlic, Super Seed	354	12.5
MR. KRISPERS	Baked Rice Krisps	BBQ*, Nacho, Sea Salt & Pepper*, Sour Cream & Onion	119	4.2
	*Dairy-Free.			
ORGRAN	Molasses Licorice		200	7
RICE WORKS	Gourmet Brown Rice Crisps	Baked Cinnamon, Parmesan & Sundried Tomato, Salsa Fresca*, Sea Salt*, Sweet Chili*, Tangy BBQ*	various sizes	
	*Dairy-Free.			
ST. CLAIRE'S ORGANICS	Organic Licorice Sweets*		43, 227, 765	1.5, 8, 21
	*Black Licorice			
TERRA	Terra Chips Original (taro, sweet potato, yucca batata, parsnip, oils and salt)		28, 213	1, 7.5
	Terra Stix (Original)		213	7.5
	Taro Chip (Original Taro)		43, 170	1.5, 6
	Sweet Potato Chips	Plain No Salt, Spiced, Sweets & Beets, Sweets & Carrots	34, 170	1.2, 6

MISCELLANEOUS SNACKS

Company	Miscellaneous Snacks	Grams	Ounces
BARKAT	Ice Cream Cones* (24)	120	4.2
	Waffle Ice Cream Cones*	150	5.3
	*Dairy-Free.		
ENER-G FOODS	Communion Wafers (50/box)	40	1.4
	Made with sweet rice flour, potato flour, potato starch. Dairy-Free.		
LET'S DO...	Gluten-Free Ice Cream Cones (12)*	34	1.2
	*Dairy-Free.		

BAKING MIXES

Company	Baking Mixes		Grams	Ounces
1-2-3 GLUTEN-FREE	Yummy Yellow Cake Mix*		495	17.4
	Cookies	Chewy Chipless Scrumdelicious Cookie Mix*	680	24
		Lindsay's Lipsmakin' Roll-Out Sugar Cookies*	612	21.6
	Aaron's Favorite Rolls*		400	14.1
	Allie's Awesome Buckwheat Pancakes*		680	24
	Devilishly Decadent Brownies*		866	30.6
	Divinely Decadent Brownies*		695	24.5
	Flour Mix*		680	24
	Meredith's Marvelous Muffin/Quickbread*		467	16.5
	Poundcakes	Delightfully Gratifying*	1.1 kg	38.7
		Peri's Perfect Chocolate*	1.1 kg	38.1
	Southern Glory Biscuits*		503	17.8
	Sweet Goodness Pan Bars*		581	20.5
	*Dairy-Free.			
ALLERGYFREE FOODS	All Purpose Breading Mix*		453	16
	Blueberry Muffin Mix*		454	16
	Cake Mix*	Chocolate, Vanilla	454	16
	Cornbread Mix*		453	16
	Pizza Crust Mix*		624	22
	Waffle & Pancake Mix*		496	17.5
	*Casein, Egg, Nut and Soy-Free.			
AMAZING GRAINS	Montina™ All-Purpose Baking Flour Blend*		680 g, 1.8 kg, 4.54 kg	24 oz., 64 oz., 10 lbs.
	Montina™ Pure Baking Flour Supplement**		340, 680	12, 24
	* White rice flour, tapioca flour and Montina™ pure flour. Dairy-Free. ** Montina™ pure flour (Indian ricegrass). Dairy-Free.			
ANDREA'S FINE FOODS	Pancake Mix*		623	22
	Super Fine Grind Flour Blend*		454	16
	*Casein-Free.			
ARROWHEAD MILLS	Gluten-Free Chocolate Chip Cookie Mix*		366	12.9
	Gluten-Free All-Purpose Baking Mix*		794	28
	Gluten-Free Brownie Mix*		496	17.5
	Gluten-Free Pancake and Baking Mix		794	28
	Gluten-Free Pancake and Waffle Mix (Wild Rice)		907	32
	Gluten-Free Pizza Crust Mix		514	18.2
	Gluten-Free Vanilla Cake Mix		592	20.9
	*Dairy-Free.			
AUTHENTIC FOODS	Bette's Gourmet Featherlight Rice Flour Blend*		1.36 kg	3 lbs.
	Bette's Gourmet Four Flour Blend*		1.36 kg	3 lbs.
	Bread Mixes	Cinnamon*, White Homestyle*	567	20
	Cake Mixes	Chocolate*, Lemon*	312	11
		Devil's Food Chocolate*, Vanilla Bean*	341	12
	*Dairy-Free.			

Company	Baking Mixes		Grams	Ounces
AUTHENTIC FOODS	Chocolate Chunk Cookie Mix*		679	24
	Falafel Mix*		567	20
	Muffin Mixes	Blueberry*	454	16
		Chocolate Chip*	482	17
	Multi Blend Gluten-Free Flour*		1.36 kg	3 lbs.
	Pancake Mix*		567 g, 3.18 kg	20 oz., 7 lbs.
	Pie Crust Mix*		341	12
	Pizza Crust Mix*		567	20
	*Dairy-Free.			
BARKAT	Bread Mix*		500	17.6
	Chocolate Muffin Mix*, Pancake & Batter Mix*		250	8.8
	Flour Mix		750	26.5
	*Dairy-Free.			
BI-AGLUT	Flour Mix		500	17.6
	Flour For Bread		1 kg	35.3
THE BIRKETT MILLS	Larrowe's Instant Buckwheat Pancake Mix		1.8 kg	64
BOB'S RED MILL	GF All-Purpose Baking Flour		624	22
	GF Brownie Mix		595	21
	GF Chocolate Cake Mix		624	22
	GF Chocolate Chip Cookie Mix		680	24
	GF Cinnamon Raisin Bread Mix		624	22
	GF Cornbread Mix		566	20
	GF Hearty Whole Grain Bread Mix		566	20
	GF Homemade Wonderful Bread Mix		454	16
	GF Pancake Mix		623	22
	GF Pizza Crust Mix		454	16
	GF Shortbread Cookie Mix		595	21
	GF Vanilla Cake Mix		540	19
	GF Wheat Free Biscuit and Baking Mix		680	24
BREADS FROM ANNA	Bread Mix (Rice & Soy Free)		588	20.8
	Bread Mix (Corn, Dairy, Rice & Soy Free)		535	18.1
	Bread Mix (Corn, Dairy, Rice, Soy & Yeast Free)		535	18.1
	Banana Bread Mix (Corn, Dairy, Rice, Soy & Yeast Free)		397	14
	Herb Bread (Corn, Dairy, Rice, & Soy Free)		606	21.4
	Pancake/ Muffin Mix	Apple, Cranberry, Maple (Corn, Dairy, Rice, & Soy Free)	396	14
	Pie Crust Mix (Corn, Dairy, Rice, Soy & Yeast Free)		265	9.4
	Pumpkin Bread Mix (Corn, Dairy, Rice, Soy, Yeast Free)		509	18
'CAUSE YOU'RE SPECIAL!	**Biscuit Mixes**	Large	510	18
		Economy	1.02 kg	36
	Bread Mixes	Traditional French	595	21
		Homestyle White	595	21
	Cake Mixes	Golden Pound	553	19.5
		Moist Lemon, Yellow – Small	419	14.8
		Moist Lemon, Yellow – Large	839	29.6
		Rich Chocolate – Small	397	14
		Rich Chocolate – Large	794	28
	All products are Casein-Free.			

Company	Baking Mixes		Grams	Ounces
'CAUSE YOU'RE SPECIAL!	Cookie Mixes	Chocolate Fudge Brownie	519	18.3
		Chocolate Chip	428	15.1
		Classic Sugar	360	12.7
	Muffin Mixes	Classic Muffin and Quickbread	394	13.9
		Lemon Poppyseed	396	13.9
		Sweet Corn Muffin	425	15
	Scone Mixes	Large	638	22.5
		Economy	1.28 kg	45
	Pancake and Waffle Mixes	Regular	553	19.5
		Economy	1.11 kg	39
	Pie Crust Mix		221	7.8
	Pizza Crust Mix		368	13
	All products are Casein-Free.			
CELIAC SPECIALTIES	CF Brownie Mix*		454	16
	Corn Bread Mix		454	16
	Gluten-Free Flour Blend		908	2 lbs.
	Muffin Mix (Flaxseed)		454	16
	Pancake Mix	Buttermilk, Flaxseed, Plain*	454	16
	*Casein-Free.			
CELIMIX (NELSON DAVID OF CANADA)	Apple Cinnamon Cake and Muffin Mix*		415	14.6
	Batter Coating Mix		240	8.5
	Bread Mixes	Flax Bread*, Potato Bread*, Rice Bread*, White Bread*	2 kg	4.4 lbs.
	Cake Mixes	Dutch Chocolate Supreme*	350	12.3
		White*	415	14.6
	Carob Cake & Loaf Mix*		415	14.6
	Cookie Mixes	Regular	300	10.6
		Shortbread*	170	6
	Dinner Roll Mix*		190	6.7
	Dutch Chocolate Supreme Brownie Mix*		400	14.1
	Hamburger Bun Mix*		190	6.7
	Lemon Loaf & Cake Mix*		415	14.6
	Muffin Mix*		430	15.2
	Pancake Mix	Regular*, Brown Rice*	600	21.2
	Pastry Mix		900	1.98 lbs.
	Pizza Crust Mix		350	12.3
	Tea Biscuit Mix		420	14.8
	Yorkshire Pudding Mix		300	10.6
	*Dairy-Free.			
CELINAL FOODS	Single Serve Mixes	GF Biscuit Mix	35	1.2
		GFDF Bread/Pizza Mix*	40	1.4
		GFDF Cornbread Mix*	52	1.8
		GF White Bread Mix	38	1.3
		GFDF White Cake Mix*	52	1.8
		GFDF Vanilla Icing*	40	1.4
	*Dairy-Free.			

Company	Baking Mixes		Grams	Ounces
CHEBE	Bread Mixes	Original, All Purpose	213	7.5
		Focaccia Italian Flatbread*	213	7.5
	Cinnamon Roll-Up Mix*		213	7.5
	Garlic Onion Bread Sticks Mix*		213	7.5
	Pizza Crust Mix*		213	7.5
	*Casein-Free. Original, All Purpose & Pizza Crust also available in bulk. Made from cassava.			
CHERRYBROOK KITCHEN	Fudge Brownie Mix		396	14
	Cake Mixes	Chocolate, Yellow	464	16.4
	Cookie Mixes	Chocolate Chip	402	14.2
		Sugar	371	13.1
	Pancake Mix		509	18
	Frosting Mixes	Chocolate	297	10.5
		Vanilla	266	9.4
	Frosting Spreads	Chocolate, Vanilla	454	16
	All products are also Dairy, Egg, Peanut and Nut-Free.			
CHOICES BEST RICE BAKERY	Brownie Mix*		364	9.5
	Pancake Mix*		336, 672	11.9, 17.6
	Pastry Mix*		454	16
	Rice Muffin Mix*		545	19.2
	Scone Mix		420	11.0
	White Rice Cake Mix*		530	18.7
	*Dairy-Free.			
DIETARY SPECIALTIES	Bread Mixes	Apple, Banana	598	21.1
		White	500	17.6
	Brownie Mix		680	24
	Cake Mixes	Chocolate, White	740	26.1
	Cornbread Mix		530	18.7
	Muffin Mixes	Blueberry	567	20
		Bran	480	16.9
	Pancake Mix		485	17.1
	All mixes are Casein-Free.			
DOWD & ROGERS	Cake Mixes	Dark Vanilla, Dutch Chocolate Golden Lemon	408	14
DUINKERKEN FOODS	Biscuit Mix*		470	16.6
	Bread Mix*		500	17.6
	Cookie Mix		426	15
	Muffin Mix		470	16.4
	Pizza Mix		477	16.8
	Waffle Mix*		420	14.8
	*Casein-Free. All mixes enriched with thiamin, riboflavin, niacin, folic acid and iron.			
EL PETO	All-Purpose Flour Mix	Regular*, Corn/Soy Free*	500g, 1 kg, 2.5, 10, 20 kg	17.5, 35 oz., 5.5, 22 & 44 lbs.
	Bread Maker Mixes	Brown Rice*, White Rice* Italian, Potato*	700 g, 2.45 kg	24.5 oz. 5.4 lbs.
	Brownie Mix*		500	17.5
	Cake Mixes	Chocolate*, Lemon*, White*	500 g, 1 kg	17.5 oz., 2.2 lbs.
	*Dairy-Free. Brownie, Cake, Muffin and Pancake Mixes also available in Corn-Free formulations.			

Company	Baking Mixes		Grams	Ounces
EL PETO	Sugar Cookie Mix*		750	26.5
	Muffin Mix*		500 g 1, 2.5 & 10 kg	17.5 oz., 2.2, 5.5 & 22 lbs.
	Pancake Mix*		500 g 1, 2.5 & 10 kg	17.5 oz. 2.2, 5.5 & 22 lbs.
	Perfect Pie Crust Mix*		500	17.5
	*Dairy-Free. Muffin and Pancake Mixes also available in Corn-Free formulations.			
ENER-G FOODS	Corn Mix*		454	16
	GF Gourmet Blend*		451	15.9
	Potato Mix* (low protein), Rice Mix*		567	20
	*Dairy-Free			
AVENA (FARMPURE FOODS) [ONLY OATS™]	Grandma's Oatmeal Cookie Mix		1 kg, 2.5 kg	35 oz., 5 lb. 8 oz.
	Muffin Mix	Cinnamon Spice, Decadent Chocolate	1 kg, 2.5 kg	35 oz., 5 lb. 8 oz.
	Whole Oat Pancake Mix		1 kg, 2.5 kg	35 oz., 5 lb. 8 oz.
	*Made with pure, uncontaminated oats.			
FOOD-TEK	**Fast & Fresh Microwave Mixes:**			
	Cake Mixes	Chocolate*, White*, Yellow*	280	9.9
		Cinnamon Coffee Cake*	320	11.3
		Double Chocolate	360	12.7
		Gooey Brownie Decadence	360	12.7
	Bread Mixes	Corn Bread*	280	9.9
		White Bread	320	11.3
	Hamburger Bun, Waffle		320	11.3
	Pizza Crust*		210	7.4
	Frostings	Chocolate, Vanilla	160	5.7
	Quick-Bake Mixes:			
	Cookie Mixes	Chocolate Chip, Double Chocolate Chip, Sugar	280	9.9
	Biscuit Mix		280	9.9
	Quick-Bake Kids Mixes:			
	Brownies		240	8.5
	Cookie Mixes	Chocolate Chip, Chocolate Sugar	104	3.7
	Chocolate Cake/Yellow Cake		184	6.5
	*Dairy-Free.			
GIFTS OF NATURE	All-Purpose Flour Blend		680 g, 1.36 kg, 4.54 kg	24 & 48 oz., 10 lbs.
	Bread Mixes	Buttermilk Cornbread	595	21
		French Bread & Pizza Crust	595 g, 4.67 kg	21 oz., 10.5 lbs.
		Sandwich White Bread and Roll	624 g, 5 kg	22 oz., 11 lbs.
	Buttermilk Biscuit & Baking Mix		539 g, 1.11 kg	19, 39

Company	Baking Mixes		Grams	Ounces
GIFTS OF NATURE	Buttermilk Pancake & Waffle Mix		624 g, 1.25 kg, 5 kg	22 & 44 oz., 11 lbs.
	Cake Mixes	Chocolate, Yellow	765	27
	Cookie Mixes	Fancy	482	17
		Triple Treat	850	30
	Fudge Brownie Mix		595	21
	Muffin Mixes	Basic	510 g, 1.53 kg	18, 54
		Cinnamon Spice, Cranberry Orange, Vanilla Poppyseed	595	21
GILLIAN'S FOODS	All Purpose Baking Mix*		454	16
	Brownie Mix*		266	9.4
	Cinnamon Bread/Roll Mix*		454	16
	French Bread Mix*		454	16
	Pizza Dough Mix*		454	16
	*Dairy-Free.			
GLUTEN-FREE BAGEL COMPANY	**Bread Mixes**	Primo White*	400	14.0
	Bread/Muffin Mixes	Banana*	590	20.8
		Blueberry*	450	16.0
		Corn*	500	17.6
		Pumpkin*	550	19.4
		Strawberry*	495	17.6
	Bagel/Soft Pretzel Mix*		830	29.4
	Pita Mix*			
	Scone Mix		330	11.6
	Donut & Donut Hole Mix*		570	20.2
	Buttermilk Pancake Mix		575	20.4
	Brownie Mix*		720	25.2
	Cake Mixes	Chocolate*	780	27.6
		White-Orange*	905	32.0
	Cookie Mixes	Chocolate Chip*	455	16.0
		Italian Ricotta Cheese	885	31.4
		Orange*	975	34.4
		Peanut Butter*	735	26.0
		Pumpkin*	975	34.4
		Brown Sugar Wafer*	735	26.0
		Cookie Jar Cut-Outs*	720	25.2
	*Dairy-Free.			
GLUTEN-FREE CREATIONS	**Baking Flour Mixes**	Basic, Enriched, Sweet Also available in bulk.	454 g, 1.36 kg	1 lb., 3 lbs.
	Bread Mixes	Almond Flax, Honey Oat*, Sandwich Bread, Seeded Multigrain	538	19
		Cinnamon Raisin	566	20
	Frosting Mixes	Chocolate, White	454	1 lb.
	Pizza Crust Mix		255	9
	Rich Brownie Mix		509	18

*Made with pure, uncontaminated oats.
Note: 1. All mixes are Dairy-Free except Sandwich Bread.
    2. All mixes are enriched with thiamin, riboflavin, niacin, folic acid, iron and calcium except the Basic Flour Baking Mix.

Company	Baking Mixes		Grams	Ounces
Gluten-Free Naturals	Cookie Blend*, Sandwich Bread Flour*		454	16
	Cornbread & Corn Muffin Mix		245	8.6
	Homemade Brownie Mix*		388	13.7
	Light & Moist Yellow Cake Mix		315	11.1
	Multi-Grain Bread Flour*		454	16
	Pancake Mix		357	12.6
	Pizzeria-Style Pizza Crust Mix*		272	9.6
	*Dairy-Free.			
Gluten-Free Pantry	**Bread Mixes**	French Bread and Pizza*	624 g, 2.27, 11.35 kg	22 oz., 5, 25 lbs.
		Favorite Sandwich Bread	624 g, 2.27, 11.35 kg	22 oz., 5, 25 lbs.
	Quick Bread, Scone & Pancake Mixes	Brown Rice Pancake & Waffle	454	16
		Muffin & Scone	425 g, 2.27, 11.35 kg	15 oz., 5, 25 lbs.
		Yankee Cornbread & Muffin*	340	12
	Dessert Mixes	Chocolate Chip Cookie & Cake*	539 g, 2.27, 11.35 kg	19 oz., 5, 25 lbs.
		Chocolate Truffle Brownie*	454 g, 2.27, 11.35 kg	16 oz., 5, 25 lbs.
		Crisp & Crumble Topping*	340	12
		Decadent Chocolate Cake*	454	16
		Old Fashioned Cake & Cookie*	425	15
		Perfect Pie Crust*	454	16
		Spice Cake & Gingerbread*	397	14
	*Dairy-Free.			
Glutino	**Cake Mixes**	Chocolate, Vanilla	375	13.2
	Muffin Mix		500	17.6
	Pancake Mix		575	20.3
Hodgson Mill	Apple Cinnamon Muffin Mix		216	7.6
	Bread Mix		454	16
	Brownie Mix		425	15
	Cake Mixes	Chocolate, Yellow	425	15
	Cookie Mix		340	12
	Multi Purpose Baking Mix		340	12
	Pancake & Waffle Mix w/Flaxseed		454	16
	Pizza Crust Mix		454	16
	All mixes are Dairy-Free.			
Hol•Grain	**Mixes**	Chocolate Chip Cookie	454	16
		Pancake & Waffle	454	16
Kaybee	Basic Bread Mix		520	18.3
	Basic Cookie Mix		370	13.1
	Basic Muffin Mix		375	13.2
	Chocolate Brownie Mix		360	12.7

Company	Baking Mixes		Grams	Ounces
KAYBEE	Corn Bread Mix		240	8.5
	Cottage Pudding		270	9.5
	Deluxe Pancake Mix		360	12.7
	No-Knead Bun Mix		320	11.3
	Pizza Crust Mix		245	8.6
	Pyrogy Dough Mix		230	8.1
	Super Easy Cake Mix		260	9.2
	Wild Rice Pancake Mix		370	13
KINNIKINNICK	**Kinni-Kwik Mixes***			
	Bread & Buns	Plain, Sunflower & Flax	1000	35.5
	Regular Mixes Breads	Candadi Yeast Free Rice, Tapioca Rice, White Rice	650	23
	Kinni-Kwik mixes require only the addition of water.			
	Cake Mixes	Angel Food	450	16
		Chocolate, Sponge, White	500	18
	Cookie Mixes		650	23
	Cornbread & Muffin Mix		650	23
	Miscellaneous	All-Purpose Celiac Flour	1000	35.5
		All-Purpose Mix	650	23
		Easy White Fibre Mix	250	9
	Muffin Mix		624	22
	Pancake & Waffle Mix		650	23
	Pastry & Pie Crust Mix		650	23
	Pizza Crust Mix		650	23
	All mixes are Casein-Free.			
KOKIMO KITCHEN	Pancake Mix*, Waffle Mix*		640	22.6
	*Dairy-Free.			
LAUREL'S SWEET TREATS	Baking Flour Mix		454 g, 2.2 kg	16 oz., 5 lbs.
	Bread Mixes	Banzo Bread*	454	16
		Good Ol' Corn Bread	510	18
	Cake Mixes	Cameron's Vanilla*	425, 850	15, 30
		Cinnamon Spice	425, 850	15, 30
		Mom's Chocolate*	354, 709	12.5, 25
	Chocolate Dream Brownie Mix		538	19
	Cookie Mixes	Chocolate Chip*	822	29
		Double Chocolate Chip	822	29
		Roll 'Em Out Sugar*	652	23
	Dinner Roll Mix		567	20
	Honey Grahamless Crackers		454	16
	Pancake Mix*		539 g, 2.2 kg	19 oz., 5 lbs.
	Pizza Dough Mix*		340	12
	All mixes are Casein-Free. *Also available in bulk.			
MANISCHEWITZ	Homestyle Potato Latke Mix		170	6
	Mini Potato Knish Mix		170	6
	Potato Kugel Mix		170	6
	Potato Pancake Mix		85, 170	3, 6
	Sweet Potato Pancake Mix		170	6

Company	Baking Mixes		Grams	Ounces
MISS ROBEN'S	Bagel Mix*		672	24
	Biscuit Mix*		364	13
	Bread Mixes	Dinner*, French*	392	14
		Homestyle*	386	14
		Noah's*	456	16.3
		Potato*	532	19
		Traditional Cornbread*	420	15
		White Sandwich*	588	21
	Cake-Like Doughnut Mix*		868	31
	Cake Mixes	One Step Angel Food*	336	12
		Carrot*	616	22
		Chocolate*, Gingerbread*	588	21
		Pound*	532	19
		White*	812	29
		Yellow*	672	24
	Chewy Brownie Mix*		423	14.9
	Cookie Mixes	Animal*	364	13
		Crunchy Chocolate Chip*	840	30
		Crunchy Chocolate Sugar*	476	17
		Crunchy Sugar*	476	17
		Crunchy Versatile*	700	25
		Mock Graham Cracker*	364	13
		Roll & Cut Gingerbread*	588	21
		Roll & Cut Sugar*	532	19
	Frosting Mixes	Milk Chocolate Buttercream*	599	21.4
		Vanilla Buttercream*	621	22.2
	Ice Cream Mixes	Chocolate FreeZ*	448	16
		Versatile FreeZ*	305	10.9
	Mock Goldfish Cracker Mix*		538	19.2
	Muffin Mixes	English Muffin*	392	14
		Versatile*	784	28
	Pancake & Waffle Mix*		336	12
	Pie Crust Mix*		308	11
	Pizza Crust	Corn Free*	409	14.6
	Mixes	Small (12")*	336	12
		Large (18")*	504	18
	Popover or Pastry Mix*		174	6.2
	Soft Pretzel Mix		364	13
	Tortilla Mix*		409	14.6
	*Dairy-Free.			
MR. RITT'S	Bread Mixes		various sizes	
	Flour Blends	Buckwheat*, White Rice*	various sizes	
	White Rice Waffle Mix		various sizes	
	*Available in Dairy-Free.			
NAMASTE FOODS	Biscuits, Pie Crust & More		1.36 kg	4 lbs.
	Blondies Mix, Brownie Mix		907	32
	Bread Mix		454	16
	All mixes are Dairy, Corn, Potato & Soy-Free. Also available in bulk.			

Company	Baking Mixes		Grams	Ounces
NAMASTE FOODS	Cake Mixes	Chocolate	822	29
		Spice Carrot	737	26
		Vanilla	765	27
	Cookie Mix		624	22
	Frosting Mix	Chocolate Fudge, Toffee Vanilla	496	17.5
	Muffin Mix	Regular	454	16
		Sugar-Free	397	14
	Perfect Flour Blend		1.36 kg	4 lbs.
	Pizza Crust Mix		765	27
	Waffle/Pancake Mix		680	24
	All mixes are Dairy, Corn, Potato & Soy-Free. Also available in bulk.			
NATURE'S OWN BAKERY	Baking Mix (All-Purpose)		900	31.7
ORGRAN	All Purpose Pastry Mix		375	13.2
	Bread Mixes	GF Bread, Alternative Grain Whole Meal Bread	450	15.9
	Cake Mixes	Chocolate, Vanilla	375	13.2
	Chocolate Mousse Mix		120	4.2
	Cornbread & Muffin Mix		375	13.2
	Custard Powder Mix, Falafel Mix		200	7
	Flour Mixes	Plain All-Purpose, Self-Raising Flour	500	17.6
		Gluten-Free Gluten Substitute	120	4.2
	Muffin Mixes	Chocolate, Lemon Poppyseed	375	13.2
	No Egg-Egg Replacer		200	7
	Pancake Mixes	Apple & Cinnamon, Buckwheat	375	13.2
	Pizza & Pastry Multi Mix		375	13.2
	All mixes are Dairy-Free.			
PAMELA'S PRODUCTS	Gluten-Free Bread & Flour Mix*		539 g, 1.8 kg	19 oz., 4 lbs.
	Gluten-Free Cornbread & Muffin Mix*		340	12
	Cake Mix	Luscious Chocolate, Classic Vanilla	595	21
	Frostings	Confetti	369	13
		Dark Chocolate, Vanilla	340	12
	Incredible Chocolate Chunk Cookie Mix		386	13.6
	Irresistible Chocolate Brownie Mix		454	16
	Ultimate Baking & Pancake Mix		680 g, 1.81 kg	24 oz., 4 lbs.
	*Dairy-Free.			
PANERISO/ KINGSMILL	Apple Crisp Mix*		275	9.7
	Rice Bread and Baking Mix		800	28.2
	Rice Bread Machine Mix		325	11.5
	Rice Cake and Cookie Mix		600	21.2
	Mixes available in bulk. *Made with pure, uncontaminated oats.			
PANNE RIZO	Classic White Cake Mix*		600	21.2
	Gluten-Free Flour Mix* (white or brown)		908 g, 2.27 kg	2 lbs., 5 lbs.
	Pizza Crust Mix*		300	10.5
	*Dairy-Free.			

Company	Baking Mixes		Grams	Ounces
The Really Great Food Company	Biscuit Mixes	Old Time	425	15
		Spinach & Cheese	284	10
	Bread Mixes	Biscuit Loaf	496	17.5
		Brown Rice Bread	595	21
		Old Fashioned Cinnamon Bread	567	20
		Dark European Bread	595	21
		French Bread/Country Farm Bread	369	13
		Home-Style Cornbread	794	28
		Irish Soda Bread	709	25
		Original White Bread	567	20
		Rye-Style Bread	539	19
	Muffin Mixes	Apple Spice, Cornbread	369	13
		English Muffin	397	14
		Maple Raisin, Sweet Muffin	369	13
		Vanilla	340	12
	Pancake Mixes	Brown Rice Flour, Classic	454 g, 1.28 kg	16, 45
	Pizza Crust Mix		454	16
	Flaky Pie Crust Mix		369	13
	Cake Mixes	Angel Food	425	15
		Aunt Tootsie's Brownie	595	21
		Aunt Tootsie's Devil's Food Cake	650	23
		Banana Bread, Pumpkin Bread	539	19
		Chocolate	650	23
		Coffee Crumb Cake	567	20
		Colonial Spice	709	25
		Gingerbread	539	19
		Grandma's Pound	567	20
		Lemon Poppy, Orange, Golden	650	23
		Pineapple	567	20
		Pumpkin Spice	539	19
		White	397	14
		Yellow	650	23
	Cookie Mixes	Anise Biscotti	425	15
		Butter	425	15
		Chocolate Crinkle	454	16
		Coconut Macaroon	425	15
		Lemon Poppyseed Biscotti	425	15
		Versatile	425 g, 1.28 kg	15, 45
	All mixes are Dairy-Free.			
The Ruby Range	All-Purpose Mix		454, 908	1, 5 lbs.
	Cake or	Double Chocolate Truffle	295	10.4
	Cupcakes	Spice	309	10.9
	Old Fashioned Cookies		360	12.7
	Southwestern Pancakes		261	9.2

Company	Baking Mixes		Grams	Ounces
SCHÄR	Classic White Bread Mix		540	19
STERK'S BAKERY	All-Purpose Flour Mix*		908 g, 2.27, 4.54 kg	2, 5, 10 lbs.
	Brownie Mix*		475	16.8
	Cake Mixes*	Banana, Carrot	650	23
		Chocolate, Lemon	400	14.1
	Pancake Mix*		1, 2 kg	2.2, 4.4 lbs.
	Pizza Mix		350	12.4
	*Dairy-Free.			
SYLVAN BORDER FARM	Bread Mix, Bread Mix (Non-Dairy)*, Classic Dark Bread Mix		454	16
	Chocolate Cake Mix		794	28
	General Purpose Flour*		908	2 lbs.
	Pancake & Waffle Mix*		340	12
	Lemon Cake Mix*		757	26.7
	*Dairy-Free.			
TOM SAWYER	All-Purpose Gluten-Free Flour*		680 g, 2.27 kg, 4.54 kg	24 oz., 5 lbs., 10 lbs.
	*Dairy-Free.			

FLOURS

✦ Some "wheat-free" flours (e.g., kamut and spelt) are **NOT** gluten-free.

✦ Some buckwheat mixes contain **wheat flour and buckwheat flour**.

✦ When purchasing bulk-bagged gluten-free flours be aware of the possibility of cross-contamination with other gluten-containing flours. Ask the store what procedures they use when bagging their various flours.

✦ A variety of gluten-free all-purpose flour mixes and flours are listed below and on the following pages. Each flour has unique properties, therefore follow recipes closely!

All-Purpose Flour Mixes

1-2-3 GLUTEN-FREE
  ✦ **Flour Mix**
    – white rice flour, tapioca flour, potato starch, xanthan gum

AMAZING GRAINS
  ✦ **Montina™ All-Purpose Baking Flour Blend**
    – white rice flour, tapioca starch flour and Montina™ Pure Flour

ANDREA'S FOODS
  ✦ **Super Fine Grind Flour Blend**
    – brown rice, tapioca starch, potato starch, xanthan gum

ARROWHEAD MILLS
  ✦ **Gluten-Free All-Purpose Baking Mix**
    – organic whole grain brown rice flour, organic potato starch, tapioca starch flour, baking powder, fava bean flour, sea salt

AUTHENTIC FOODS
  ✦ **Bette's Gourmet Featherlight Rice Flour Blend**
    – white rice flour, tapioca flour, cornstarch, potato flour

All-Purpose Flour Mixes CONT'D.

AUTHENTIC FOODS

✦ **Bette's Gourmet Four Flour Blend**
 – garfava flour, sorghum flour, corn flour, cornstarch, tapioca flour

✦ **GF Classical Blend**
 – brown rice flour, potato starch, tapioca flour

✦ **Multi Blend Gluten-Free Flour**
 – brown rice flour, sweet rice flour, tapioca flour, corn starch, potato starch, xanthan gum

BARKAT

✦ **Flour Mix**
 – maize (corn) starch, rice starch, soya whole meal, guar gum, sweet whey powder, skimmed milk powder, lecithin

BI-AGLUT

✦ **Flour (Farina) Mix**
 – maize (corn) starch, potato flour, rice starch, carob seed flour, dextrose, powdered lactose-free skimmed milk, sodium caseinate

✦ **Flour for Bread**
 – maize (corn) starch, potato flour, skimmed milk powder, glucose, thickeners, guar flour, salt of zinc, Vitamin B_1

BOB'S RED MILL

✦ **GF All-Purpose Baking Flour**
 – garbanzo flour, potato starch, tapioca flour, sorghum flour, fava bean flour

CELIAC SPECIALTIES

✦ **Gluten-Free Flour Blend**
 – rice flour, potato starch, tapioca starch

EL PETO

✦ **All-Purpose Flour Mix**
 – cornstarch, white rice flour, xanthan and/or guar gum

✦ **All-Purpose Flour Mix (Corn-Free/Soy-Free)**
 – potato starch, white rice flour, xanthan and/or guar gum

ENER-G FOODS

✦ **Gluten-Free Gourmet Blend**
 – white rice flour, potato starch, tapioca starch

GIFTS OF NATURE

✦ **All-Purpose Flour Blend**
 – brown rice flour, potato starch flour, white rice flour, Montina™ pure, sweet rice flour, tapioca flour, xanthan gum

GILLIAN'S FOODS

✦ **All Purpose Baking Mix**
 – rice flour, potato starch flour and tapioca flour

GLUTEN-FREE CREATIONS

✦ **Basic Baking Mix**
 – white rice flour, tapioca starch, arrowroot, xanthan gum and gelatin

✦ **Enriched Baking Mix**
 – tapioca starch, brown rice flour, white rice flour, sweet rice flour, rice bran, xanthan gum, citric acid, niacin, iron, thiamin, riboflavin, folic acid and tricalcium phosphate

✦ **Sweet Baking Mix**
 – sorghum flour, white rice flour, tapioca starch, xanthan gum, niacin, iron, thiamin, riboflavin, folic acid and tricalcium phosphate

All-Purpose Flour Mixes CONT'D.

GLUTEN-FREE PANTRY

✦ **Beth's All-Purpose Gluten-Free Baking Flour**
  – rice flour, potato starch, tapioca starch, guar gum, salt

GOOD EATZ

✦ **Flour Mix with Xanthan Gum**
  – rice flour, potato starch, tapioca starch, corn starch, chickpea flour, sorghum flour, xanthan gum

HODGSON MILL

✦ **Multi Purpose Baking Mix**
  – whole grain millet flour, whole grain garbanzo flour, whole grain brown rice flour, xanthan gum

KINNIKINNICK

✦ **All-Purpose Celiac Flour**
  – white rice flour, potato starch, tapioca starch, sodium carboxymethylcellulose, guar gum

✦ **All-Purpose Mix**
  – white rice flour, tapioca starch, potato starch, sugar, fructooligosaccharide, gluco delta lactone, dextrose, whole egg powder, sodium bicarbonate, egg white powder, pea fiber, rice bran extract, sodium carboxymethylcellulose, pea protein, salt, fructose

LAUREL'S SWEET TREATS

✦ **Gluten-Free Baking Flour Mix**
  – white rice flour, potato starch, tapioca flour

MISS ROBEN'S

✦ **Bette Hagman's Original Flour Mix**
  – white rice flour, potato starch, tapioca starch

NATURE'S OWN BAKERY

✦ **Baking Mix (All-Purpose)**
  – flaked corn, soy flakes, organic millet meal, organic sunflower seeds, flax meal, garfava flour

ORGRAN

✦ **Plain All-Purpose Flour Mix**
  – maize starch, tapioca flour, rice flour, guar gum, methylcellulose

✦ **Self-Raising Flour**
  – maize starch, tapioca flour, rice flour, glucono delta lactone, sodium bicarbonate, guar gum

✦ **Gluten-Free Gluten Substitute**
  – superfine rice flour, pea extract, maize starch, potato starch, guar gum, methylcellulose, carboxmethylcellulose, monoglycerides

PANNE RIZO

✦ **Gluten-Free Flour Mix**
  – white rice flour, potato starch, tapioca flour OR
    brown rice flour, potato starch, tapioca flour

THE REALLY GREAT FOOD COMPANY

✦ **All-Purpose Rice Flour Mix**
  – white rice flour, potato starch, cornstarch, xanthan gum

THE RUBY RANGE

✦ **All-Purpose Mix**
  – rice flour, mesquite meal, potato starch flour, teff flour, tapioca flour, baking powder, baking soda, salt

All-Purpose Flour Mixes CONT'D.

STERK'S BAKERY
- ✦ **All-Purpose Flour Mix**
  - – brown rice flour, corn flour, guar gum

SYLVAN BORDER FARM
- ✦ **General Purpose Flour Mix**
  - – potato starch, white rice flour, brown rice flour, amaranth flour, quinoa flour, white cornmeal, garbanzo bean flour, soy flour

TOM SAWYER
- ✦ **All-Purpose Gluten-Free Flour**
  - – white rice, sweet rice and tapioca flours, xanthan gum and gelatin

Bean, Chickpea, Lentil and Pea Flours

BETTE'S GOURMET FOUR FLOUR BLEND (garfava flour, sorghum flour, cornstarch, tapioca starch)
- ✦ Authentic Foods
- ✦ Miss Roben's

BLACK BEAN FLOUR
- ✦ Bob's Red Mill

CHICKPEA FLOUR (garbanzo bean flour)
- ✦ Authentic Foods
- ✦ Bob's Red Mill
- ✦ Gifts of Nature
- ✦ Gillian's Foods
- ✦ Northern Quinoa Corporation

EASY WHITE FIBRE MIX (pea fibre, inulin, cellulose)
- ✦ Kinnikinnick

GARBANZO BEAN FLOUR (see chickpea flour)

GARBANZO BEAN FLOUR AND FAVA BEAN FLOUR
- ✦ Authentic Foods (developed original mixture called "Garfava Flour")
- ✦ Bob's Red Mill
- ✦ El Peto
- ✦ Miss Roben's ("Garfava")

GREEN LENTIL FLOUR
- ✦ Northern Quinoa Corporation

GREEN PEA FLOUR
- ✦ Bob's Red Mill
- ✦ Northern Quinoa Corporation

LIMA BEAN FLOUR
- ✦ Gifts of Nature

PEA HULL FIBRE
- ✦ Kinnikinnick

ROMANO BEAN FLOUR (cranberry bean or whole bean)
- ✦ El Peto

WHITE BEAN FLOUR
- ✦ Bob's Red Mill

YELLOW PEA FLOUR
- ✦ Northern Quinoa Corporation
- ✦ Best Cooking Pulses

Flours

ALMOND FLOUR OR ALMOND MEAL
- ✦ Authentic Foods
- ✦ Bob's Red Mill
- ✦ Dowd & Rogers
- ✦ Miss Roben's

AMARANTH FLOUR
- ✦ Bob's Red Mill
- ✦ El Peto
- ✦ Northern Quinoa Corporation
- ✦ Nu-World Amaranth/Nu-World Foods (also carry Toasted Amaranth Bran Flour, Puffed Amaranth, Amaranth Pre-Gel Powder)

ARROWROOT STARCH
- ✦ Authentic Foods
- ✦ Bob's Red Mill
- ✦ El Peto
- ✦ Miss Roben's
- ✦ Nelson David

BUCKWHEAT BRAN
- ✦ Minn-Dak Growers, Ltd. – "Farinetta"

BUCKWHEAT FLOUR
- ✦ Aliments Trigone Inc. (Cream of the Crop)
- ✦ Arrowhead Mills
- ✦ The Birkett Mills
- ✦ Bob's Red Mill
- ✦ Hodgson Mill
- ✦ Minn-Dak Growers, Ltd.
- ✦ Miss Roben's
- ✦ Nelson David

CHESTNUT FLOUR
- ✦ Dowd & Rogers

COCONUT FLOUR
- ✦ Bob's Red Mill
- ✦ Miss Roben's

CORN FLOUR
- ✦ Authentic Foods
- ✦ Bob's Red Mill
- ✦ El Peto
- ✦ Kinnikinnick
- ✦ Nelson David

CORNMEAL
- ✦ Arrowhead Mills
- ✦ Bob's Red Mill
- ✦ El Peto
- ✦ Gifts of Nature
- ✦ Kinnikinnick
- ✦ Native Seeds

CORN GRITS
- ✦ Bob's Red Mill

FLAX SEED MEAL (Ground Flax)
- ✦ Arrowhead Mills
- ✦ Bob's Red Mill
- ✦ CanMar Grain Products Ltd.
- ✦ El Peto
- ✦ Hodgson Mill
- ✦ Miss Roben's
- ✦ Nature's Path
- ✦ Nelson David
- ✦ Omega Nutrition ("Nutri-Flax")

HAZELNUT FLOUR
- ✦ Bob's Red Mill

Flours CONT'D.

Mesquite Flour
- ✦ Casa deFruta
- ✦ Native Seeds
- ✦ The Ruby Range

Millet Flour
- ✦ Arrowhead Mills
- ✦ Bob's Red Mill
- ✦ El Peto
- ✦ Nu-World Amaranth/Nu-World Foods

Montina™ Flour
- ✦ Amazing Grains

Oat Bran (Pure, Uncontaminated)
- ✦ Avena (FarmPure Foods) [Only Oats™]

Oat Flour (Pure, Uncontaminated)
- ✦ Cream Hill Estates (Lara's)
- ✦ Avena (FarmPure Foods) [Only Oats™]

Potato Flour
- ✦ Authentic Foods
- ✦ Bob's Red Mill
- ✦ Club House
- ✦ Duinkerken Foods
- ✦ El Peto
- ✦ Ener-G Foods
- ✦ Gillian's Foods

Potato Starch Flour
- ✦ Authentic Foods
- ✦ Bob's Red Mill
- ✦ 'Cause You're Special!
- ✦ Duinkerken Foods
- ✦ El Peto
- ✦ Ener-G Foods
- ✦ Gifts of Nature
- ✦ Gillian's Foods
- ✦ Gluten-Free Bagel Company
- ✦ Kinnikinnick
- ✦ Manischewitz
- ✦ Miss Roben's
- ✦ Nelson David
- ✦ The Really Great Food Company

Quinoa Flour
- ✦ Ancient Harvest
- ✦ Bob's Red Mill
- ✦ El Peto
- ✦ Northern Quinoa Corporation – "NorQuin" brand
- ✦ Nu-World Amaranth/Nu-World Foods

Rice Bran
- ✦ Bob's Red Mill
- ✦ El Peto
- ✦ Ener-G Foods
- ✦ Kinnikinnick

Rice Flour (Brown)
- ✦ Authentic Foods
- ✦ Bob's Red Mill
- ✦ El Peto
- ✦ Ener-G Foods
- ✦ Gifts of Nature
- ✦ Gillian's Foods
- ✦ Kinnikinnick
- ✦ Lundberg Family Farms
- ✦ Miss Roben's
- ✦ Nelson David
- ✦ The Really Great Food Company

Rice Flour (Sweet)
- ✦ Authentic Foods
- ✦ Bob's Red Mill
- ✦ El Peto
- ✦ Ener-G Foods
- ✦ Gifts of Nature
- ✦ Kinnikinnick
- ✦ Lundberg
- ✦ Miss Roben's
- ✦ The Really Great Food Company

Flours CONT'D.

RICE FLOUR (White)
- ✦ Arrowhead Mills
- ✦ Authentic Foods
- ✦ Bob's Red Mill
- ✦ 'Cause You're Special!
- ✦ Club House
- ✦ Duinkerken Foods
- ✦ El Peto
- ✦ Ener-G Foods
- ✦ Gifts of Nature
- ✦ Gillian's Foods
- ✦ Gluten-Free Bagel Company
- ✦ Gluten-Free Pantry
- ✦ Kinnikinnick
- ✦ Miss Roben's
- ✦ Nelson David
- ✦ The Really Great Food Company

SORGHUM FLOUR
- ✦ Authentic Foods
- ✦ Bob's Red Mill
- ✦ El Peto
- ✦ Miss Roben's
- ✦ Nu-World Amaranth/Nu-World Foods
- ✦ Twin Valley Mills

SOY FLOUR
- ✦ Arrowhead Mills
- ✦ Eden Foods
- ✦ El Peto
- ✦ Kinnikinnick
- ✦ Nelson David

TAPIOCA STARCH FLOUR
- ✦ Authentic Foods
- ✦ Bob's Red Mill
- ✦ 'Cause You're Special!
- ✦ Duinkerken Foods
- ✦ Edward & Son's Trading Co.
- ✦ El Peto
- ✦ Ener-G Foods
- ✦ Gifts of Nature
- ✦ Gillian's Foods
- ✦ Gluten-Free Bagel Company
- ✦ Kinnikinnick
- ✦ Miss Roben's
- ✦ Nelson David
- ✦ The Really Great Food Company

TEFF FLOUR
- ✦ Bob's Red Mill
- ✦ Nu-World Amaranth/Nu-World Foods
- ✦ The Ruby Range
- ✦ The Teff Company

NOTE: Gluten-Free Bakeries, Specialty Stores and Distributors and health food stores (see pages 321 to 338) also carry many of the flours from the companies listed above.

GRAINS

AMARANTH
- ✦ Arrowhead Mills
- ✦ Bob's Red Mill
- ✦ El Peto
- ✦ GoGo Quinoa
- ✦ Inca Organics
- ✦ Native Seeds
- ✦ Northern Quinoa Corporation
- ✦ Nu-World Amaranth/Nu-World Foods
- ✦ Shiloh Farms

Grains CONT'D.

BUCKWHEAT (Whole Groats, Roasted Groats [Kasha], or Grits)

- ✦ Arrowhead Mills
- ✦ The Birkett Mills
- ✦ Bob's Red Mill
- ✦ Eden Foods
- ✦ Minn-Dak Growers, Ltd.
- ✦ Northern Quinoa Corporation
- ✦ Shiloh Farms

FLAX (Whole Seed or Ground, Milled Meal)

- ✦ Arrowhead Mills
- ✦ Bob's Red Mill
- ✦ CanMar Grain Products Ltd.
- ✦ El Peto
- ✦ Gluten-Free Pantry
- ✦ Hodgson Mill
- ✦ Nature's Path
- ✦ Nelson David
- ✦ Northern Quinoa Corporation
- ✦ Omega Nutrition

MILLET

- ✦ Arrowhead Mills
- ✦ Bob's Red Mill
- ✦ Eden Foods
- ✦ El Peto
- ✦ Northern Quinoa Corporation
- ✦ Shiloh Farms

OATS (Gluten-Free, Pure Uncontaminated)

- ✦ Bob's Red Mill
- ✦ Cream Hill Estates (Lara's)
- ✦ Avena (FarmPure Foods) [Only Oats™]
- ✦ Gifts of Nature
- ✦ Gluten-Free Oats®

QUINOA (Golden or Black Seed)

- ✦ Ancient Harvest
- ✦ Arrowhead Mills
- ✦ Bob's Red Mill
- ✦ Eden Foods
- ✦ El Peto
- ✦ GoGo Quinoa
- ✦ Inca Organics
- ✦ Northern Quinoa Corporation – "NorQuin" brand
- ✦ Shiloh Farms

SORGHUM (GRAIN)

- ✦ Shiloh Farms
- ✦ Twin Valley Mills

TEFF (GRAIN)

- ✦ Bob's Red Mill
- ✦ Shiloh Farms
- ✦ The Teff Company

PASTAS

✦ Some "**wheat-free**" pastas are made from **kamut** or **spelt** and are **NOT** gluten-free.

✦ Some buckwheat pastas contain buckwheat flour and **wheat flour** and are **NOT** gluten-free.

✦ Gluten-free pastas are made from amaranth, corn, legumes, potato, quinoa, rice or soy. However, check ingredient labels to make sure that no **wheat**, **spelt** or **kamut** has been added to these gluten-free ingredients.

Company	Pasta		Grams	Ounces
ALLERGAROO	Pasta Dinners*	Chili Mac, Spyglass Noodles, Spaghetti	227	8
	*Ready-made in microwavable pouch. Dairy and Soy-Free.			

Company	Pasta		Grams	Ounces
ANCIENT HARVEST	Elbows, Garden Pagodas, Linguine, Rotelle, Shells, Spaghetti, Veggie Curls		227 g, 4.5 kg	8 oz., 10 lbs.
	Quinoa and corn flour pasta.			
ANDEAN DREAM	**Quinoa Pasta***	Fusilli, Macaroni, Spaghetti	227	8
	*Made from organic quinoa and rice flours.			
ANNIE CHUN'S	**Rice Noodles**	Maifun	227	8
	PAD THAI RICE NOODLES	Original	227	8
ANNIE'S HOMEGROWN	Gluten-Free Rice Pasta & Cheddar Macaroni & Cheese		170	6
	White rice pasta.			
BARKAT	**Buckwheat Pasta***	Penne, Spirals	250	8.8
	*Also contains corn and rice flours.			
	Corn Pasta	Animal, Alphabet, Macaroni, Tagliatelle, Spaghetti, Spirals	500	17.6
BI-AGLUT	**PastaMia** Bucatini, Ditalini, Fusilli, Linguine, Maccheroncini, Penne, Pipe, Rigatoni, Sedani, Spaghetti		500	17.6
	Maize (corn) starch, potato and lupin flour.			
	Gemmine, Micron, Stelline		250	8.8
	Maize (corn) starch, potato and lupin flour.			
	Lasagna**, Tagliatelle*		250	8.8
	Sedani*		500	17.6
	* Maize (corn) and tapioca starch, eggs, milk protein, carrot pulp, carob seed flour. ** Maize (corn) starch, eggs, potato flour, milk protein.			
	Fusilli, Penne, Spaghetti		500	17.6
	Tagliatelle		250	8.8
	Maize (corn) and milk protein.			
BIONATURAE	Elbows, Fusilli, Penne, Spaghetti		340	12
	Organic pasta made with rice, potato & soy.			
CELIMIX	Brown Rice Elbows, Shells, Spaghetti		350	12.3
DE BOLES	Corn Elbows		340	12
	Corn Spaghetti		227	8
	Multi Grain*	Penne, Spaghetti	226	8
	*Brown rice, white rice, rice bran, amaranth flour, quinoa flour. Enriched with thiamin, niacin, riboflavin, iron and folic acid.			
	Rice	Angel Hair, Fettuccine, Penne, Spaghetti, Spirals	227	8
	Rice	Lasagna	284	10
	Rice Plus Golden Flax*	Angel Hair, Spirals	226	8
	*Enriched with thiamin, niacin, riboflavin, iron and folic acid.			
	GF Rice Shells & Cheddar		206	7.25
	GF Rice Elbow Style Pasta & Cheese		206	7.25
DIETARY SPECIALTIES	Elbows, Porridge, Spaghetti, Spirals		500	17.6

Company	Pasta		Grams	Ounces
EDEN FOODS	Bifun (Rice Pasta)		100	3.5
	Harusame (Mung Bean Pasta)		70	2.4
	Kuzu Pasta		100	3.5
ENER-G FOODS	**White Rice**	Lasagna, Macaroni, Small Shells	454	16
		Spaghetti	446	15.8
		Vermicelli	298	10.5
GILLIAN'S FOODS	Fettucini, Fusilli, Penne, Spaghetti		454	16
	Rice, Rice Bran.			
GLUTEN FREE & FABULOUS	**Quinoa Pasta**	Macaroni & Cheese, Quinoa with Marinara	185	6.5
GOGO QUINOA	**Amaranth Pasta**	Penne	227	8
	Quinoa Pasta	Fusilli, Macaroni, Spaghetti	227	8
HODGSON MILL	**GF Brown Rice Pasta***	Angel Hair, Elbows, Lasagna, Linguine, Penne, Spaghetti	227	8
	*Brown rice flour and golden milled flaxseed.			
LE VENEZIANE	Anellini, Ditalini, Eliche, Fettucce, Penne Rigate, Pipe Rigate		250	8.8
	Spaghetti		500	17.6
	*Corn-based pasta (corn flour or cornmeal).			
LUNDBERG	**Organic Brown Rice Pasta**	Elbow, Penne	340	12
		Rotini, Spaghetti	284	10
MRS. LEEPER'S	**Brown Rice Pasta**	Alphabets, Elbows*, Penne*, Kids Shapes, Spaghetti, Vegetable Twists	340	12
	Corn Pasta	Elbows*, Rotelli, Spaghetti, Vegetable Radiatore	340	12
	Pasta & Sauce Mixes**	Beef Lasagna (corn lasagna)	182	6.4
		Beef Stroganoff (rice pasta)	210	7.4
		Cheeseburger Mac (rice pasta)	236	8.3
		Chicken Alfredo (rice pasta)	200	7
		Creamy Tuna (corn lasagna)	210	7.4
		Mac & Cheese (rice pasta)	323	11.6
	*Available in bulk. **Serve as a side dish or meal. Ready in 5 minutes.			
NAMASTE FOODS	Say Cheez Pasta Meal (Dairy/Casein-Free)		255	9
	Pisavera Pasta Meal		255	9
	Taco Shells Pasta Meal		248	8.75
	Rice pasta and seasoning packet.			
NORTHERN QUINOA CORPORATION	Elbows		340	12
	Spaghetti		454	16
	Spirals		227	8
	Organic brown rice & quinoa pasta sold as "Norquin".			
ORGRAN	**Gourmet Corn Pasta**	Corn & Vegetable Shells, Corn & Vegetable Spirals,	250	8.8
	Gourmet Rice Pasta	Garlic & Parsley Rice Shells, Rice Pasta Spirals, Vegetable Rice Penne, Vegetable Rice Spirals	250	8.8

Company	Pasta		Grams	Ounces
ORGRAN	Gourmet Rice & Corn Pasta	Rice & Corn Vegetable Animal Shapes, Rice & Corn Rison Garlic Herb	200	7
	Essential Fibre*	Penne, Spirals	250	8.8
		*Brown rice flour, cornmeal, resistant cornstarch, rice bran, psyllium.		
	Multigrain Pasta	Multigrain with Amaranth Spirals*, Multigrain with Quinoa Penne**	250	8.8
		*Corn, rice, millet, amaranth. **Corn, rice, millet, quinoa.		
	Ris O Mais*	Macaroni, Penne, Spirals, Tortelli	250	8.8
		Mini Lasagna Sheets	200	7
		Spaghetti Noodles	375	13.3
		*Rice & corn pasta.		
	Stoneground Pasta	Buckwheat Spirals, Rice & Millet Spirals	250	8.8
	Pasta and Sauce (Canned)	Alternative Grain Pasta Meal	420	14.8
		Spaghetti in Tomato Sauce	220	7.8
		Spirals in Sauce	218	7.7
	Pasta & Sauce Tomato Basil		120	4.2
PASTAMAIZA	Corn Pasta Elbows, Penne, Spaghetti, Vege Radiatore		454	16
PASTARISO	All-Natural Brown Rice*	Elbows, Penne, Rotini, Spaghetti, Vegetable Rotini	454	16
	Organic Brown Rice*	Angel Hair, Elbows, Fettucini, Lasagna, Linguine, Penne, Rotini, Vegetable Rotini, Shells, Spaghetti, Spinach Spaghetti, Vermicelli	227	8
	Rice Pasta & Cheese Dinners	Rice Mac & White Cheddar, Rice Mac & Yellow Cheddar	168	6
		Rice Mini Shells & White Cheddar, Rice Mini Shells & Yellow Cheddar	142	5
		White Rice Mac & Yellow Cheddar	168	6
	*Most shapes available in bulk.			
PASTATO	Fortified Potato Pasta*	Elbows, Penne, Spaghetti	284	10
	Cheese Dinners	Potato Mac & White Cheddar, Potato Mac & Yellow Cheddar	168	6
		Potato Mini Shells & White Cheddar, Potato Mini Shells & Yellow Cheddar	142	5
	*Potato flour, white rice flour, quinoa flour, ground flax, psyllium husks, FOS (prebiotic) Vitamins B_1, B_2, B_3, B_6, folic acid, pantothenic acid, iron, magnesium.			
RIZOPIA	Brown Rice	Elbows*, Fettuccine*, Fusilli*, Penne*, Shells*, Spaghetti*, Spinach Brown Rice, Spirals*	454	16
		Lasagne	340	12
	*Available in bulk.			

Company	Pasta		Grams	Ounces
RIZOPIA	Brown Rice (organic)	Elbows*, Fantasia, Fettuccine*, Fusilli*, Penne*, Spaghetti*	454	16
	Spinach Brown Rice Spaghetti*		454	16
	Vegetable Brown Rice Fusilli*		454	16
	White Rice	Spaghetti*	454	16
	Wild Rice (organic)	Elbows*, Fusilli*, Penne*, Radiatore*, Shells*, Spaghetti*	454	16
	*Available in bulk.			
ROAD'S END ORGANICS	GF Cheddar Penne & Cheese*, GF Alfredo Mac & Cheese*		170	6
	*Dairy-Free.			
SCHÄR	Anellini, Fusilli, Multigrain Penne, Penne, Spaghetti, Tagliatelle		340	12
THAI KITCHEN	Dry Rice Noodles	Stir-Fry Rice	397	14
		Thin Rice	250	8.8
	Stir-Fry Rice Noodles with Sauce	Lemongrass & Chili	150	5.3
		Original Pad Thai	255	9.0
		Pad Thai with Chili	170	6.0
		Thai Peanut	156	5.5
	NOODLE CARTS	Pad Thai, Thai Peanut, Roasted Garlic, Toasted Sesame	64	2.25
	Take Out Meals*	Ginger and Sweet Chili, Original Pad Thai, Thai Basil and Chili	167	5.9
	*Microwavable rice noodles with sauce.			
TINKYADA	Elbows*, Fusilli*, Penne*, Shells*, Spaghetti*, Spirals*		454	16
	Grand Shells*		227	8
	Lasagna* or Lasagna**		280	10
	Spinach Rice Spaghetti*, Vegetable Rice Spirals*		340	12
	Elbows**, Penne**, Spaghetti**, Spirals**		340	12
	Spaghetti***		454	16
	Fettuccini*, Little Dreams*		397	14
	*Brown rice with rice bran. **Organic brown rice. ***White rice. All pasta available in bulk 4.54 kg (10 lbs.).			

ENTRÉES AND SIDE DISHES

Company	Entrées & Side Dishes	Grams	Ozs.	Serves
ALLERGYFREE FOODS	Chicken Filets*	340	12	NA
	Chicken Tenderloins*	453	16	NA
	Chicken Nuggets*	679	24	NA
	Chicken Wings*	566	20	NA
	*Casein, Egg, Nut and Soy-Free.			

Company	Entrées & Side Dishes		Grams	Ozs.	Serves
ALPINEAIRE FOODS	Brown Rice (Instant)		57, 227	2, 8	2, 8
	Chicken Gumbo		156	5.6	2
	Mountain Chili		170, 340	6, 12	2, 4
	Santa Fe Black Beans & Rice		184	6.5	2
	Note: Also have many other products that are gluten-free.				
AMY'S KITCHEN	Asian Meals (Stir-Frys)	Asian Noodle Stir-Fry*	284	10	
		Thai Stir-Fry*	269	9.5	
	Bowls	Baked Ziti*, Mexican Casserole, Mexican Casserole (light in sodium), Teriyaki*, Tortilla Casserole & Black Beans	269	9.5	
		Brown Rice & Vegetables*, Brown Rice & Vegetables (light in sodium)*, Santa Fe Enchilada	283	10	
		Brown Rice/Black-Eyed Peas & Veggies*	255	9	
	Organic Chilies	Black Bean*, Medium*, Medium (light in sodium)*, Medium with Vegetables*, Spicy*, Spicy (light in sodium)*, Southwestern Black Bean*	416	14.7	
	Enchiladas	Black Bean Vegetable*, Black Bean Vegetable (light in sodium)*	269	9.5	
		Black Bean Whole Meal*	284	10	
		Cheese	255	9	
		Cheese Whole Meal	255	9	
	Indian Meals	Mattar Paneer (reg & light in sodium)	284	10	
		Mattar Tofu*	269	9.5	
		Palak Paneer	284	10	
		Paneer Tikka	269	9.5	
		Vegetable Korma*	269	9.5	
	Miscellaneous	Baked Ziti Kids Meals*	227	8	
		Bistro Burger*	284	10	
		Black Bean Tamale Verde*	291	10.3	
		Cheese Tamale Verde*	291	10.3	
		Garden Vegetable Lasagna	291	10.3	
		Mexican Tamale Pie*	227	8	
		Rice Crust Cheese Pizza	340	12.0	
		Rice Crust Spinach Pizza*	397	14	
		Rice Mac & Cheese	255	9	
		Roasted Vegetable Tamale*	323	11.4	
		Shepherd's Pie*	227	8	
		Shepherd's Pie (light in sodium)*	227	8	
		Non-Dairy Rice Crust Pizza*	170	6	
		Tofu Scramble (Plain*, Mexican)	255	9	
	*Dairy-Free.				

Company	Entrées & Side Dishes		Grams	Ozs.	Serves
ANDREA'S FINE FOODS	**Pizza** (6" Individual)	Cheese, Sausage, Pepperoni, Veggi	198	7	1
	Pizza (12" Large)	Cheese, Canadian Bacon, Pepperoni, Sausage, Veggi	764	27	–
	Pizza cannot be shipped. Available in store only.				
ANNIE CHUN'S	**RICE EXPRESS***	Black Pearl Rice, Multigrain Rice, Sprouted Brown Rice	178	6.3	
		Sticky White Rice	209	7.4	
	*Microwavable and ready in 1 minute.				
APETITO	**Special Diet Frozen Entrées** (Indivdual Complete Meals)	Apple Braised Pork*	300	10.6	1
		Beef and Vegetable Casserole*	275	10	1
		Country Chicken with Gravy	285	10	1
		Lemon Herbed Fish	245	8.7	1
		Pot Roast with Rice & Peas*	255	9	1
		Sweet & Sour Hawaiian Chicken*	310	11	1
		Turkey with Gravy	270	9.5	1
	Portioned into a 3-compartment tray. *Also available in 250 g (8.8 oz) foil container with the protein portion only and no side dishes.				
	Special Diet Frozen Entrées (Bulk)**	Apple Braised Pork, Beef & Vegetable Casserole, Sweet & Sour Hawaiian Chicken, Turkey with Gravy	1 kg	35.3	
		Pot Roast with Rice & Peas	1.3 kg	45.9	
	**Available in foil trays.				
CELIAC SPECIALTIES	Lasagna		454	16	
	Mac & Cheese		227	8	
	Pizza – cheese (10")		679	24	
	Pizza – cheese (individual)		227	8	
	Pot Pies	Beef Flavored, Chicken Flavored	454	16	
CHOICES BEST RICE BAKERY	Spinach & Onion Quiche		275	9.7	
	Veggie Pot Pie		NA	NA	
DIETARY SPECIALTIES	**Entrées**	Linguini with Meat Sauce	454	16	
		Potato, Onion & Cheese Pierogies	454	16	
		Potato & Onion Pierogies	454	16	
		Spaghetti & Meatballs	454	16	
	Filled Pasta	Cheese Ravioli, Meat Ravioli*, Spinach & Cheese Ravioli, Stuffed Shells & Tomato Sauce	454	16	
	Pizza	Cheese (8")	340	12	3
	*Casein-Free.				
DR. PRAEGER'S	GF California Veggie Burger		312	11	4
	GF Potato Crusted Filet Fish Sticks		368	13	14 pcs.
	GF Potato Crusted Fish Fillets		340	12	6 pcs.
	GF Potato Crusted Fishies		340	12	25 pcs.
	GF Potato Littles	Broccoli, Potato, Spinach, Sweet Potato	340	12	
	GF Sweet Potato Pancakes		382	13.5	6 pcs.

Company	Entrées & Side Dishes		Grams	Ozs.	Serves
EVERYBODY EATS	Pizza – Tomato Mozzarella (11")		908	2 lbs.	2
	Ravioli	Beef, Chicken*, Cheese, Spinach-Ricotta	454	1 lb.	
	*Dairy-Free.				
FOODS BY GEORGE	Lasagna		340	12	
	Pizza (Cheese)		255	9	1
gf MEALS	**Entrées***	American Turkey Meatloaf	NA	NA	2-4
		Asian Style Orange Chicken	NA	NA	2
		Autumn Chicken	NA	NA	2
		Bombay Beef Curry	NA	NA	2
		Chicken Tenders	454	1 lb.	2-4
		Greek Chicken and Rice	NA	NA	2
		Home-Run Slider Burgers	NA	NA	2-4
		Macaroni & Beef	NA	NA	2-4
		Make Your Own Pizza Kit (4 mini pizzas)	NA	NA	2-4
		Maple Blueberry Chicken Sausage	NA	NA	2-4
		Meatballs	454	1 lb.	2-3
		No Soy Mac & Cheese	NA	NA	2-3
		Turkey Breakfast Sausage Patties	NA	NA	2-4
		Turkey Burger Macaroni	NA	NA	2
		Turkey Burger Patties	NA	NA	2-4
		Turkey Chili with White Beans	NA	NA	2
		Turkey Meatballs	454	1 lb.	2-3
	*All are Casein-Free.				
GLUTEN FREE & FABULOUS	**Pizza**	Cheese, Pepperoni, Pesto Margherita, Spinach Feta, Vegetable Margherita	283	10	
GLUTINO	**GF Frozen Chicken Entrées**	Chicken Pad Thai*	200	7.1	1
		Chicken Ranchero*, Chicken Penne Alfredo, Chicken Pomodoro	260	9.2	1
	Mac & Cheese (3 cheese)		300	10.6	1
	Penne Alfredo		300	10.6	1
	Pizza	Pizza Duo Cheese, Spinach Feta	175	6.2	1
	Brown Rice Pizza Crust	BBQ Chicken, Spinach Soy Cheese, 3 Cheese	176	6.2	1
	*Dairy-Free				
GLUTENFREEDA FOODS	**Burritos**	Breakfast, Chicken & Cheese, Vegetarian Bean & Cheese, Vegetarian & Dairy-Free*	113	4	1
	*Dairy-Free				

Company	Entrées & Side Dishes		Grams	Ozs.	Serves
IAN'S NATURAL FOODS	**Breakfast***	WFGF French Toast Sticks	284	10	
	Fish*	WFGF Battered Fish	200	7	
		WFGF Fish Sticks	227	8	
	Chicken*	WFGF Chicken Nuggets	227	8	
		WFGF Chicken Patties	200	7	
		WFGF Chicken Finger Meal	200	7	
	Turkey*	WFGF Popcorn Turkey Corndogs	227	8	
	Pasta*	WFGF Mac and No Cheese	227	8	
		WFGF Mac and Meat Sauce	227	8	
	Pizza*	WFGF French Bread Pizza with Soy Cheese	227	8	
	Miscellaneous*	WFGF Alphatots	340	12	
	Shelf-Stable	WFGF Pasta Kit	452	16	
		WFGF Pizza Kit	508	18	

*Frozen. Frozen and Shelf-Stable products are Casein and Egg-Free.

Company	Entrées & Side Dishes		Grams	Ozs.	Serves
LUNDBERG	**Brown Rice Couscous**	Plain	284	10	1
		Mediterranean Curry, Roasted Garlic & Olive Oil	198	7	1
		Savory Herb	193	6.8	1
	Heat & Eat Organic Brown Rice Bowls	Countrywild, Long Grain, Short Grain	210	7.4	1

Note: Sesame Teriyaki contains wheat and is not gluten-free.
Microwave. Ready to eat in 90 seconds.

	Risottos: Eco-Farmed	Butternut Squash	164	5.8	4
		Cheddar Broccoli	167	5.9	4
		Creamy Parmesan, Garlic Primavera, Italian Herb	156	5.5	4
	Risottos: Organic	Alfredo	156	5.5	4
		Florentine, Tuscan	163	5.75	4
		Porcini Mushroom	167	5.9	4

Company	Entrées & Side Dishes	Grams	Ozs.	Serves
MANISCHEWITZ	Lentil Pilaf Mix	191	6.75	4
MARSAN FOODS	**Balanced Cuisine Single Serve Meals** (12 trays/case)			
	Beef Strips*	250	8.8	
	Chicken Korma	325	11.5	
	Country Chicken Casserole	250	8.8	
	Pork Goulash	325	11.7	
	Rotisserie Style Chicken with Vegetables*	300	10.6	
	Shepherd's Pie (regular)*	325	11.5	
	Tilapia Almondine	275	11.5	
	Tilapia Mediterranean	325	11.5	
	Vegan Chana Masala*	275	9.7	
	Vegan Shepherd's Pie*	325	11.5	
	Western Omelet	250	8.8	
	Balanced Cuisine Entrées & Sides (Bulk) (4x2 kg pouches)			
	Beef Stew*, Beef Chili*, Chicken Cacciatore*, Rice Pilaf*, Plain Rice*, Vegan Chana Masala*, Vegan Tuscan Bean*	2 kg	70.7	

*Dairy-Free.

Company	Entrées & Side Dishes		Grams	Ozs.	Serves
MY OWN MEALS	Beef Stew, Chicken & Black Beans, Mediterranean Chicken, My Kind of Chicken, Old World Stew		283	10	1
	Casein-Free. Fully cooked meals – heat and serve.				
NATURE'S HILIGHTS	Rice Crust Pizza (Soy Cheese Style)		312	11	2
NU-WORLD AMARANTH	Amaranth Side Serves	Garlic-Herb, Savory-Herb, Spanish Tomato	75	2.63	
THE ORGANIC BISTRO	Frozen Whole Meals	Chicken Citron*	298	10.5	
		Ginger Chicken*	305	10.75	
		Jamaican Shrimp Cakes*	298	10.5	
		Pasta Putanesca*	312	11	
		Savory Turkey	312	11	
		Sockeye Salmon Cakes*	284	10	
		Spiced Chicken Morocco*	298	10.5	
		Wild Salmon*	292	10.3	
	*Dairy-Free.				
PANNE RIZO	Macaroni and Cheese		390	13.8	1
	Mini Pizzola	Various flavors	200	7	1
	Panini	Tuna Melt	310	11	1
		Oven Roasted Turkey	225	8	1
	Pot Pies	Chicken, Tomato Vegetable	300	10.6	1
PURFOODS/ FRESH STARTS GLUTEN-FREE MEALS (Available April 2010)	Omelettes	Denver Style with Turkey Ham & Potatoes	NA	NA	NA
		Vegetable	NA	NA	NA
		Western Style with Turkey Ham & Potatoes	NA	NA	NA
	Miscellaneous Breakfast	Breakfast Skillet with Turkey Ham & Scrambled Egg*	NA	NA	NA
		Buckwheat Banana & Walnut Pancakes with Honey & Turkey Sausage	NA	NA	NA
		Ranch Skillet with Scrambled Eggs & Cheddar Cheese	NA	NA	NA
		Southwestern Skillet (Scrambled Eggs, Salsa & Cheddar Cheese)	NA	NA	NA
		Banana Chocolate Almond Shake & Pumpkin Seeds*	NA	NA	NA
	Beef	Chili Rub Beef Steak with Candied Sweet Potatoes, Sauteed Vegetables and Feta Cheese	NA	NA	NA
		Beef Chili Tostada with Salsa	NA	NA	NA
		Herb Rubbed Beef Steak with Quinoa Loaf & Sauteed Carrots*	NA	NA	NA
		London Broil with Butternut Squash, Mashed Potatoes, Asparagus & Pesto	NA	NA	NA
	Fish	Baked Cod with Thyme & Black Bean Salad*	NA	NA	NA
	*Dairy-Free.				

Company	Entrées & Side Dishes		Grams	Ozs.	Serves
PURFOODS/ FRESH STARTS GLUTEN-FREE MEALS	Poultry	Chicken Vesuvio (Chicken Breast with New Potatoes & Peas)*	NA	NA	NA
		Grilled Chicken Breast with Herb Potatoes & Broccoli*	NA	NA	NA
		Lemon Herb Chicken with Wild Rice & Broccoli	NA	NA	NA
		Lemon Herb Chicken Breast with Roasted Red Potatoes and Green Beans with Peppers*	NA	NA	NA
		Oven Roasted Turkey with Savory Sweet Potatoes & Gingered Carrots/Onions*	NA	NA	NA
		Turkey Bolognese over Rice Noodles	NA	NA	NA
		Vegetable Ratatouille with Baked Chicken Breast*	NA	NA	NA
	Pork	Port Ragout with Spicy Roasted Vegetables & Baked Sweet Potato*	NA	NA	NA
		Roasted Pork Loin, Candied Sweet Potatoes & Gingered Carrots/Onions	NA	NA	NA
	Salads	BBQ Chicken w/Tomato & Zucchini Salad*	NA	NA	NA
		Grilled Turkey & Wild Rice Salad*	NA	NA	NA
		Quinoa & Garbanzo Salad with Moroccan Carrots*	NA	NA	NA
	Vegetarian	3 Bean Vegetarian Chili with Quinoa Loaf & Sauteed Carrots	NA	NA	NA
		Vegetable Curry with Chick Peas & Brown Rice*	NA	NA	NA
		Vegetarian Red Beans & Rice*	NA	NA	NA
	*Dairy-Free.				
RICE EXPRESSIONS	Precooked Frozen Rice (organic)	Brown Rice, Long Grain Rice, Thai Jasmine	852	30	Three packages/box.
		Brown Rice Pilaf, Tex Mex Rice	568	20	Two packages/box.
TASTE ADVENTURE	Quick Cuisine "Entrées"	Black Beans & Rice Santa Fe Fiesta	170	6	4
		Lentil & Rice Bombay Curry	170	6	4
		Louisiana Red Bean Jambalaya	170	6	4
	Quick Cooking Chilies	Black Bean, Five Bean, Lentil, Red Bean	156	5.5	2
THAI KITCHEN	Jasmine Rice Mixes	Lemongrass & Ginger, Roasted Garlic & Chili, Spicy Thai Chili, Thai Yellow Curry	198	7	
		Sweet Chili & Onion	227	8	

SOUPS

✦ Most canned soups are **NOT** gluten-free as they contain **wheat flour, barley, noodles,** hydrolyzed plant or vegetable protein (**HPP** or **HVP**) made from **wheat**.

✦ Bouillon cubes and soup broths often contain **wheat flour** or **HPP** or **HVP** made from wheat and are **NOT** gluten-free.

✦ Soup stock can be made from meat or poultry bones and a variety of vegetables.

Company	Soups		Grams	Ounces
ALPINEAIRE FOODS	Cream of Broccoli, Creamy Potato Cheddar, Kernel's Corn Chowder		various	
AMY'S KITCHEN	Organic Canned Soups	Black Bean Vegetable*	411	14.5
		Chunky Tomato Bisque (reg; light sodium)	411	14.5
		Chunky Vegetable*	405	14.3
		Cream of Tomato (reg; light sodium)	411	14.5
		Curried Lentil*	411	14.5
		Fire Roasted Southwestern Vegetable*	405	14.3
		Lentil (reg; light sodium)*	411	14.5
		Lentil Vegetable (reg; light sodium)*	411	14.5
		Split Pea (reg; light sodium)*	400	14.1
		Summer Corn & Vegetable	411	14.5
		Thai Coconut*	400	14.1
		Tuscan Bean & Rice*	400	14.1
	*Dairy-Free.			
CELIFIBR	Soup Base	Vegetarian Beef, Vegetarian Chicken, French Onion Vegetable Medley	454	1 lb.
	Soup Cubes*	Vegetarian Beef, Vegetarian Chicken, Vegetable Medley	60	2
	*6 cubes/box.			
CELINAL FOODS	GFDF Broth Mixes*	Beef, Chicken	6	0.2
		*Single serve mixes. Dairy-Free.		
COOK IN THE KITCHEN	Dried Soup Mixes	Harvest Garden Vegetable	156	5.5
		Mediterranean Lentil Soup	156	5.5
		Dilled Tomato	156	5.5
		Welsh Potato	156	5.5
CUISINE SANTÉ	Stock*	Beef Flavored**, Chicken**, Vegetable**	908	2 lbs.
		*1 can yields 16 gallons. 12 cans/case. **Also available in low sodium.		
	Soup Mix*	Sweet Corn, Tomato	849	30 oz. cans
		*1 can yields 2.5 gallons. 12 cans/case.		
	Note: Stock and Soup Mixes are free of Gluten, Casein, Egg, Nut, Soy and MSG.			
EDWARD & SON'S TRADING CO.	Miso-Cup (Organic Instant)	Japanese Restaurant Style	82	2.9
		Organic Reduced Sodium	29	1.0
		Organic Traditional with Tofu	36	1.3
		Original Golden	70	2.5
		Savory Seaweed	70	2.5
EL PETO	Soup Concentrates* (Dry Mixes)	Beef Broth, Onion, Tomato, Tomato Vegetable	300	10.6
		Chicken Broth, Vegetable	280	9.9
	*Dairy-Free.			

Company	Soups		Grams	Ounces
GoGo Quinoa	**Quinoa Instant Soup**	Quinoa Cream*, Quinoa & Vegetable*	130	4.6
	*Dairy-Free. Cooks in 3 minutes.			
Imagine	**Garden Natural Creamy Soups***	Broccoli, Butternut Squash, Portobello Mushroom**, Potato Leek, Corn & Lemongrass, Tomato, Tomato Basil	473, 946 mL	16, 32
		Acorn Squash & Mango, Sweet Pea, Sweet Potato	946 mL	32
	*All soups are Dairy-Free. **All soups are organic except Portobello Mushroom.			
	Organic Cooking Stocks	Beef*, Chicken*, Vegetable*	946 mL	32
	Organic Garden Natural Broths	Beef*, Free Range Chicken*, Vegetable*	946 mL	32
		No Chicken	946 mL	32
	*Also available in low sodium.			
Kettle Cuisine	**Gluten-Free Frozen Soup**	Angus Beef Steak Chili with Beans*, Chicken Soup with Rice Noodles*, Chicken Chili with White Beans, Grilled Chicken & Corn Chowder, New England Clam Chowder, Organic Carrot & Corriander*, Organic Mushroom & Potato, Roasted Vegetable*, Three Bean Chili*, Tomato Soup with Garden Vegetables*	283	10
	*Dairy-Free. All soups are packed in a microwavable bowl.			
Manischewitz	**Borscht**	Clear, No Sodium, Reduced Sodium, Reduced Calorie, Shredded Beets	936	33
	Schav		936	33
Marsan Foods	**Balanced Cuisine** (4 x 2 kg pouches)	Country Vegetable*, Cream of Carrot, Cream of Cauliflower, French Onion*, Turkey Rice*	2 kg	70.7
	*Dairy-Free.			
Orgran	Garden Vegetable Soup for Cup		24	0.8
	Tomato Soup for Cup		36	1.3
	Soups are Dairy-Free. 2 soup packets per box.			

Company	Soups		Grams	Ounces
PACIFIC FOODS	Broths	Beef*, Free Range Chicken*	946 mL	32
	Organic Broths	Free Range Chicken*, Vegetable*	240, 946 mL	8, 32
		Beef*, Mushroom*	946 mL	32
		Low Sodium Chicken*	240, 946 mL	8, 32
		Low Sodium Beef*, Low Sodium Vegetable*	946 mL	32
	Organic Concentrated Broths (Foodservice)	Chicken*, Vegetable*	946 mL	32
	Organic Condensed Soups	Cream of Celery, Cream of Chicken, Cream of Mushroom	340 mL	12
	All Natural Soups	Cashew Carrot Ginger*, Curried Red Lentil* Spicy Black Bean*	454, 946 mL	16, 32
		Chipotle Sweet Potato, Rosemary Potato, Thai Sweet Potato*	500 mL	17.6
	All Natural Soups (Organic)	Creamy Butternut Squash*, Creamy Roasted Red Pepper & Tomato, Creamy Tomato, French Onion	454, 946 mL	16, 32
	All Natural Soups Light Sodium (Organic)	Creamy Butternut Squash*, Creamy Tomato, Creamy Roasted Red Pepper & Tomato	946 mL	32
	Artisian Inspired Soups (Organic)	Savory Chicken & Wild Rice*, Savory White Bean with Bacon, Spicy Chicken Fajita*, Split Pea with Bacon & Swiss Cheese	411	14.5
	*Dairy-Free.			
SAVORY CHOICE	Broth Concentrates (Consumers)*	Beef, Chicken, Turkey, Vegetable	12	0.4
	*Available in a 12 gram stick pouch (12 in a package). Contains 770 mg sodium/serving.			
	Reduced Sodium Broth Concentrates (Consumers)*	Beef, Chicken, Vegetable	9.6	0.34
	*Available in a 9.6 gram stick pouch (4 in a package). Contains 360 mg sodium/serving.			
	Broth Concentrates (Foodservice)*	Beef, Chicken, Turkey, Veal, Vegan (beef type), Vegan (chicken type), Vegetable	4.5 L	152
	*Available in 4.5 litre Bag-in-Box. Each box makes 27-29 gallons of single strength broth. Contains 770 mg sodium/serving.			

Company	Soups		Grams	Ounces
SAVORY CHOICE	Clean & Healthy Reduced Sodium Broth Concentrates (Foodservice)*	Beef, Chicken, Vegetable	9.6	0.3
		*Available in 9.6 gram stick pouch (200 stick pouches/box). Add 240 mL (1 cup) water to make single strength broth. Contains 360 mg sodium/serving.		
	Low Sodium Stock Pot In-A-Pouch (Foodservice)	Chicken Broth Concentrate*	500	17.6
		Broth Concentrate**–Beef, Chicken	100	3.53
		*Add to 40 liters of water. Each pouch makes 10 gallons of single strength broth. **Add to 7.6 liters of water. Each pouch makes 2 gallons of single strength broth.		
SIMPLY ASIA	Rice Noodle Soup Bowls	Garlic Sesame, Sesame Chicken, Spring Vegetable	70	2.5
TASTE ADVENTURE	Dried Soups	Black Bean	130	4.6
		Curry Lentil	170	6
		Golden Pea	142	5
		Navy Bean	156	5.5
		Split Pea, Sweet Corn Chowder	142	5
THAI KITCHEN	Heat & Serve Soups (canned)	Coconut Ginger, Hot & Sour	397	14
	Instant Rice Noodle Soup Bowls	Lemon Grass & Chili, Mushroom, Roasted Garlic, Spring Onion, Thai Ginger	70	2.4
	Instant Rice Noodle Soups	Bangkok Curry, Garlic & Vegetable, Lemon Grass & Chili, Spring Onion, Thai Ginger	45	1.6

COATINGS AND CRUMBS

Company	Coatings & Crumbs		Grams	Ounces
ANDREA'S FINE FOODS	Seasoned Bread Crumbs		227	8
	Seasoned Croûtons		85	3
BARKAT	Sage & Onion Stuffing Mix*		250	8.8
	*Dairy-Free.			
CELIAC SPECIALTIES	Graham Cracker Crumbs*		227	8
	Seasoned Bread Crumbs*		227	8
	*Casein-Free.			
CHOICES BEST RICE BAKERY	Brown Rice Bread Crumbs	Flaxseed, Italian, Multiseed, Plain, Quinoa Multigrain	340	12
	Brown Rice Bread Croûtons		100	3.5
DIETARY SPECIALTIES	Rice Crumbs		454	16
EL PETO	Gluten-Free Bread Crumbs*		500	17.5
	Gluten-Free Stuffing*		280	10
	*Dairy-Free.			
ENER-G FOODS	Bread Crumbs (Stuffing)		284	10

Company	Coatings & Crumbs	Grams	Ounces
GILLIAN'S FOODS	**Bread Crumbs*** Cajun Style, Italian, Plain	340	12
	*Dairy-Free.		
GLUTEN-FREE BAGEL COMPANY	**Bread Crumbs*** Plain, Herb	454	16
	*Dairy-Free.		
GLUTEN-FREE CREATIONS	Bread Crumbs*, Mock Graham Cracker Crumbs	227	8
	*Dairy-Free. Crumbs are enriched with thiamin, niacin, riboflavin, folic acid, iron and calcium.		
GLUTEN-FREE PANTRY	Olive Oil & Garlic Croûtons	142	5
HOL•GRAIN	Brown Rice Bread Crumbs	113	4
	Chicken Coating Mix	227	8
IAN'S NATURAL FOODS	Gluten-Free Stuffing*	336	12
	*Dairy-Free.		
KINNIKINNICK	Panko Style Bread Crumbs*	340	12
	Bread Cubes*	227	8
	Crispy Chicken Coating Mix*	500	18
	Chocolate Cookie Crumbs*	300	10.5
	Graham Style Cracker Crumbs*	300	10.5
	*Casein-Free.		
LAUREL'S SWEET TREATS	All Purpose Batter	340	12
MARY'S GONE CRACKERS	**Gone Crackers Crumbs** – Original*, Caraway*, Savory Blend*	456	16
	*Dairy-Free.		
MISS ROBEN'S	Bread & Batter Coating Mix	170, 510	6, 18
NATURE'S OWN BAKERY	Bread Crumbs	275	9.7
ORGRAN	All-Purpose Crumbs*, Corn Crispy Crumbs*	300	10.6
	Coating & Stuffing Mix*	120	4.2
	*Dairy-Free.		
PANERISO/ KINGSMILL	Herb & Garlic Croûtons*	175	6.2
	Rice Bread Crumbs*	500	17.6
	*Dairy-Free.		
PANNE RIZO	Plain Rice Crumbs	250	8.8
	Herb Croûtons	160	5.6
SCHÄR	Gluten-Free Bread Crumbs	250	8.8
WHOLE FOODS GF BAKEHOUSE	Stuffing Cubes (seasonal)	227	8
	Croûtons	227	8

GRAVY MIXES

Company	Gravy Mixes	Grams	Ounces
ALLERGYFREE FOODS	**Gravy Mixes*** Beef, Chicken, Country Pepper Steak	227	8
	*Dairy-Free.		
BARKAT	Vegetable Gravy Mix*	250	8.8
	*Dairy-Free.		

Company	Gravy Mixes		Grams	Ounces
CELINAL FOODS	GFDF Gravy Mixes*	Beef, Chicken	10 g	0.35 oz.
	*Single serve mixes. Dairy-Free.			
CUISINE SANTÉ	"Au jus" Clear Gravy*		908	2 lbs.
	*1 can yields 8 gallons. 12 cans/case. Note: Free of Gluten, Dairy, Soy, Egg, Nut and MSG.			
GLUTINO	Brown Gravy Mix		159	5.6
ORGRAN	Gravy Mix*		200	7
	*Dairy-Free.			
ROAD'S END ORGANICS	Gravy Mixes*	Golden, Savory Herb, Shiitake Mushroom	28.3	1
	*Dairy-Free.			

SAUCES

Company	Sauces		Grams	Ounces
CUISINE SANTÉ	Demi-Glace/Brown Sauce Mix*		908	2 lbs.
	*1 can yields 4 gallons. 12 cans/case. Free of Gluten, Dairy, Soy, Egg, Nut and MSG.			
	White Roux Base for Soups and Sauces*		594	21
	*1 can yields 2.6 gallons. 12 cans/case. Free of Gluten, Dairy, Soy, Egg, Nut and MSG.			
MR. SPICE	Garlic Steak Sauce, Ginger Stir Fry Sauce, Honey BBQ Sauce, Honey Mustard Sauce, Hot Wing! Sauce, Indian Curry Sauce, Sweet & Sour Sauce, Tangy Bang! Hot Sauce, Thai Peanut Sauce		298	10.5
PREMIER JAPAN	Wheat Free Sauces*	Hoisin, Teriyaki	251 mL	8.5
	*Casein-Free.			
ROAD'S END ORGANICS	Gluten-Free Alfredo Sauce Mix*		31, 454	1.1 oz., 1 lb.
	Gluten-Free Chreese Mix*	Cheddar Style, Alfredo	31, 454	1.1 oz., 1 lb.
	*Dairy-Free.			
SAVORY CHOICE	Demi-Glace	Beef*	500	17.6
	*Can be made with water or wine. Comes in 500 gram pouch that makes 3 cups. 6 pouches/case.			
	Demi-Glace	Veal*	4.5 L	152
	*Available in a 4.5 liter Bag-in-Box. Each box makes 28.4 liters.			
THAI KITCHEN	Curry Pastes	Green Curry, Red Curry, Roasted Red Chili	112	4
	Sauces	Premium Fish, Less Sodium Fish	200 mL	7
		Original Pad Thai, Peanut Satay, Spicy Thai Chili, Sweet Red Chili	227 mL	8
THE WIZARD'S	Wheat-Free Sauces	Hot Stuff	147 mL	5
		Worcestershire	251 mL	8.5

SOY SAUCES

Company	Soy Sauces	Grams	Ounces
CELINAL FOODS	GF Soy Sauce*	8	0.28
	*Single serve packet.		
EDEN FOODS	Organic Tamari Soy Sauce (Imported)	148, 296, 592 mL	5, 10, 20
	Organic Tamari Soy Sauce (Brewed in USA)	296, 529 mL	10, 20
KARI-OUT	Panda Soy Sauce (Low Sodium Gluten-Free)	small individual packets	
LIFESOURCE	**Wheat-Free/Gluten-Free Tamari Soy Sauce** Original, Oriental Ginger, Shitake Mushroom, Spicy Garlic	500	17.6
SAN-J	Organic Wheat-Free Tamari Soy Sauce (Gold Label)	284, 567 mL	10, 20
	Organic Lite Tamari Soy Sauce (25% less salt)*	284, 567 mL	10, 20
	Note: San-J regular tamari and lite tamari soy sauces contain wheat. *In USA called "Reduced Sodium Wheat-Free Tamari".		

SPREADS

Company	Spreads	Grams	Ounces
NO NUTS	Golden Peabutter	510	18

DAIRY/NON-DAIRY BEVERAGES

✦ Some non-dairy beverages are **NOT** gluten-free as they contain **barley malt, barley malt extract, barley malt flavoring,** or **regular oats**:

– **Eden Soy Beverages** all contain gluten EXCEPT "Eden Blend" and "Eden Soy Unsweetened".

– **Pacific Foods Non-Dairy Oat Beverage** contains **regular oats**.

Lactose-Reduced Dairy Products

DAIRY EASE (USA)
✦ Refrigerated (8 oz.) – Reduced Fat (2%), Fat-Free
✦ Refrigerated (32 oz.) – Reduced Fat (2%), Fat-Free
✦ Refrigerated (64 oz.) – Whole, Reduced Fat (2%), Fat-Free

LACTAID MILK (CANADA)
✦ Refrigerated (1 litre) – skim, 2%
✦ Refrigerated (2 & 4 litres) – skim, 1%, 2%

LACTAID MILK (USA)
✦ Refrigerated (half gallon) – Fat-Free, Low-Fat (1%), Reduced Fat (2%), Whole, Chocolate Low Fat (1%), Calcium Enriched [Fat-Free, Low-Fat (1%), Reduced Fat (2%), Whole]
✦ Refrigerated (half gallon) Organic – Fat-Free, Reduced Fat (2%)
✦ Refrigerated (single serve) – Fat-Free, Chocolate Low Fat (1%)

Lactose-Reduced Dairy Products CONT'D.

LACTEEZE MILK (CANADA)
- ✦ Refrigerated (1 litre) – Skim, 1% and 2%
  - (2 litre) – 1% and 2%
- ✦ Shelf-Stable (1 litre) – Skim, 1%, 2%, Chocolate

Soy Beverages

EDEN FOODS "SOY UNSWEETENED"
- ✦ Shelf-Stable (32 oz./946 mL)

IMAGINE FOODS "SOY DREAM" NON-DAIRY BEVERAGES
- ✦ Shelf-Stable
  - Soy Dream Classic Vanilla (32 oz/946mL)
  - Soy Dream Enriched – Original*, Vanilla* (8, 32 and 64 oz/240, 946 mL and 1.89 litre),
    - Chocolate* (8 and 32 oz/240 and 946 mL)
- ✦ Refrigerated (64 oz.)
  - Soy Dream Enriched – Original*, Vanilla*
    * Enriched with Calcium and Vitamins A, D, E and B_{12} in USA
    * Enriched with Calcium and Vitamins A, D, B_2, B_{12} and Zinc in Canada

IMAGINE FOODS "KIDZ DREAM" SMOOTHIES
- ✦ Shelf-Stable (8 oz/240 mL) – Berry Blast, Orange Cream
    * Made with soy milk, juice and enriched with Calcium and Vitamin D.

PACIFIC FOODS "NON-DAIRY SOY BEVERAGES"
- ✦ Shelf-Stable (8 oz./240 mL)
  - Enriched Soymilk – Plain*, Chocolate*, Vanilla*
    * Enriched with Calcium and Vitamins A and D.
- ✦ Shelf-Stable (32 oz./946 mL)
  - Organic Original Soy – Unsweetened
  - Select Soy – Low-Fat Plain, Low-Fat Vanilla
  - Ultra Soy – Plain*, Vanilla*
    * Enriched with Calcium and Vitamins A, D, E, B_2, B_6 and B_{12}.
- ✦ Shelf-Stable (32 oz./946 mL)
  - Soy Blenders* – Plain, Vanilla
    * For use in coffee, latte, and chai beverages formulated for the foodservice industry.

SOYA WORLD "SO GOOD FORTIFIED" (CANADA)*
- ✦ Shelf-Stable (250 mL) – Chocolate, Strawberry, Vanilla
- ✦ Shelf-Stable (1 litre) – Original, Fat-Free Original, Fat-Free Vanilla
- ✦ Refrigerated (946 mL) – Decadent Chocolate, Trim
- ✦ Refrigerated (1.89 litres) – Original, Chocolate, Fat-Free Original, Fat-Free Vanilla,
    - No Sugar Added Original, Omega DHA Original**, Omega DHA Vanilla**, Strawberry, Vanilla
- ✦ Refrigerated (2.84 litres) – Original
    * Fortified with Calcium, Iron, Phosphorus, Potassium, Zinc and Vitamins A, C, D, B_6, B_{12}, Thiamin, Riboflavin, Niacin, Folacin and Pantothenate.
    ** Contains flaxseed oil.

Soy Beverages CONT'D.

SOYA WORLD "SO NICE SOY BEVERAGE" (CANADA)*
- ✦ Shelf-Stable (250 mL/8 oz.) – Chocolate, Mocha, Original, Vanilla
- ✦ Shelf-Stable (946 mL/32 oz.) – Organic Natural**, Original, Chocolate, Vanilla
- ✦ Refrigerated (946 mL/32 oz.) – Chocolate Passion, Original Delight, Vanilla Bliss, Noel Nog
- ✦ Refrigerated (1.89 litres/64 oz.) – Original, Chocolate, Vanilla, Unsweetened, Plus Prebiotic Fibre***, Plus Omega-3****

  * All flavors except organic natural are fortified/enriched with Calcium, Zinc and Vitamins A, C, D, B_6, B_{12}, Thiamin, Riboflavin, Niacin, Folacin and Pantothenate.
  ** Natural is non-fortified/enriched.
  *** Contains chicory fibre.   **** Contains flaxseed oil and hemp oil.

SOYA WORLD "SO NICE SOYMILK" (USA)*
- ✦ Refrigerated (64 oz.) – Chocolate, Original, Vanilla
- ✦ Refrigerated (64 oz.) – Omega Plus Original**, Omega Plus Vanilla**

  * Fortified with Calcium, Zinc, Thiamin, Riboflavin, Niacin, Folic Acid, Pantothenic Acid and Vitamins A, D, B_6, B_{12}.
  ** Contains flaxseed oil.

SUNRISE SOYA BEVERAGE (CANADA)
- ✦ Refrigerated (1.89 and 3.95 litres) – Sweetened*, Light Fortified**
- ✦ Refrigerated (1.89 and 3.95 litres) – Unsweetened*
- ✦ Refrigerated (1.89 litres) – Organic Unsweetened*

  * Non-fortified.
  ** Fortified with Thiamin, Riboflavin, Niacin, Folacin, Pantothenate, Zinc, Calcium and Vitamins A, D, B_6 and B_{12}.

WHITE WAVE SILK SOY BEVERAGES (CANADA)*
- ✦ Refrigerated (946 mL) – Original Plain, Vanilla
- ✦ Refrigerated (1.89 litres) – Original Plain, Light Plain, Chocolate, Vanilla, Light Vanilla, DHA Omega-3**, Unsweetened***

  * Fortified with Calcium, Zinc and Vitamins A, B_2, B_{12} and D.
  ** Contains flaxseed oil.   *** Contains FOS (Prebiotic)

WHITE WAVE SILK SOY MILK (USA)
- ✦ Refrigerated (11 oz./330 mL, Single Serve) – Chocolate*, Vanilla*
- ✦ Refrigerated (32 oz./946 mL) – Original Plain*, Chocolate*, Vanilla*, Nog, Light Original (Chocolate, Plain Vanilla)
- ✦ Refrigerated (64 oz./1.89 litres) – Original Plain*, Unsweetened*, Chocolate*, Light Original Plain*, Light Chocolate*, Light Vanilla*, Organic (Original*, Unsweetened*, Vanilla*), DHA Omega-3 and Calcium**, Heart Health***
- ✦ Shelf-Stable (8.25 oz./244 mL) – Chocolate*, Original*, Vanilla*, Very Vanilla*
- ✦ Shelf-Stable (32 oz./946 mL) – Chocolate*, Original Plain*, Unsweetened*, Vanilla*

  * Enriched with Calcium and Vitamins A, B_2, B_{12} and D.
  ** Enriched with Calcium, Zinc, Folic Acid and Vitamins A, B_2, B_6, B_{12}, C, D and E and flax oil.
  *** Enriched with Calcium, Vitamins A, B_2, B_{12} and D, and plant sterols.

SOY YOGURTS

SOYA WORLD "SO NICE" YOGURTS (CANADA)
- ✦ Refrigerated Carton (175 g) – Peach, Strawberry, Vanilla
- ✦ Refrigerated Carton (440 g) – Plain, Peach, Vanilla, Strawberry

White Wave Silk Cultured Yogurts*
- ✦ Refrigerated Carton (32 oz./908 g) – Plain, Vanilla
- ✦ Refrigerated Carton (6 oz./170 g) – Banana Strawberry, Black Cherry, Blueberry, Key Lime, Peach, Plain Raspberry, Strawberry, Vanilla
  - * Enriched with Calcium.

Rice Beverages

Amazake Rice Shakes*
- ✦ Refrigerated (8 oz.) – Almond Shake
- ✦ Refrigerated (16 oz.) – Oh So Original, Almond Shake, Chocolate Almond, Cool Coconut, Go Hazelnuts, GoGo Green, Tiger Chai**, Vanilla Gorilla**
- ✦ Refrigerated (32 oz.) – Almond Shake
  - * All made with organic brown rice. Vanilla Gorilla also contain soy protein.
  - ** Enriched with vitamins and minerals.

Good Karma Foods Organic Ricemilk
- ✦ Shelf-Stable (32 oz./946 mL) – Chocolate, Original, Unsweetened, Vanilla
  - * Enriched with Calcium, Vitamins A, B_{12}, and D.

Pacific Foods Non-Dairy Rice Beverages*
- ✦ Shelf-Stable (32 oz.)
  - • Low Fat Rice – Plain, Vanilla
    - * Enriched with Calcium and Vitamins A and D.

Other Beverages

Blue Diamond "Almond Breeze" Non-Dairy Beverage*
- ✦ Refrigerated (64 oz./1.89 liters) – Chocolate, Original, Unsweetened Vanilla, Vanilla
- ✦ Shelf-Stable (32 oz./946 mL) – Chocolate**, Original**, Vanilla**
  - * Enriched with Vitamins A, D, and E and Calcium.
  - ** Available in regular and unsweetened.

Eden Foods "Edenblend" Brown Rice & Soy Beverage
- ✦ Shelf-Stable (8.45 and 32 oz./250 mL and 946 mL)

Imagine "Almond Dream"*
- ✦ Shelf-Stable (32 oz./946 mL and 64 oz./1.89 liters) – Original, Unsweetened
  - * Enriched with Vitamins A, B_{12}, D, E and Calcium.

Pacific Foods Almond Beverages*
- ✦ Shelf-Stable (32 oz. and 64 oz.) – Low-Fat Sweetened
  - • Original, Vanilla
- ✦ Shelf-Stable (32 oz.) – Organic Unsweetened
  - • Low-Fat Original, Low-Fat Vanilla
- ✦ Shelf-Stable (8 oz.) – Low-Fat Sweetened
  - • Chocolate, Vanilla
    - * Enriched with Calcium, Vitamins A, B_2, and D.

Other Beverages CONT'D.

PACIFIC FOODS HAZELNUT NON-DAIRY BEVERAGE*
- ✦ Shelf-Stable (32 oz.) – Original, Chocolate
- ✦ Shelf-Stable (8 oz.) – Chocolate
    - * Enriched with Calcium, Vitamins A, B_2 and D.

SILK "TRUE ALMOND" (CANADA)*
- ✦ Refrigerated (64 oz./1.89 liters) – Dark Chocolate, Original
    - * Enriched with Vitamins A, B_{12}, D, Riboflavin and Zinc.

SILK "PURE ALMOND MILK" (USA)
- ✦ Refrigerated (64 oz./1.89 liters) – Dark Chocolate*, Original**, Unsweetened**, Vanilla**
    - * Enriched with Vitamins A, B_{12}, C, D, E, Riboflavin, Calcium, Iron, Copper, Magnesium, Manganese and Zinc.
    - ** Enriched with Vitamins A, D, E, Riboflavin, Calcium, Copper, Iron, Magnesium, Manganese, Phosphorous and Zinc.

VANCES DARIFREE NON-DAIRY BEVERAGE (POTATO BASED SUBSTITUTE) USA*
- ✦ Dry Mix Potato Based Milk Substitute – Original
    - • 21 g Single Serve Sample yields 8 oz.
    - • 19.5 oz. Can yields 6 quarts
    - • 25 lb. Box yields 115 quarts
- ✦ Dry Mix Potato Based Milk Substitute – Chocolate
    - • 33 g Single Serve Sample yields 8 oz.
    - • 23.3 oz. Can yields 5 quarts
    - • 25 lb. Box yields 86 quarts
        - * Enriched with Calcium, Folic Acid, Biotin, Pantothenic acid, Vitamins A, B_1, B_2, B_3, B_6, B_{12}, C, D, E and K.

BEER

- ✦ Regular beer, ale and lagers are **NOT** gluten-free, as they are made from barley.
- ✦ There are several gluten-free products on the market (see below).

Company	Beer		Grams	Ounces
ANHEUSER-BUSCH	Redbridge Beer (4.8%)*		340 mL	12
	*Sorghum			
BARD'S TALE	Bard's Gold*		341 mL	12
	*Sorghum			
BI-AGLUT	76 Beer*		330 mL	11.7
	*Buckwheat			
GREEN'S GLUTEN-FREE BEER	**Ale***	Herald (4%)	500 mL	16.9
	Beer*	Discovery Amber (6%), Endeavour Double Dark (6%), Mission Amber (6%), Pathfinder Dubbel Dark (7%), Quest Tripel Blonde (8.5%)	500 mL	16.9
	Lager*	Pioneer (5%), Trailblazer Low Carb (4.7%)	500 mL	16.9
	*Millet, brown rice, buckwheat, sorghum.			

Company	Beer	Grams	Ounces
LAKEFRONT BREWERY	New Grist Beer*	340 mL	12
	*Sorghum and rice.		
LA MESSAGÈRE	Gluten-Free Beer (4.7%)*	341 mL	12
	*Rice and buckwheat.		

FROZEN DESSERTS

Company	Frozen Desserts		Grams	Ounces
GOOD KARMA FOODS	**Organic Rice Divine Frozen Desserts***	Banana Fudge, Carrot Cake, Chocolate Chip, Chocolate Peanut, Butter Fudge, Coconut Mango, Key Lime Pie, Mint Chocolate Swirl, Mudd Pie, Very Vanilla, Very Cherry	473	16
	Organic Rice Divine Chocolate Covered Bars*	Chocolate Chocolate, Very Vanilla	266 mL	9
	Note: 3 bars/box.			
	*Dairy-Free.			
IMAGINE FOODS	**Soy Dream Non-Dairy Dessert***	Butter Pecan, French Vanilla, Green Tea, Mocha Fudge Swirl	473 mL	16
		Chocolate, Strawberry Swirl, Vanilla, Vanilla Fudge Swirl	946 mL	32
	*Dairy-Free.			
PHILLY SWIRL	**Original Italian Ice Swirls*** (cups)	Banana Berry, Cotton Candy, Hurricane, Paradise Punch, Rainbow, Sunburst	712 mL	24
	Swirl Stix* (14/box)	Banana Split, Cotton Candy, Orange Dream, Paradise Punch, Rainbow, Razzle Dazzle	624 mL	21
	Sugar-Free Swirl Stix* (12/box)	Cotton Candy, Hurricane, Orange Dream, Paradise Punch	2.08 L	70
	Swirl Popperz* (8/box)	Cotton Candy, Cherry Melon, Orange Dream, Rainbow	712 mL	24
	Fudge Swirl Stix (12/box)	Fudge & Caramel, Fudge & Chocolate, Fudge & Vanilla	624 mL	21
	Fruit & Cream Stix	Berry & Vanilla, Cherry & Vanilla, Orange & Vanilla, Strawberry & Vanilla	624 mL	21
	*Dairy-Free.			
SOYA WORLD	**So Good Non-Dairy Frozen Dessert***	Boysenberry Swirl, Butterscotch Swirl, Chocolate Supreme, Creamy Vanilla, Simply Strawberry	946 mL	32
	*Dairy-Free.			

COMPANY DIRECTORY

The following directory is divided into three categories:

1) MANUFACTURERS OF GLUTEN-FREE PRODUCTS

- These include gluten-free specialty manufacturers and companies who produce gluten-free products exclusively, and other companies who manufacture both gluten-free and gluten-containing products, in addition to other items.

- Company contact information; an overview of the company and their products; options for purchasing the products (including retail or specialty stores) and whether they can be ordered directly from the company via phone, fax, mail, email and/or internet along with shipping information. Ordering directly from the company will be denoted by a symbol ✦.

2) GLUTEN-FREE BAKERIES AND/OR BISTROS, CAFES, DELIS

- These include gluten-free specialty bakeries and bakeries with an attached bistro, cafe or deli.

- Company contact information; the type of products made and whether they can only be purchased in the store or also ordered via phone, fax, mail, email and/or internet including shipping information; and if available from other retail stores.

3) GLUTEN-FREE SPECIALTY STORES AND DISTRIBUTORS

- These include specialty stores who exclusively sell gluten-free products and/or allergen free products; they may also have an attached bistro, café or deli. The distributors handle gluten-free products only or sell both gluten-free and other items.

- Company contact information; types of products sold or distributed; how they can be purchased (in-store only or order direct by phone, fax, mail, email and/or internet and shipping information).

The information was exhaustively researched from sources believed to be reliable at the time of printing and recorded from August-December 2009. It should be noted that this is not an all-inclusive list. The author assumes no liability for any errors, omissions or inaccuracies in this section.

Manufacturers of Gluten-Free Products

✦ = Products can be ordered directly from company

1-2-3 Gluten-Free Inc., 125 Orange Tree Drive, Orange, OH, USA 44022
✦ Phone: 216-378-9233   FAX: 216-378-9234
  Email: kim@123glutenfree.com   www.123glutenfree.com

- Gluten-free specialty company; dedicated GF facility; products certified by Gluten-Free Certification Organization (GFCO).
- Produce "1-2-3 Gluten-Free" baking mixes (biscuits, brownies, cakes, cookies, muffins, pancakes, rolls).
- Available in retail stores.
- Order direct by phone, fax, mail or internet; shipping charges based on weight; ships via FedEx Ground or USPS.

Allergaroo, Allergy Friendly Foods, P.O. Box 790, Springfield, MO, USA 65801
✦ Phone: 417-799-1875   FAX: 417-863-0402
  Email: info@allergaroo.com   www.allergaroo.com

- Produce gluten, dairy and soy-free pasta (ready made in a microwavable pouch).
- Pasta made in a dedicated GF facility; pasta and sauce combined using shared and dedicated equipment that is thoroughly cleaned.
- Available in retail stores and gluten-free specialty companies.
- Order direct by internet.

AllergyFree Foods, 310 West Hightower Drive, Dawsonville, GA, USA 30534
✦ Phone: 706-265-1317   FAX: 706-265-1281
  Email: info@allergyfreefoods.com   www.allergyfreefoods.com

- Manufacture a variety of products in their dedicated facility that is free of the major allergens (tree nuts, peanuts, soy, milk, egg, fish, shellfish, wheat), barley and rye. Some products made in other facilities that also have the same strict allergen quality control procedures to prevent cross-contamination.
- President of the company has food allergies.
- Products include cookies, entrées and mixes.
- Available in retail stores.
- Order direct by internet; shipping charges based on weight; ships via UPS.

AlpineAire Foods, TyRy Inc., P.O. Box 1799, Rocklin, CA, USA 95677
  Phone: 800-322-6325/866-322-6325   FAX: 916-624-1604
✦   916-624-6050
  Email: info@aa-foods.com   www.aa-foods.com

- Fully prepared meals, side dishes, vegetables, fruits, desserts, beverages, soups, rice and legumes that are freeze-dried and specially packaged for a long shelf life. No preservatives or MSG. These instant foods are in re-sealable, lightweight, foil pouches (stable for 1 year) and can be prepared in the pouch by adding hot water. Also available in cans (stable for 5-20 years).
- Many products are gluten-free.
- Available in retail stores.
- Order direct by phone, fax or internet; shipping charges based on weight; ships via UPS Ground.

Amazake, Grainaissance Inc., 1580 - 62nd St., Emeryville, CA, USA 94608
    Phone: 800-472-4697/510-547-7256   FAX: 510-547-0526
    Email: amazake@grainaissance.com   www.grainaissance.com

- Produce dairy-free, low-fat shakes from organic brown rice. Contains no added sweeteners. Some flavors contain soy protein, nuts and/or are enriched with vitamins and minerals.
- All flavors are gluten-free except Mocha Java and Gimme Green.
- Available in retail stores.

Amazing Grains, LLC, P.O. Box 919, Pablo, MT, USA 59855
    Phone: 877-278-6585/406-675-3536   FAX: 406-675-3537
    Email: customercare@amazinggrains.com   www.montina.com
                                         www.amazinggrains.com

- Specialize in Montina™ products made from Indian ricegrass that is grown by its members and milled, processed and packaged in a dedicated GF facility. The ricegrass is tested for gluten before it enters the milling facility. Certified by the Gluten-Free Certification Organization (GFCO).
- Available as Montina™ Pure Baking Supplement (Montina flour) and Montina™ All Purpose Flour Blend (white rice flour, tapioca flour and Montina flour).
- Available in retail stores.
- Order direct by phone, fax,mail or internet; shipping charges based on weight; ships via UPS Ground.

Amy's Kitchen Inc., Box 449, Petaluma, CA, USA 94953
    Phone: 707-578-7270   FAX: 707-578-7995
    Email: amy@amyskitchen.com   www.amyskitchen.com

- Organic, vegetarian, prepared natural meals (e.g., pot pies, entrées, pizzas, whole meals, Asian and Indian meals, skillet meals, burritos, pocket sandwiches, veggie burgers, snacks, toaster pops, soups, chilies, refried beans, pasta sauces and salsas).
- A variety of products (over 75) are gluten-free and some are also dairy-free.
- Gluten-free products made in a shared facility. Strict quality control procedures used to prevent cross-contamination.
- Available in retail stores.

Ancient Harvest Quinoa Corporation, Box 279, 222 E. Redondo Beach Blvd., Unit B, Gardena, CA, USA 90248
    Phone: 310-217-8125   FAX: 310-217-8140
    Email: quinoacorp@quinoa.net   www.quinoa.net

- Organic quinoa products include quinoa grain, flour, cereal flakes, pastas (quinoa flour and corn flour) and polenta (quinoa and cornmeal) which are gluten-free.
- Regular supergrain organic pasta (whole-wheat and quinoa flour) is **NOT** gluten-free.
- Available in retail stores.
- Order direct by internet; shipping charges based on weight; ships via UPS Ground.

Andean Dream, LLC., P.O. Box 411404, Los Angeles, CA, USA 90041
✦ Phone: 310-281-6036
Email: andeancookies@aol.com   www.andeandream.com
- Produce quinoa cookies and pasta made in a dedicated GF facility in Bolivia.
- All products are gluten, casein, soy and nut-free.
- Available in retail stores and gluten-free distributors.
- Order direct by internet; shipping charges based on weight, ships via USPS, FedEx or UPS.

Andrea's Fine Foods, 759 Spirit of St. Louis Blvd. Chesterfield, MO, USA 63005
✦ Phone: 877-671-0051/636-536-9953   FAX: 636-536-9660
Email: andrea@andreasfinefoods.com   www.andreasfinefoods.com
- Gluten-free specialty company; dedicated GF facility.
- Produce a variety of baked products (breads, buns, cakes, cookies, cupcakes, muffins, pizza, pizza crust and rolls), flours and other items.
- Also carry other companies' products.
- Shop in person or order direct by phone, fax, email or internet; shipping charges based on weight; ships via FedEx or USPS.

Annie Chun's Inc., 4340 Redwood Highway, Suite B60, San Rafael, CA, USA 94903
✦ Phone: 866-972-6879/415-479-8272   FAX: 415-479-8274
Email: info@anniechun.com   www.anniechun.com
- Asian sauces, noodles (chow mein, rice, soba), meal kits (noodles and sauces) and rice dishes.
- Rice noodles and Rice Express (microwavable rice) are gluten-free. Rice products made in a facility that only produce rice.
- Available in retail stores.
- Order direct by phone or internet; shipping charges based on amount purchased; ships via UPS.

Annie's Homegrown Inc., 580 Gateway Drive, Napa, CA, USA 94559
✦ Phone: 800-288-1089/630-343-0240
Email: bernie@annies.com   www.annies.com
- Produce pasta, macaroni and cheese dinners, pasta meals, Cheddar snacks, cookies and cereals.
- One product is gluten-free (Gluten-Free Rice Pasta and cheese) and is produced in a dedicated GF facility.
- Available in retail stores.
- Order direct by internet; shipping charges based on weight; ships via FedEx Ground.

Apetito, (formerly Private Recipes) 12 Indell Lane, Brampton, ON, Canada L6T 3Y3
Phone: 800-268-8199/905-799-1022   FAX: 800-561-9778/905-799-2666
Email: info@apetito.ca   www.apetito.ca
- Manufacturer of a wide range of frozen products in various textures for home use, hospitals, long-term care, Meals on Wheels and other institutions.
- Products (cereals, desserts, entrées, gravies, thickened juices, sauces, side dishes, soups) available in bulk and portioned formats.
- Produce a line of gluten-free complete meals (also suitable for lactose-free and renal diets) in bulk and individual trays. Dedicated production periods where equipment and packaging lines are thoroughly cleaned.
- Foodservice organizations purchase Apetito products through distributors (e.g., Sysco, GFS, Summit Foods, Flanagans, Shalit Foods). Consumers can purchase products through local Meals on Wheels Agency.

Arico Natural Foods Company, P.O. Box 910602, San Diego, CA, USA 92191
✦   Phone: 866-595-8917/858-880-9389   FAX: 858-408-9222
     Email: info@aricofoods.com   www.aricofoods.com
- Gluten-free specialty company; extensive cleaning and sanitization process in their shared manufacturing facility to prevent cross-contamination. Products are tested for gluten and dairy using highly sensitive ELISA tests.
- Produce gluten-free, dairy-free cookies (made from organic brown rice flour) and cassava chips in various flavors.
- Available in retail stores.
- Order direct by phone, fax,mail or internet; shipping charges based on weight; ships via UPS Ground or USPS.

Arrowhead Mills, Hain-Celestial Group, Consumer Relations Department,
              4600 Sleepytime Drive, Boulder, CO, USA 80301
     Phone: 800-434-4246   FAX: 303-581-1520
✦   Phone Orders: 866-595-8917
     Email: consumerrelations@hain-celestial.com   www.arrowheadmills.com
- Wide variety of products (cereals, flours, mixes, legumes, seeds, pastas).
- Many products are gluten-free and are tested for gluten.
- Available in retail stores.
- Order direct by phone or internet; shipping charges based on weight; ships via UPS Ground.

Aunt Gussies Cookies and Crackers, 141 Lanza Ave., Garfield, NJ, USA 07026
     Phone: 800-422-6654/973-340-4480   FAX: 973-340-3501
     Email: info@auntgussies.com   www.auntgussies.com
- Produce a variety of breads, biscotti, brownies, cookies, crackers and English muffins.
- Many products are gluten-free and are made in a dedicated GF facility. Products certified by Gluten-Free Certification Organization (GFCO).
- Available in retail stores.

Authentic Foods, 1850 W. 169th St., Suite B, Gardena, CA, USA 90247
✦   Phone: 800-806-4737/310-366-7612   FAX: 310-366-6938
     Email: sales@authenticfoods.com   www.authenticfoods.com
- Gluten-free specialty company; a dedicated GF facility.
- A variety of "Authentic Foods" wheat-free and gluten-free baking mixes, flours and baking supplies. Mixes contain Garfava™ flour (chickpeas and fava beans) developed by founder of this company.
- Also carry other companies' products (cereals, pasta, snacks) and books.
- Available in retail stores.
- Order direct by phone, fax or internet; shipping charges based on weight; ships via UPS Ground or USPS.

Bakery On Main, 2836 Main Street, Glastonbury, CT, USA 06033
✦   Phone: 860-895-6622   FAX: 860-895-6624
     Email: info@bakeryonmain.com   www.bakeryonmain.com
- Produce a variety of granola cereals and bars including a line of gluten-free products which are tested for gluten. Gluten-free products are made in a separate dedicated area of the shared facility. Products certified by Gluten-Free Certification Organization (GFCO).
- Available in retail stores.
- Order direct by phone or internet; shipping charges based on weight; ships via UPS.

Barbara's Bakery, 3900 Cypress Dr, Petaluma, CA, USA 94954
    Phone: 707-765-2273   FAX: 707-765-2927
    Email: info@barbarasbakery.com   www.barbarasbakery.com

- Produce a line of natural cereals and snacks (chips, crackers, cookies and snack bars). Several cereals and snack foods are gluten-free.
- Available in retail stores.

Bard's Tale Beer Company, LLC, P.O. Box 24835, Minneapolis, MN, USA 55424-0835
    Phone: 877-440-2337   FAX: 816-222-0413
    Email: info@bardsbeer.com   www.bardsbeer.com

- Produce a gluten-free beer made from malted sorghum called "Bard's Gold" which is available in 12 oz. bottles that are sold in six-packs and cases of four six-packs.
- Both founders of the company have celiac disease.
- Rigid quality control procedures are utilized to prevent cross-contamination.
- Available from select distributors (see website for retail locations and distributors) in the USA and Canada.

Barkat, Gluten-Free Foods Ltd., Unit 270 Centennial Ave., Elstree, Borehamwood,
        Hertfordshire WD6 3SS, England
    Phone: 44 20 8953 4444   FAX: 44 20 8953 8285
    Email: info@glutenfree-foods.co.uk   www.glutenfree-foods.co.uk

- Gluten-free specialty company; dedicated GF facility.
- Produce a variety of "Barkat" products (breads, rolls, pizza crusts, cereals, pasta, pretzels, cakes, cookies, ice cream cones and mixes).
- Available from gluten-free distributors in North America and from health food stores and pharmacies in the U.K. and Europe.
- Order direct by internet in the U.K.

Bi-Aglut, H.J. Heinz Co., Via Cascina Bel Casule 7, Milan, Italy
    Phone: 39 02 52561 (from N.A.)   FAX: 39 02 5256 2396
          800-318357 (Toll-free in Italy)
    Email: info@biaglut.com   www.biaglut.com

- Gluten-free specialty company; dedicated GF facility; products tested for gluten.
- Produce a variety of breads, crackers, cookies, mixes, muffins, pasta and frozen desserts.
- Sold under three brand names "SfornaGusto," "DolciSfizi" and "PastaMia".
- Available from gluten-free specialty stores.
- Distributed in North America by Quattrobimbi.

Bionaturae, Euro-USA Trading Co. Inc., P.O. Box 98, 5 Tyler Drive,
        North Franklin, CT, USA 06254
    Phone: 860-642-6996   FAX: 860-642-6990
    Email: info@bionaturae.com   www.bionaturae.com

- Organic food company that produces olive oil, balsamic vinegar, fruit spreads, tomato products and two lines of pasta (one is gluten-free made from rice, potato and soy).
- Gluten-free pasta made in a shared facility. The company is one of the select few in Italy authorized by the Italian Ministry of Health to produce gluten-free pasta. Product is tested for gluten during each production cycle and also tested in the USA by an independent lab. Pasta certified by Gluten-Free Certification Organization (GFCO).
- Available in retail stores.

The Birkett Mills, 163 Main Street, Penn Yan, NY, USA 14527

✦ Phone: 315-536-3311   FAX: 315-536-6740
Email: custserv@thebirkettmills.com   www.thebirkettmills.com

- One of the world's largest millers of buckwheat products.
- Process all buckwheat products in a self-contained mill dedicated solely to buckwheat grain. No other items are processed in their buckwheat milling systems. After milling, buckwheat products are packaged on totally dedicated equipment.
- They also do random testing for gluten in their products using the enzyme immunoassay that tests at sensitivity levels of 20 ppm.
- Gluten-free products include Pocono (cream of buckwheat, buckwheat groats, buckwheat flour, Kasha) and Larrowe (Instant buckwheat pancake mix).
- Available in retail stores.
- Order direct by phone, fax, mail or internet; shipping charges based on weight; ships via UPS Ground.

Blue Diamond Growers, 1802 C Street, Sacramento, CA, USA 95814

✦ Phone: 800-987-2329/916-442-0771   FAX: 916-446-8461
Email: feedback@bdgrowers.com   www.bluediamond.com

- World's largest tree nut processing and marketing company specializing in a variety of almond products (nuts, nut thins and "Almond Breeze" non-dairy beverage).
- Most products are gluten-free. Nut thins are made in a shared facility, equipment is thoroughly cleaned; products are tested for gluten.
- Available in retail stores.
- Order direct by phone or internet; shipping charges based on weight; ships via UPS.

Bob's Red Mill Natural Foods Inc., 13521 SE Pheasant Court, Milwaukie, OR, USA 97222

✦ Phone: 800-553-2258/503-654-3215   FAX: 503-653-1339
800-349-2173 (mail orders)   www.bobsredmill.com

- Mill and manufacture a very extensive line of whole-grain natural foods using flint-hard quartz millstones.
- Produce a large variety of products (baking ingredients, cereals, dried fruits, flours, mixes, nuts, legumes, seeds, soup mixes, spices/herbs and sweeteners). Many of these products are gluten-free. They also sell baking equipment and books.
- Gluten-free specialty products and many grains are milled in a separate dedicated gluten-free production facility and are batch-tested using the ELISA test for gluten in Bob's Red Mill laboratory.
- Process pure, uncontaminated oats (steel cut and rolled). Oats are grown on dedicated fields which have no wheat, rye or barley for at least three years. All equipment used in planting, harvesting, transporting and processing is dedicated and/or cleaned to prevent cross-contamination. Oats are tested using the R5 ELISA test after harvesting and processing.
- Available in retail stores and in the Bob's Red Mill retail store.
- Order direct by phone, fax, mail or internet; shipping charges based on weight; ships via UPS Ground.

Breads From Anna, Gluten Evolution LLC., 358 West Side Drive, Iowa City, IA, USA 52246

✦ Phone: 877-354-3886/319-354-3886　　FAX: 319-358-9920

Email: info@breadsfromanna.com　　www.breadsfromanna.com

- Gluten-free specialty company; dedicated gluten-free and nut-free facility.
- Products created by the owner who has celiac disease and is a graduate of a culinary school.
- Variety of gluten-free mixes (breads and pie crust) made from bean flours, Montina™, millet, tapioca and arrowroot that are high in protein and fiber.
- Available in retail stores.
- Order direct by phone, fax or internet; shipping charges based on amount purchased; ships via UPS Ground.

BumbleBar Foods Inc., 3808 N. Sullivan Road, Building 12, Suite P, Spokane, WA, USA 99216

✦ Phone: 509-924-2080　　FAX: 509-931-5000

Email: info@bumblebar.com　　www.bumblebar.com

- Produce organic snack bars made with sesame and flax seeds, and other ingredients. All bars are gluten and dairy-free and made in a dedicated GF facility.
- Available in retail stores.
- Order direct by phone, fax, email or internet; shipping charges based on weight; ships via UPS or USPS.

Canbrands Specialty Foods (see PaneRiso/Kingsmill)

Candy Tree, Health Flavors Ltd., 1944 Route 22, P.O. Box 551, Brewster, NY, USA 10509

✦ Phone: 877-380-3422/845-278-8164　　FAX: 845-278-6277

Email: healthflavors@gmail.com

- Produce a variety of organic corn-based candies (toffee, lollipops, licorice) including a line of wheat-free/gluten-free licorice (black and red).
- Gluten-free products are tested for gluten.
- Available in retail stores.
- Order direct by internet from various distributors.

CanMar Grain Products Ltd., 2480 Sandra Schmirler Way, Regina, SK, Canada S4W 1B7

✦ Phone: 866-855-5553/306-721-1375　　FAX: 306-721-1378

www.roastedflax.com

- Mill and manufacture regular and organic GF roasted flax products (whole seed and milled, ground flax) in a dedicated gluten-free facility.
- Retail products sold under the name "Flax For Nutrition" available in family size and bulk.
- Available in retail stores.
- Order direct by phone, fax, email, mail or internet; flat shipping rate; ships via FedEx Ground.

Casa deFruta, 10021 Pacheco Pass Highway, Hollister, CA, USA 95023
✦ Phone: 800-543-1702/408-842-7282   FAX: 408-842-0248
    Email: info@casadefruta.com   www.casadefruta.com

- Specialty store with a variety of products including fresh and dried fruits, nuts, chocolates, meats, cheese, wine, sauces and mesquite flour.
- Largest importer of mesquite flour in the US.
- USDA organic, kosher mesquite flour is available in packages direct for retail, retail packages for wholesale distribution, 22 lbs. (10 kg) for restaurants and in pallet quantities for manufacturers.
- Available in the Casa deFruta retail store or order direct by phone or internet; shipping charges based on amount purchased; ships via UPS Ground.

'Cause You're Special!, P.O. Box 316, Phillips, WI, USA 54555
    Phone: 866-669-4328/715-339-6959   FAX: 603-754-0245
✦ Email: info@causeyourespecial.com   www.causeyourespecial.com
                                    www.glutenfreegourmet.com

- Gluten-free specialty company; dedicated GF facility; products tested for gluten.
- A variety of "Cause You're Special" gluten-free, casein-free baking mixes (breads, biscuits, cakes, cookies, muffins, pancakes, pie crusts, pizza crusts, scones), flours and other baking ingredients. Also carry beverages and gravy mixes.
- Available in some retail stores.
- Order direct by phone, fax or internet; shipping charges based on amount purchased; ships via UPS (all available services) and USPS Priority Mail.

Celiac Specialties, LLC, 1928 Star Batt Drive, Suite D, Rochester Hills, MI, USA 48309
✦ Phone: 586-598-8180
    Email: contact-us@celiacspecialties.com   www.celiacspecialtiesshop.com

    39799 Grand River, Novi, MI, USA 48375
    Phone: 248-987-2348

- Gluten-free specialty company; dedicated gluten-free and nut-free facility; products tested for gluten.
- Produce breads, brownies, cakes, cupcakes, cereals, cookies, cookie dough, crumbs, croûtons, donuts, frosting, entrées, mixes, muffins, pasta, pies, pizza, pizza crusts.
- Also carry other companies' products (e.g., Glutino, Maxwell's, Schär).
- Available in some retail stores.
- Shop in person or order direct by internet; shipping charges based on amount purchased; ships via UPS.

CelifibR, Maplegrove Gluten-Free Foods, 13112 Santa Anna Ave., Unit A2-A3, Fontana, CA, USA 92337
✦ Phone: 909-823-8230   FAX: 909-823-2708
    Email: info@maplegrovefoods.com   www.maplegrovefoods.com

- Gluten-free bouillon cubes and soup base mix. Made with organic vegetables and cold pressed sunflower oil. Does not contain MSG or sulphites. Made in a dedicated GF facility.
- Available in retail stores.
- Order direct by internet.

Celimix (see Nelson David of Canada)

Celinal Foods, 689 Talamini Road, Bridgewater, NJ, USA 08807

✦ Phone: 908-704-7017   FAX: 908-566-0774
    Email: info@celinalfoods.com   www.celinalfoods.com

- Gluten-free specialty company that provides single serve and easy to prepare products (with a 2-year shelf life) for hospitals, nursing homes, schools, prisons and individuals needing emergency supplies.
- Gluten-Free Foodservice Starter Kits includes microwave mixes (bread, cornbread, biscuit), oven mix (cake), cake frosting mix, soup bases, pasta, instant gravy mix, soy sauce, gluten-free tent cards and three day sample menus with nutrient breakdown, recipes and in service education.
- All products made in a dedicated GF facility and are batch-tested for gluten.
- Order direct by phone, mail or internet.

Chebe, Prima Provisions Co., 1840 Lundberg Drive, Spirit Lake, IA, USA 51360

✦ Phone: 800-217-9510/712-336-4211   FAX: 712-336-4217
    Email: info@chebe.com   www.chebe.com

- Produce mixes (bread, bread sticks, cinnamon rolls, pizza dough) and frozen dough (bread sticks, pizza and sandwich buns) made from manioc flour and manioc starch (also known as tapioca, yucca or cassava).
- All products are free of gluten, soy, potato, yeast, nuts and MSG. Most mixes are also casein-free.
- Made in a dedicated GF facility.
- Available in some retail stores.
- Order direct by phone, mail or internet; flat rate shipping charge; ships via UPS Ground.

CheeCha, CadCan Marketing and Sales Inc., 3412 9th Street SE.,
        Calgary, AB, Canada T2G 3C3

✦ Phone: 877-243-3242/403-287-6731   FAX: 403-287-6732
    Email: info@cheecha.ca   www.cheecha.ca

- Produce "Cheecha Krackles" (puffed potato/wheat based snacks) and "CheeCha Potato Puff Snacks (gluten-free) in various flavors.
- CheeCha Potato Puff Snacks are produced on a dedicated gluten-free line and are batch tested for gluten.
- Available in retail stores.
- Order direct by phone, fax, mail or internet; shipping charges based on weight; ships via UPS Ground.

Cherrybrook Kitchen, Inc., 20 Mall Road, Burlington, MA, USA 01803

✦ Phone: 866-458-8225/781-272-0400   FAX: 781-272-4460
    Email: info@cherrybrookkitchen.com   www.cherrybrookkitchen.com

- Produce a variety of cookies, frostings and baking mixes that are all dairy, egg, peanut and nut-free.
- Some products are also gluten-free (cookies, cake frosting spreads and mixes – brownie, cake, cookie, frosting, pancake).
- Equipment is thoroughly cleaned and tested to prevent coss-contamination. Products are tested for peanuts, dairy, egg and gluten by an independent certified lab.
- Available in retail stores.
- Order direct by internet; shipping charges based on weight; ships via FedEx Ground.

Club House, McCormick Canada, P.O. Box 5788, London, ON, Canada N6A 4Z2
    Phone: 800-265-2600/519-432-1166   www.clubhouse.ca

- Large variety of products (baking ingredients, food extracts and colors, dry sauces and seasoning mixes, spices).
- Many products are gluten-free (e.g., spices, potato flour, rice flour).
- Contact company for a listing of gluten-free products.

Cook in the Kitchen, P.O. Box 961, White River Junction, VT, USA 05001
✦   Phone: 800-474-5518/802-333-4141   FAX: 802-304-3454
    Email: info@cookinthekitchen.com   www.cookinthekitchen.com

- Produce a variety of products (e.g., soups and mixes). Soups (4 flavors) are gluten-free and made in a shared facility where equipment is thoroughly cleaned.
- Available in some retail stores.
- Order direct by phone, fax, mail or internet; shipping charges based on amount purchased; ships via UPS Ground.

Cream Hill Estates Ltd., 9633 rue Clément, Lasalle, QC, Canada H8R 4B4
✦   Phone: 866-727-3628/514-363-2066   FAX: 514-363-1614
    Email: info@creamhillestates.com   www.creamhillestates.com

- Gluten-free specialty company that mill and manufacture pure, uncontaminated oat products in a dedicated GF facility and are certified by the Gluten-Free Certification Organization (GFCO). Also certified kosher.
- Their seed quality meets established standards of purity as specified by the Canadian Seed Grower's Association and regulated under the Canada Seeds Act. The oats are planted in fields that have not grown any wheat-related cereal crops for at least the three previous years. The fields are monitored for purity by crop inspectors from the Canadian Food Inspection Agency. The equipment used in planting, harvesting, transporting, processing and packaging is dedicated and/or cleaned to guarantee pure-oat production with no cross-contamination.
- The harvested crop is analyzed for purity using certified seed labs and the highly sensitive R5-ELISA test.
- Oat products sold under the name Lara's (rolled oats, whole-grain oat flour and whole oats, both heat treated and raw) are available in family-size and bulk quantities.
- Supply pure, uncontaminated oats in bulk to gluten-free bakeries and manufacturers.
- Family member of the company has celiac disease.
- Available in retail stores and online stores.
- Order direct by phone, fax or internet; shipping charges based on weight; ships via UPS (in the USA) and UPS (in Canada).

Cream of The Crop, Aliments Trigone Inc., 93 rue de l'Aqueduc,
                St.Francois de Montmagny, QC, Canada G0R 3A0
    Phone: 877-259-7491/418-259-7414   FAX: 418-259-2417
    Email: bio@alimentstrigone.com   www.alimentstrigone.com

- Producer of organic products (green and black buckwheat, hemp, kamut, spelt and fresh garlic).
- Buckwheat products (flour, grits [sold as "cream of buckwheat"] and groats) are processed in a separate production area and are laboratory tested for gluten.
- Available in retail stores.

Crunchmaster, TH Foods, Inc., 2154 Harlem Road, Loves Park, IL, USA 61111

✦ Phone: 800-896-2396/815-636-9500　　　　FAX: 815-636-8400
　Email: crunchmasterguru@thfoods.com　　　　www.crunchmaster.com

- Produce baked rice crackers in a variety of flavors.
- Made in a shared facility; products certified by the Gluten-Free Certification Organization (GFCO).
- Available in retail stores and amazon.com.
- Order direct by internet; shipping charges based on weight; ships via FedEx Ground.

Cuisine Santé, Haco Ltd., CH-3073 Guemligen, Switzerland

✦ Phone: 41 (0) 31 950 11 11　　　　FAX: 41 (0) 31 950 15 15
　Email: cuisine.sante@haco.ch　　　　www.haco.ch

USA Distributor:
Swiss Chalet Fine Foods, 9455 NW-40 Street Road, Miami, FL, USA 33178
Phone: 305-592-0008
Phone orders: 800-347-9477 ext. 5316　　　　FAX: 305-702-5395
Email orders: order@scff.com　　　　FAX Orders: 305-592-1651
　　　　　　　　　　　　　　　　　　　　www.scff.com

- Swiss Chalet Fine Foods distribute specialty foods to the foodservice industry including products from Haco Ltd., a Swiss company.
- Haco produces a variety of dehydrated products (soup bases, sauce mixes, seasonings, side dishes, desserts) including a line of products called "Cuisine Sante" that are free of gluten, lactose, allergens, hydrogenated fats, artificial flavors and MSG.
- Products made in a shared facility and every production batch of every product is tested for gluten. Certified by the Gluten-Free Certification Organization (GFCO).
- Order direct by phone, fax or email. Internet ordering coming soon.

Dairy Ease (Land O Lakes), White Wave Foods Company, Consumer Affairs,
　　　　　　　　12002 Airport Way, Broomfield, CO, USA 80021
　Phone: 800-878-9762/303-635-4000
　www.dairyease.com　　　　www.landolakes.com　　　　www.whitewave.com

- Lactose free milks available in fat-free, fat reduced (2%) and whole in refrigerated forms.
- All products are gluten-free.
- Available in retail stores.

De Boles, Hain-Celestial Group, Consumer Relations Department,
4600 Sleepytime Drive, Boulder, CO, USA 80301
Phone: 800-434-4246   FAX: 303-581-1520
Email: consumerrelations@hain-celestial.com   www.deboles.com

- Produce a variety of pastas (wheat, rice and corn).
- Corn and rice pastas in a variety of shapes are gluten-free. Equipment is thoroughly cleaned and products are tested for gluten.
- Available in retail stores.

Dietary Specialties, 8 South Commons Road, Waterbury, CT, USA 06704
✦   Phone: 888-640-2800/973-884-4402   FAX: 973-884-5907
Email: info@dietspec.com   www.dietspec.com

- Gluten-free specialty company; dedicated GF facility.
- Produce "Dietary Specialties" baking mixes (breads, cakes, muffins, pancakes), as well as ready-to-eat frozen products (e.g., desserts, pastas, pie shells and pizza) and English muffins.
- Also produce low protein products.
- Available in retail stores.
- Order direct by phone, fax, mail or internet; shipping charges based on amount purchased.
- Grocery items shipped via UPS Ground service and frozen items shipped express with freezer packs within contiguous USA.

Dowd & Rogers Inc., 1400 Kearns Blvd., Park City, UT, USA 84060
Phone: 800-669-8877   FAX: 800-767-8514
Email: info@dowdandrogers.com   www.dowdandrogers.com

- Gluten-free specialty company.
- Produce "Dowd & Rogers" gluten-free/soy-free cake and brownie mixes made from white rice, Italian chestnut and tapioca starch flours. Also sell Italian chestnut flour and almond flour in resealable pouches.
- Ingredients and final products tested for gluten.
- Available in retail stores and from www.glutenfreemall.com

Dr. Praeger's Sensible Foods, 9 Boumar Place, Elmwood Park, NJ, USA 07407
✦   Phone: 877-772-3437/201-703-1300   FAX: 201-703-9333
Email: info@drpraegers.com   www.drpraegers.com

- A variety of kosher products (appetizers, breaded fish, gefilte fish, minced fish, prepared pancakes, pizza bagels, vegetables, veggie burgers) that are low in saturated fat, cholesterol and sugar. All foods are certified kosher.
- Produce a line of gluten-free products (fish sticks, pancakes, potato littles and veggie burgers).
- Available in retail stores.
- Order direct by phone, fax or internet; shipping charges based on flat fee; ships via Overnight Express; frozen products shipped in a container with dry ice.

Duinkerken Foods Inc., 57 Watts Ave., Charlottetown, P.E.I., Canada C1E 2B7
✦ Phone: 902-569-3604   FAX: 902-569-3342
  Email: info@duinkerkenfoods.com   www.duinkerkenfoods.com

- Gluten-free specialty company, dedicated GF facility, ingredients purchased from dedicated facilities.
- Produce a variety of baking mixes (bread, biscuit, cookie, muffin, pizza and waffle) that are enriched with thiamin, riboflavin, niacin, iron and folic acid. Also sell baking flours.
- Available in retail stores.
- Order direct by mail, phone, fax or internet; shipping based on weight; ships via Canada Post.

Eden Foods Inc., 701 Tecumseh Rd, Clinton, MI, USA 49236
✦ Phone: 888-424-3336/517-456-7424   FAX: 517-456-6075
  Email: info@edenfoods.com   www.edenfoods.com

- Oldest natural food company in North America.
- Extensive line of organic products (e.g., beans, condiments, fruits/juices, grains, oils, pasta, sauces, snack foods, soy beverages). Many products are gluten-free which are tested for gluten.
- Available in retail stores.
- Order direct by phone, fax, mail or internet; shipping charges based on amount purchased; ships via FedEx Ground or USPS.

Edward & Son's Trading Company, Inc., Box 1326, Carpinteria, CA, USA 93014
✦ Phone: 805-684-8500   FAX: 805-684-8220
  Email: edwardsons@aol.com   www.edwardandsons.com
       or info@edwardandsons.com

- Produce a variety of natural and organic vegetarian foods under the brand names: Edward & Son's, Let's Do, Let's Do Organic, Native Forest, Premier Japan, Road's End Organics and The Wizard's.
- Brown rice snaps, rice toast, bouillon cubes and instant soups, gravy mixes, some pasta and sauces, gummi candies and one brand of ice cream cones are gluten-free.
- Road's End Organics gluten-free products and Miso Cup made in a dedicated GF facility and are tested for gluten by an independent lab.
- Brown rice snaps and sauces produced in a shared facility and are tested for gluten by an independent lab.
- Available in retail stores.
- Order direct by phone, fax, email, mail or internet; shipping charges based on weight; ships via FedEx Ground or USPS.

El Peto Products Ltd., 65 Saltsman Dr., Cambridge, ON, Canada N3H 4R7
✦ Phone: 800-387-4064/519-650-4614   FAX: 519-650-5692
  Email: sales@elpeto.com   www.elpeto.com

- Gluten-free specialty company; dedicated gluten-free facility.
- Wide variety of "El Peto" baked products (breads, buns, cakes, cookies, muffins, pies, pizza crusts), cereals, mixes, flours, grains and soups.
- Also carry other companies' products (e.g., Barkat, CelifibR, GoGo Quinoa, Pastariso, Pastato, Tinkyada) and books.
- Available in retail stores and the El Peto retail store.
- Order direct by phone, fax, email or mail; shipping charges based on weight; ships via UPS Ground.

Ener-G Foods, Box 84487, Seattle, WA, USA 98124

✦   Phone: 800-331-5222/206-767-6660   FAX: 206-764-3398
     Email: customerservice@ener-g.com   www.ener-g.com

- Gluten-free specialty company; dedicated GF and dairy-free facility and kosher certified facility.
- Very large variety of "Ener-G" shelf-stable gluten-free baked products (breads, buns, rolls, English muffins, pizza crust, cakes, cookies, crackers), baking ingredients, flours, mixes, pastas and snacks.
- Available in retail stores.
- Order direct by phone, fax or internet; shipping charges based on amount purchased; ships via FedEx or UPS Ground or USPS.

Enjoy Life, Enjoy Life Natural Brands, 3810 N. River Road, Schiller Park, IL, USA 60176

     Phone: 888-503-6569/847-260-0300   FAX: 847-260-0306
     Email: info@enjoylifefoods.com   www.enjoylifefoods.com

- Gluten-free specialty company; dedicated facility free of gluten, dairy, egg, soy, peanut, tree nut, corn and potato; kosher certified facility; products certified by Gluten-Free Certification Organization (GFCO).
- A variety of "Enjoy Life" products (bagels, granola cereals, "Perky's" cereals, cookies, snack bars, trail mix, chocolate bars and chocolate chips).
- Available in retail stores.

EnviroKidz, Nature's Path Foods Inc., 9100 Van Horne Way,
          Richmond, BC, Canada V6X 1W3

✦   Phone: 888-808-9505/604-248-8777   FAX: 604-248-8760
     Email: consumer_services@naturespath.com   www.envirokidz.com

- Variety of organic cereals, snack bars, cookies and waffles.
- Many products are gluten-free. All products are casein-free (except the chocolate crispy rice bar).
- Specific manufacturing processes are utilized to prevent cross-contamination. All gluten-free products are regularly tested for gluten. GF cereals and snack bars are certified by the Gluten-Free Certification Organization (GFCO).
- Available in retail stores.
- Order direct by phone or internet; shipping charges based on amount purchased; ships via UPS Ground.

Eragrain, HB Specialty Foods, Hydroblend, Inc., 1801 North Elder, Nampa, ID, USA 83687

     Phone: 877-467-7441/208-467-7441   FAX: 208-467-2220
     Email: customerservice@hydroblendinc.com   www.hydroblendinc.com

- Manufacturer of batters and breadings. Also produce a gluten-free line called "Eragrain" made with teff (frozen bread). Gluten-free products done in a separate dedicated facility. Products tested for gluten using ELISA.
- Available in some retail stores and gluten-free distributors (Glutenfreemall.com and GardenSpot Distributors).

Erewhon, Attune Foods, 535 Pacific Ave., 3rd Floor, San Francisco, CA, USA 94133
  Phone: 800-641-4508/415-486-2101

www.attunefoods.com

- Produce a variety of cereals that do not contain artificial colors, flavors, preservatives or hydrogenated oils. Some cereals are gluten-free.
- Equipment is thoroughly cleaned and strict allergen quality control procedures are used prior to production of gluten-free cereals. Products tested for gluten.
- Available in retail stores.

Everybody Eats, Inc., 294 Third Ave., corner of Carroll St., Brooklyn, NY, USA 11215
  ✦ Phone: 718-369-7444
  Email: everybodyeats@hotmail.com   www.everybodyeats-inc.com

- Gluten-free specialty company; dedicated gluten-free and nut-free facility.
- Produce bagels, baguettes, breads, brownies, cakes, cookies, rolls and entrées (pizza and ravioli).
- Co-owner has celiac disease.
- Available in some retail stores.
- No retail storefront but products that are pre-ordered can be picked up at the kitchen facility from M-F. Walk in sales on Saturdays.
- Order direct by mail, phone, email or internet; shipping charges based on weight; ships via UPS. Fresh pasta and pizza products are shipped frozen in styrofoam container with ice packs.

Avena (formerly FarmPure Foods™), 316 - 1st Ave. East, Regina, SK, Canada S4N 5H2
  ✦ Phone: 866-461-3663/306-757-3663   FAX: 306-757-1218
                                             www.onlyoats.com
                                             www.onlyoats.ca

- Operate a dedicated GF facility committed to processing pure, uncontaminated oat products.
- Owned by pedigreed seed growers across western Canada who follow a very rigid set of guidelines in pedigreed seed production, crop production best management practices, harvesting, cleaning, storage and logistics of oats that meet rigid quality standards.
- Quality protocol starts with variety specific pedigreed seeds planted on fields which have not grown any cereal crops containing gluten for a minimum of three years. Fields are maintained as per standards set out by the Canadian Seed Growers Association. The entire processing facility is oat dedicated. All oat deliveries, as well as all associated product ingredients, are tested before entering the plant, during and after processing using the R5-ELISA test.
- Facility and products are certified by the Gluten-Free Certification Organization (GFCO). Base products are also kosher certified. All products are allergen-free.
- Produce base products (regular and quick oat flakes, oat flour, oat bran and steel cut oat pearls), breakfast blends and ready mixes (cookies, muffins and pancakes).
- Supply in bulk to independent gluten-free bakers, processors and the foodservice sector. Also supply wholesale to gluten-free private label manufacturers, as well as grocery distributors.
- Available in retail stores under the brand name Only Oats™.
- Order direct by internet; ships via international ground courier service or Canada Post.

Food For Life Baking Company, Box 1434, Corona, CA, USA 92878
Phone: 800-797-5090/951-279-5090   FAX: 951-279-1784
Email: info@foodforlife.com   www.foodforlife.com

- Wholesale bakery that produces a variety of "Food For Life" specialty breads, buns, and tortillas. Some breads and the corn & rice tortillas are gluten-free.
- Gluten-free products are made on a dedicated line and in a separate area of the plant; products are tested for gluten.
- Available in retail stores.

Foods By George LLC, 3 King St., Mahwah, NJ, USA 07430
✦ Phone: 201-612-9700   FAX: 201-684-0334
Email: info@foodsbygeorge.com   www.foodsbygeorge.com

- Gluten-free specialty company; dedicated GF facility; products tested for gluten by an independent lab.
- A variety of "Foods By George" baked products (biscotti, brownies, cakes, muffins, tarts), pizza and lasagna.
- Available in retail stores and in person at the Foods By George store.
- Order direct by internet; shipping charges based on amount purchased; ships via UPS Ground, or 2nd day air. Products shipped frozen in a styrofoam cooler with dry ice and gel packs.

Food-Tek, Inc., 50 Intervale Road, Boonton, NJ, USA 07005
✦ Phone: 800-648-8114/973-257-4000   FAX: 973-257-5555
Email: info@foodtek.com   www.foodtek.com

- Food product development and manufacturing company. Produce a variety of confectionary items including a line of gluten-free mixes (bread, brownie, bun, cake, cookie, pizza crust and waffle) that are enriched with B vitamins.
- "Fast & Fresh" (microwave mixes) and "Quick-Bake" (oven mixes) are packed in small serving sizes and many have mixing cups and/or baking trays.
- Gluten-free products made on dedicated lines. Products tested for gluten.
- Available in retail stores and amazon.com
- Order direct by phone, fax or internet; ships via DHL Ground.

gf Meals, Your Dinner Secret, 20929 Ventura Blvd., #22, Woodland Hills, CA, USA 91364
✦ Phone: 888-700-5610/818-888-6338   FAX: 818-888-6336
Email: info@gfmeals.com   www.gfmeals.com

- Gluten-free specialty company; dedicated gluten and casein-free facility.
- Offer frozen, ready-to-cook entrées, side dishes, sauces and baked goods that are gluten and casein-free. Baked goods produced by The Sensitive Baker, a dedicated gluten and casein-free bakery.
- Also carry other companies' products (dips, dressings, flavored oils and sauces).
- Shop in person or order direct by mail, phone, fax, email or internet; shipping charges based on amount purchased; ships via UPS in special insulated containers with dry ice.

Gifts of Nature Inc., P.O. Box 956, Polson, MT, USA 59860

✦ Phone: 888-275-0003/406-883-3730   FAX: 406-883-3731
Email: info@giftsofnature.net   www.giftsofnature.net

- Gluten-free specialty company; dedicated GF facility.
- Produce a variety of "Gifts of Nature" mixes (biscuits, breads, brownies, cakes, cookies, muffins, pancakes, pizza) and sell flours and baking ingredients including Montina™.
- Also manufacture pure, uncontaminated oats in a dedicated GF facility that is certified by the Gluten-Free Certification Organization (GFCO).
- Oats are produced by a Grower Cooperative that grow oats on dedicated fields and use dedicated equipment for harvesting, cleaning and transportation. Products are ELISA tested for purity after harvest and then processed (cleaned and rolled) in the Grower Cooperative dedicated facility that is GFCO certified. Packaged into large tote bags and shipped to Gifts of Nature facility where they are re-tested and packaged for sale.
- Available in some retail stores.
- Order direct by phone, mail or internet; shipping charges based on weight; ships via UPS.

Gillian's Foods, Inc., 82 Sanderson Ave., Lynn, MA, USA 01902

✦ Phone: 781-586-0086   FAX: 781-586-0087
Email: chefbob@gilliansfoods.com   www.gilliansfoods.com

- Gluten-free specialty company; dedicated GF facility.
- Variety of "Gillian's" baked products (breads, brownies, cookies, pies, pie crusts, pizza crusts, pizza dough, rolls), bread crumbs and pastas. Also sell flours and mixes.
- Available in retail stores.
- Order direct by phone, fax or internet; shipping charges based on weight; ships via UPS (Ground, Next or 2nd day air or 3rd day select); frozen products shipped in a stryofoam container with an ice pack.

Gluten Free & Fabulous™, 7323 East Valley View Road, Scottsdale, AZ, USA 85250

✦ Phone: 480-947-7315   FAX: 480-946-9402
Email: info@glutenfreefabulous.com   www.glutenfreefabulous.com

- Gluten-free specialty company; dedicated GF facility; products tested by ELISA for gluten. Family member has celiac disease.
- Produce cookies, crackers, pasta dinners (made from quinoa), pizza and pizza crusts.
- Available in retail stores.
- Order online from amazon.com

Gluten-Free Bagel Company, RR3, Box 117 EE, Meshoppen, PA, USA 18630

✦ Phone: 888-458-8360/570-965-2767   FAX: 570-965-0929
Email: diane@glutenfreebagelcompany.com   www.glutenfreebagelcompany.com

- Gluten-free specialty company; dedicated GF facility.
- Produce ready-to-eat gluten-free baked products (breads, bagels, soft pretzels, rolls, cakes, brownies and cookies), baking mixes (breads, bagels, soft pretzels, cakes, cookies, brownies, muffins, scones) and flours.
- Order direct by phone, mail or internet; shipping charges based on weight; ships via USPS Priority Mail.

Gluten-Free Naturals, LLC, P.O. Box 1626, Cranford, NJ, USA 07016

✦ Phone: 866-761-6147/917-885-3087

Email:sales@gfnfoods.com　　　　　　　www.gfnfoods.com

- Gluten-free specialty company; products made in a dedicated GF area of a shared facility and are tested for gluten using an ELISA test.
- Produce gluten-free mixes (bread, brownie, cake, cookie, pancake and pizza).
- Available in retail stores.
- Order direct by phone, mail or internet; shipping charges based on weight; ships via UPS Ground.

Gluten-Free Oats®, 578 Lane 9, Powell, WY, USA 82435

✦ Phone: 888-941-9922/307-754-7541　　　FAX: 307-754-7043

Email:sales@glutenfreeoats.com　　　　　www.glutenfreeoats.com

- Gluten-free specialty company that mill and manufacture pure, uncontaminated oats (rolled oats and oat groats) that are certified by the Gluten-Free Certification Organization (GFCO).
- Maintain their own certified seed and personally contract with farmers who do not grow any wheat, rye or barley on the land for the last two years. Use combines for gluten-free oats or non-gluten crops only. The fields and equipment are monitored and inspected by Gluten-Free Oats® and Wyoming Seed Certification Service.
- The harvested crop is analyzed for purity using R5 ELISA test at the mill and by the University of Nebraska Food Allergy and Resource Program.
- The equipment used in transporting, processing and packaging is dedicated to prevent cross-contamination.
- The three owners of the company have celiac disease.
- Available in retail stores.
- Order direct by phone, fax or internet; shipping charges based on weight; ships via UPS Ground.

Glutenfreeda Foods, Inc., P.O. Box 487, Burlington, WA, USA 98233

✦ Phone: 360-755-1300　　　　　　　　FAX: 360-755-1303

Email: jessica@glutenfreeda.com　　　　www.glutenfreedafoods.com

- Gluten-free specialty company; dedicated GF facility.
- Produce "Real Cookies™" frozen pre-formed cookie dough, instant oatmeal cereals and granola (using gluten-free oats), burritos and organic ice cream sandwiches.
- Available in retail stores, amazon.com and glutenfreemall.com.

Gluten-Free Pantry, Glutino Food Group, 2055 Boulevard Dagenais West, Laval, QC, Canada H7L 5V1

✦ Phone: 800-291-8386　　　　　　　　FAX: 450-963-0137

Email: pantry@glutenfree.com　　　　　www.glutenfree.com

- Gluten-free specialty company; dedicated GF facility.
- Produce "Gluten-Free Pantry" mixes (breads, cakes, cookies, muffins, pastry, pancakes and scones).
- Available in retail stores.
- Order direct by phone, fax or internet; shipping charges based on weight; ships via UPS Ground or Air.

Glutino Food Group, 2055 Boulevard Dagenais West, Laval, QC, Canada   H7L 5V1
✦   Phone: 800-363-3438/450-629-7689   FAX: 450-629-4781
Email: pantry@glutenfree.com   www.glutino.com
                                             www.glutenfree.com

- Gluten-free specialty company; dedicated GF facility.
- Wide variety of "Glutino" baked products (bagels, breads, buns, cakes, cookies, muffins, pizza crusts), crackers, mixes, pretzels, snack bars and entrées.
- Many of their products made in a dedicated GF facility and tested for gluten. Some products made in a shared facility in a dedicated area and on dedicated equipment. Products are tested for gluten.
- Available in retail stores and the Glutino retail store.
- Order direct by phone, fax or internet; shipping charges based on weight; ships via UPS Ground or UPS Air.

GoGo Quinoa, Compagnie 2 Ameriks, CP 344 Succ. Snowdon,
                Montreal, QC, Canada   H3X 3Y1
✦   Phone: 514-249-5103   FAX: 866-847-6906
Email: info@gogoquinoa.com   www.gogoquinoa.com

- Produce a variety of organic quinoa and amaranth based products manufactured in a dedicated GF facility in Bolivia and Montreal; products tested for gluten using ELISA test.
- Quinoa products (puffed cereals, flakes, whole grain [black, red, white], pasta, snacks, soups, burger mix and risotto).
- Amaranth products (puffed cereal, pasta, whole grain).
- Available in retail stores and from gluten-free companies.
- Order direct by internet; shipping charges based on weight; ships via Canada Post.

Good Eatz and Good Eatz Green Cafe, 701 Penn Ave., West Reading, PA, USA   19611
✦   Phone: 610-670-4885   FAX: 610-670-4885
Email: goodeatz@comcast.net   www.goodeatz.org

- Gluten-free specialty company; dedicated GF facility; products tested for gluten using ELISA test.
- Produce brownies, cakes, cookies, loaves, tarts and other baked goods.
- Good Eatz Green Cafe open for breakfast, lunch and dinner. Features meals and snacks for special dietary needs (gluten-free, dairy-free, vegetarian and vegan).
- Available in retail stores.
- Order direct by internet; shipping charges based on weight; ships via FedEx or UPS.

Good Karma Food Technologies Inc., 1622 S. Gaffey St., Suite 208,
                San Pedro, CA, USA   90731
Phone: 800-550-6731/310-547-0000   FAX: 310-547-0010
Email: loren@goodkarmafoods.com   www.goodkarmafoods.com

- Produce organic brown rice frozen desserts/novelties and rice milk that are gluten and casein-free, vegan and kosher.
- Available in retail stores.

Green's Gluten-Free Beer, 9 Briar Rhydding, Baildon Shipley, West Yorkshire, England BD17 7JW

Phone: 44 1274 714664   FAX: 44 1274 714601

Email: info@glutenfreebeers.co.uk   www.glutenfreebeers.com

US and Canadian Importer:

Merchant duVin, 18200 Olympic Ave. South, Tukwila, WA, USA 98188

Phone: 253-656-0320   FAX: 253-872-5530

Email: info@merchantduvin.com   www.merchantduvin.com

- Produce gluten-free ales, beers and lagers made from millet, brown rice, buckwheat and sorghum that have 6-8.5% alcohol in 16.9 oz. (500 mL) bottles.
- Available in some retail stores, liquor stores, grocery and health food stores.

Health Valley, Hain-Celestial Group, Consumer Relations Department, 4600 Sleepytime Drive, Boulder, CO, USA 80301

Phone: 800-434-4246   FAX: 303-581-1520

Email: consumerrelations@hain-celestial.com   www.healthvalley.com

- A variety of natural health-food products (e.g., chilies, soups, broths, cereals, crackers, cookies, snack bars). Some cereals are gluten-free.
- Available in retail stores.
- Order direct by phone or internet; shipping charges based on weight; ships via FedEx or USPS.

Heaven Scent Natural Foods, Eco Heaven LLC, Dept. 50207, Box 803338, Chicago, IL, USA 60680

Phone: 630-701-8801   FAX: 888-252-7997

Email: info@eco-planet.net   www.ecoheavenllc.com

- Natural food company that produces bread crumbs, cookies, croûtons and crispy rice and marshmallow bars. The bars are gluten and dairy-free.
- Available in retail stores.

Hodgson Mill, 1100 Stevens Ave., Effingham, IL, USA 62401

Phone: 800-347-0105   FAX: 217-347-0198

Email: customerservice@hodgsonmill.com   www.hodgsonmill.com

- Whole grain milling company using a stone grind milling process.
- Sell a variety of flours, mixes, baking ingredients and pastas. Somemixes and pastas are gluten-free. Gluten-free mixes and pastas use gluten-free ingredients that are tested for gluten using the ELISA test and are produced and packaged in an isolated gluten-free room within the facility.
- Available in retail stores.
- Order direct by phone, fax, mail or internet; shipping charges based on amount purchased; ships via UPS Ground.

Hol•Grain, Conrad Rice Mill Inc., P.O. Box 10640, New Iberia, LA, USA 70562

Phone: 800-551-3245/337-364-7242   FAX: 337-365-5806

Email: info@conradricemill.com   www.conradricemill.com

- Oldest rice mill in North America.
- A variety of rice mixes, sauces, seasonings, snacks, soups, spices and wheat-free/ gluten-free products. Brown rice crackers, brown rice bread crumbs, chocolate chip cookie mix, pancake/waffle mix and plain rice are gluten-free.
- Available in retail stores.
- Order direct by phone or internet; shipping charges based on amount purchased; ships via UPS Ground.

Holly's Oatmeal, 241 Northside Drive, Torrington, CT, USA 06790
✦ Phone: 860-618-0090   FAX: 860-618-3008
Email: info@hollysoatmeal.com   www.hollysoatmeal.com

- Produce 2 lines of whole-grain porridge (regular and gluten-free varieties). The gluten-free oatmeal (available in plain and cranberry) is a mixture of pure, uncontaminated oats, quinoa flakes, amaranth, flax, whole-grain brown rice, corn, sorghum and buckwheat.
- Gluten-free oatmeal produced in a separate dedicated room and on dedicated equipment. Product is tested for gluten using ELISA test.
- Available in some retail stores and amazon.com
- Order direct by phone, fax, mail or internet; shipping charges based on weight; ships via DHL.

Ian's Natural Foods, 360 Merrimack Street, Building 9, Suite 320, Lawrence, MA, USA 01843
Phone: 800-543-6637/978-989-0601   FAX: 978-989-0602
Email: customerservice@iansnaturalfoods.com   www.iansnaturalfoods.com

- Produce an extensive line of natural and organic frozen and shelf-stable foods including a variety of wheat-free, gluten-free products. Many are also casein, egg and soy-free.
- Gluten-free products manufactured in a shared facility on separate days and equipment is thoroughly cleaned to prevent cross-contamination. Ingredients and final products are tested for gluten using the ELISA test.
- Available in retail stores.
- Order direct by internet; shipping charges based on weight; minimum $75.00 order; $10.00 handling fee on frozen foods; ships via FedEx next day air.

Imagine Foods, Hain-Celestial Group, Consumer Relations Department, 4600 Sleepytime Drive, Boulder, CO, USA 80301
Phone: 800-434-4246   FAX: 303-581-1520
Email: consumerrelations@hain-celestial.com   www.imaginefoods.com
                                        www.tastethedream.com

- Natural and organic products include beverages (Almond Dream, Kidz Dream, Rice Dream, Soy Dream), frozen desserts and novelties (Rice Dream, Soy Dream) and soups and broths (Imagine). Most of the products are gluten-free.
- Available in retail stores and some online stores.

Inca Organics, 155 Pine Tops Drive, Athens, GA, USA 30606
Phone: 866-328-4622/706-549-8947   FAX: 240-282-2589
Email: marjorie@incaorganics.com   www.incaorganics.com

- Bulk wholesaler of certified South American organic quinoa and black amaranth.
- Sell to distributors and food manufacturers in bulk quantities.

Jennies, Red Mill Farms Inc., 290 S. 5th St., Brooklyn, NY, USA 11211
✦ Phone: 888-294-1164/718-384-2150   FAX: 718-384-2988
Email: info@macaroonking.com   www.macaroonking.com

- Produce gluten-free coconut macaroons and "low carb" coconut macaroons in various flavors, as well as "omega-3 energy bars" made with coconut and seeds (flax, pumpkin, sunflower).
- Dedicated GF facility.
- Available in retail stores.
- Order direct by internet; shipping charges based on weight; ships via UPS Ground.

Kari-Out Company, 399 Knollwood Road, Suite 309, White Plains, NY, USA 10603
    Phone: 800-433-8799/914-580-3200   FAX: 914-580-3248
    Email: amsales@kariout.com   www.kariout.com

- Manufacturer of take-out packaging containers, cleaning supplies and food ingredients (sauces, spices, seasonings).
- Produce "Panda Brand" gluten-free, low-sodium soy sauce available in individual packets, sold in bulk (350 packets/case) to distributors.
- Available to restaurants and other foodservice facilities.
- Consumers can order in a case lot from specific distributors. Contact Kari-Out to locate nearest distributor.

Kaybee, Box 629, Cudworth, SK, Canada S0K 1B0
✦   Phone: 306-256-3951   FAX: 306-256-3424
    Email: kaybee@sasktel.net   www.kaybeeglutenfree.ca

- Gluten-free specialty company; dedicated gluten-free facility.
- Variety of "Kaybee" gluten-free mixes (bread, buns, cakes, cookies, muffins, pancakes, pizza crusts, puddings, and perogies).
- Available in retail stores.
- Order direct by phone or fax. Shipping is free for orders of 18 packages or more; shipping parcels under 24 packages is a flat rate of $10.00 in Canada and $15.00 (U.S. funds) in USA.

Kettle Cuisine, 270 Second Street, Chelsea, MA, USA 02150
    Phone: 877-302-7687/617-884-1219   FAX: 617-884-1041
    Email: contactus@kettlecuisine.com   www.kettlecuisine.com

- Produce a large variety of soups for retail and foodservice including a line of frozen gluten-free soups (single-serve, microwavable).
- Gluten-free soups are made under strict manufacturing procedures to prevent cross-contamination and each batch is tested for gluten. Products certified by Gluten-Free Certification Organization (GFCO).
- Available in retail stores and from www.glutenfreemall.com

Kingsmill Foods (see PaneRiso/Kingsmill)

Kinnikinnick Foods, 10940 - 120 Street, Edmonton, AB, Canada T5H 3P7
✦   Phone: 877-503-4466/780-424-2900   FAX: 780-421-0456
    Email: info@kinnikinnick.com   www.kinnikinnick.com

- Gluten-free specialty company; dedicated gluten-free and nut-free facility.
- On-site quality control lab that tests for gluten using the highly sensitive ELISA test.
- Very large variety of "Kinnikinnick" baked products (bagels, breads, bread crumbs, cookie crumbs, buns, cakes, cereal, cookies, donuts, muffins, pizza crust, waffles) and baking mixes, as well as flours. All products are dairy-free/casein-free except cheese bread.
- Carry a variety of products from other companies (cereals, crackers, pasta), as well as Toastabags (reuseable toaster bags).
- Available in retail stores and the Kinnikinnick retail store.
- Order direct by phone, fax or internet; shipping charges are a $10 flat rate for Canadian orders (of any value) and $10 (U.S. funds) for USA orders (valued up to $200); ships UPS Air.

Kitchen Table Bakers, 41 Princeton Drive, Syosset, NY, USA 11793
    Phone: 800-486-4582/516-931-5113   FAX: 516-932-5467
    Email: info@kitchentablebakers.com   www.kitchentablebakers.com

- Produce all parmesan gourmet wafer crisps in various flavors that are all gluten-free.
- Made in a shared facility; dedicated gluten-free equipment and baking pans; products tested for gluten.
- Available in retail stores and some online stores.

Kokimo Kitchen Ltd., 2771 County Road 25, Castleton, ON, Canada K0K 1M0
    Phone: 888-344-7977/905-344-7960   FAX: 905-344-7961
    Email: amazing@kokimokitchen.com   www.kokimokitchen.com

- Gluten-free specialty company; dedicated gluten-free facility.
- Produce "Kokimo" mixes (pancakes, waffles and eggless French toast) made from buckwheat, cornmeal, brown rice, millet and Asian bean flours. Mixes are also dairy and egg-free. Available in family size and bulk quantities.
- Available in some retail stores.

Lactaid, McNeil Consumer Health Care, Guelph, ON, Canada N1K 1A5
      McNeil Nutritionals, 7050 Camp Hill Rd., Ft. Washington, PA, USA 19034
    Phone: 800-522-8243 (USA)   www.lactaid.com
    Phone: 800-563-1515 (Canada)

- Lactaid® brand of dairy products are made with lactose-reduced milk. Available as refrigerated milk (regular, organic, eggnog), cottage cheese, ice cream and evaporated milk.
- "Lactaid tablets", "Lactaid caplets" and "Lactaid drops" can be used when consuming milk and milk products.
- All products are gluten-free.
- Available in retail stores.

Lacteeze,
  Farmer's Dairy, P.O. Box 8118, Halifax, NS, Canada B3K 5Y6
    Phone: 800-565-1626/902-835-4005   FAX: 800-565-1945
    Email: customer.service@farmersdairy.ca   www.farmersdairy.ca

Gay Lea Foods, 5200 Orbitor Drive, Mississauga, ON, Canada L4W 5B4
    Phone: 800-268-0508/905-283-5300   www.gayleafoods.com

- "Lacteeze" (lactose-reduced milk) is available in shelf-stable and refrigerated forms.
- "Lacteeze" drops and tablets/caplets.
- All products are gluten-free.
- Available in retail stores.

Lakefront Brewery, Inc., 1872 N. Commerce Street, Milwaukee, WI, USA 53212
    Phone: 414-372-8800   FAX: 414-372-4400
    Email: info@lakefrontbrewery.com   www.lakefrontbrewery.com
                             www.newgrist.com

- Produce a variety of ales, beers and lagers including a gluten-free beer called "New Grist" made from sorghum, rice, hops and yeast (made from molasses) available in 12 oz. bottles.
- New Grist is tested for gluten prior to fermentation and before bottling.
- Available in some bars, restaurants, grocery and liquor stores.

La Messagère, Les bières de la Nouvelle-France, 90 Rivière aux Écorces Road,
Saint-Alexis-des Monts, QC, Canada J0K 1V0
Phone: 819-265-4000   FAX: 819-265-4020
Email: info@lesbieresnouvellefrance.com   www.lesbieresnouvellefrance.com

- Microbrewery that produces a variety of beers including LaMessagère, a gluten-free beer (blonde ale) made from rice and buckwheat.
- Available in liquor stores across Canada and in some specialty stores in 341 mL bottles.

Lärabar, Humm Foods Inc., P.O. Box 18932, Denver, CO, USA 80218
✦ Phone: 877-527-2227/720-945-1155   FAX: 720-941-1158
Email: info@larabar.com   www.larabar.com

- Variety of nutrition energy bars (made from dried fruits, nuts and spices), chocolate snack bars called Jôcolat (made from dates, nuts and cocoa) and JamFrakas snack bars (made from dried fruits, nuts, honey and crisp rice).
- All bars are gluten, dairy and soy-free.
- Dedicated gluten-free facility; products certified by the Gluten-Free Certification Organization (GFCO).
- Available in retail stores.
- Order direct by phone, fax or internet; shipping charges based on flat rate; ships via FedEx Ground.

Lara's (see Cream Hill Estates)

La Tortilla Factory, 3300 Westwind Blvd., Santa Rosa, CA, USA 95403
✦ Phone: 800-446-1516/707-586-4000   FAX: 707-586-4017
Email: info@latortillafactory.com   www.latortillafactory.com

- Produce a variety of wraps and tortillas including a line of gluten-free products that are certified by the Gluten-Free Certification Organization (GFCO).
- Made from whole-grain millet flour and dark or ivory teff flour that contains 3 grams fiber per wrap.
- La Tortilla "Sonoma" Gluten-Free Wraps have no preservatives and must be frozen/ refrigerated.
- La Tortilla "Smart and Delicious" Gluten-Free Wraps are shelf-stable.
- Available in retail stores.
- Order direct via phone, mail, fax or internet; shipping charges based on weight; ships via FedEx Ground or air.

Laurel's Sweet Treats Inc., 8172 SW Durham Road, Tigard, OR, USA 97224
✦ Phone: 866-225-3432/503-443-3803   FAX: 503-968-5237
Email: sales@glutenfreemixes.com   www.glutenfreemixes.com

- Gluten-free specialty company; dedicated GF facility.
- Variety of baking mixes (breads, brownies, cakes, crackers, cookies, pancakes, pizza dough, rolls), all-purpose batter mix and cake decorating supplies. All baking mixes are dairy-free. Also produce ready-to-eat baked products.
- Order direct by phone, fax, email or internet; shipping charges based on weight; ships via FedEx or flat rate USPS.

Leda Nutrition, P.O. Box 714, Mudgeeraba B.C. QLD, Australia 4213
✦ Email: info@ledanutrition.com   www.ledanutrition.com
- Gluten-free specialty company; dedicated gluten-free and dairy-free facility.
- Produce gluten-free, dairy-free nutrition snack bars made from gluten-free flour mixture (chickpea, corn, tapioca, rice and soy [in some bars]) and dried fruits. Also produce gluten-free biscuits, cookies and slices.
- Available in retail stores.
- Order direct by internet; contact company for shipping arrangements for international orders.

Let's Do…, Edward & Son's Trading Company, Inc., P.O. Box 1326, Carpinteria, CA, USA 93014
✦ Phone: 805-684-8500   FAX: 805-684-8220
    Email: edwardsons@aol.com   www.edwardandsons.com
         or info@edwardandsons.com
- Produce a line of confectionary items free of gluten and major allergens including ice cream cones and sprinkelz.
- Available in retail stores.
- Order direct by phone, fax, email, mail or internet; shipping charges based on weight; ships via FedEx Ground or USPS.

Le Veneziane, Molino di Ferro, s.r.l., Via Artesini 27, 31050 Fanzolo di Vedelago (TV), Italy
✦ Phone: 39 04 23.487035   FAX: 39 04 23.476226
                                              www.molinodiferro.com
                                              www.quattrobimbi.com
- Produce gluten-free corn-based items (cookies, pasta, polenta) made in a dedicated GF facility.
- Distributed by Quattrobimbi Imports in USA.
- Available in some retail stores and gluten-free specialty stores.
- Order direct by internet from www.quattrobimbi.com; shipping charges based on weight; ships via FedEx or UPS.

LifeSource, LifeMax Natural Foods Distribution Inc., 1773 Bayly St., Pickering, ON, Canada L1W 2Y7
    Phone: 877-543-3629/905-831-5433   FAX: 905-831-4333
    Email: info@lifemax.ca   www.lifemax.ca
- Wheat-free, gluten-free tamari soy sauces.
- Available in retail stores.

Lundberg Family Farms, P.O. Box 369, 5370 Church St., Richvale, CA, USA 95974
✦ Phone: 530-882-4551   FAX: 530-882-4500
    Email: info@lundberg.com   www.lundberg.com
- Family-owned farm that grows and produces brown rice, specialty rice varieties and brown rice products.
- A variety of products (rice, rice cakes, rice snacks, rice syrup, rice cereal, rice pasta, rice side dishes). Most of these products are also organic and gluten-free.
- Available in retail stores.
- Order direct by mail or internet; shipping charges based on weight; ships via UPS.

Manischewitz, R.A.B. Food Group, LLC., One Harmon Plaza, 10th Floor,
Secaucus, NJ, USA 07094

✦ Phone: 908-654-1098/201-553-1100   FAX: 201-583-1793 (Deborah)
Email: deborah.ross@manischewitz.com   www.manischewitz.com

- Largest USA manufacturer of processed kosher foods (gefilte fish, pastas, soups and soup mixes, snack foods, tams and crackers, matzos, potato and other mixes).
- Also produce products especially for Passover.
- A variety of products are gluten-free.
- Available in retail stores.
- Order direct by internet; shipping charges based on weight; ships via FedEx.

MapleGrove Gluten-Free Foods (see CelifbR, Pastamaiza, Pastariso and Pastato)

Mariposa Baking Company, 5427 Telegraph Ave., Unit D3, Oakland, CA, USA 94609

✦ Phone: 510-595-0955   FAX: 510-595-0966
Email: info@mariposabaking.com   www.mariposabaking.com

- Gluten-free specialty company; dedicated GF facility; products tested for gluten using ELISA test.
- Produce bagels, biscotti, breads, brownies, cakes, cookies, muffins, pizza crusts. Many products are also casein-free.
- Available in some retail stores.
- Shop in person in the Cafe Mariposa & Bakeshop.
- Order direct by phone, fax, mail or internet; shipping charges based on amount purchased; ships via FedEx Ground or USPS (Priority).

Marsan Foods, 160 Thermos Road, Toronto, ON, Canada M1L 4W2

Phone: 416-755-9262   FAX: 416-755-6790
Email: sean@marsanfoods.com   www.marsanfoods.com

- Manufacturer of frozen entrées, soups and other products for retail grocery, foodservice and healthcare.
- Healthcare products applicable to cold plating; high in protein; fat and sodium controlled for most diets.
- Gluten-free products available under "Balanced Cuisine" and "Purée Essential". Single serve and bulk sizes.
- Available through distributors (e.g., Sysco, GFS, Summit Foods).

Mary's Gone Crackers, P.O. Box 965, Gridley, CA, USA 95948

✦ Phone: 888-258-1250/530-846-5100   FAX: 530-846-5500
Email: info@marysgonecrackers.com   www.marysgonecrackers.com

- Produce gluten-free, high fiber crackers, cracker crumb and snacks made from organic brown rice, quinoa, flax, sesame seeds and gluten-free tamari sauce.
- Dedicated GF and nut-free facility; also organic and kosher certified.
- Available in retail stores.
- Order direct by phone or internet; shipping charges based on weight; ships via FedEx Ground.

Minn-Dak Growers, Ltd., 4034 - 40th Ave. N., P.O. Box 13276, Grand Forks, ND, USA 58208

✦ Phone: 701-746-7453   FAX: 701-780-9050
Email: info@minndak.com   www.minndak.com

- A processor, contractor and marketer of buckwheat to the domestic and international food ingredients industry. Dedicated GF facility.
- Has the newest and largest dedicated buckwheat milling facility in North America.
- Buckwheat products include flour, Farinetta™ (buckwheat bran), groats, grits and kasha.
- Also processes safflower, sunflower seeds and mustard seeds.
- Order direct by phone, fax, mail or internet; shipping charges based on weight; ships via UPS Ground.

Miss Roben's, Allergy Grocer, LLC, 7135 Minstrel Way, Suite 101, Columbia, MD, USA 21045

✦ Phone: 888-476-3350/410-309-9343   FAX: 410-290-5689
Email: info@allergygrocer.com   www.allergygrocer.com

- Gluten-free specialty company; dedicated facility free of gluten, dairy, peanuts, tree nuts, eggs, soy, sesame and latex.
- Produce "Miss Roben's" gluten-free mixes (bagels, breads, brownies, cakes, cookies, crackers, frostings, muffins, pancakes, pie and pizza crusts, pretzels and tortillas).
- Order direct by phone, fax, or internet; shipping charges based on amount purchased; free shipping on orders over $100.00; ships via UPS Ground or USPS.

Mochi, Grainaissance Inc., 1580 - 62nd Street, Emeryville, CA, USA 94608
Phone: 800-472-4697/510-547-7256   FAX: 510-547-0526
Email: amazake@grainaissance.com   www.grainaissance.com

- Produce a bake and serve rice puff snack made from brown rice in a variety of flavors. All flavors are gluten-free (except "mugwort") and dairy-free.
- Available in retail stores in the refrigerated section.

Mr. Krispers, TH Foods, Inc., 2154 Harlem Road, Loves Park, IL, USA 61111
✦ Phone: 815-636-9500   FAX: 815-636-8400
Email: crunchmasterguru@thfoods.com   www.mrkrispers.com

- Baked whole grain chips made from brown rice and corn in a variety of flavors.
- Made in a shared facility; products certified by the Gluten-Free Certification Organization (GFCO). Available in retail stores and amazon.com
- Order direct by internet; shipping charges based on weight; ships via FedEx Ground.

Mr. Spice, Healthy Foods, 20 Silva Lane, Newport, RI, USA 02842
✦ Phone: 800-728-2348/401-848-7700   FAX: 401-848-7701
Email: customerservice@mrspice.com   www.mrspice.com

- Produce a variety of sauces that do not contain any gluten, dairy, preservatives, added salt or sulfites.
- Available in retail stores.
- Order direct by phone, fax, email or internet; shipping charges based on weight; ships via UPS Ground.

Mr. Ritt's Gluten-Free, 453 North 2nd Street, Millville, NJ, USA 08332
✦ Phone: 856-825-8770   FAX: 856-825-8776
Email: mrritt@aol.com   www.mrritts.org

- Gluten-free specialty company.
- Produce a variety of baking mixes (bread, waffle) and flour blends.
- Order direct by internet.

Mrs. Leeper's, Inc., Liberty Richter, a division of World Finer Foods, 300 Broadacres Drive, Bloomfield, NJ, USA   07003

✦ Phone: 800-225-1449/973-338-0300   FAX: 973-338-0382
Email: survey@worldfiner.com   www.mrsleepers.com

- Produce brown rice and corn pastas including pasta and sauce mix entrées.
- Available in retail stores.
- Order direct by internet; shipping charges based on weight; ships via FedEx or USPS.

Mrs. May's Naturals, Inc., 860 E. 238th Street, Carson, CA, USA   90745

✦ Phone: 877-677-6297/310-830-3130   FAX: 310-830-3045
Email: info@mrsmays.com   www.mrsmays.com

- Produce snacks made from dried fruit, nuts and/or seeds. Sweetened with rice malt which is gluten-free. All products are gluten and casein-free.
- Products tested for gluten using ELISA test.
- Available in retail stores.
- Order direct by phone or internet; shipping charges are a flat rate; ships via UPS Ground or USPS.

My Own Meals, Inc., P.O. Box 334, Deerfield, IL, USA   60015

✦ Phone: 847-948-1118   FAX: 847-948-0468
Email: sales@myownmeals.com   www.myownmeals.com

- Produce fully cooked single serve meals (in individual trays) in vacuum-sealed packages that requires no refrigeration.
- All meals are kosher and are free of soy, fish, shellfish and MSG.
- Some products are also gluten and dairy-free.
- Available in retail stores and from some gluten-free companies.
- Contact company for ordering information.

Namaste Foods, P.O. Box 3133, Coeur D'Alene, ID, USA   83816

✦ Phone: 866-258-9493/208-772-6325   FAX: 208-772-4318
Email: admin@namastefoods.com   www.namastefoods.com

- Gluten-free specialty company; dedicated GF facility.
- Produce a variety of mixes (breads, brownies, cakes, cookies, muffins, pancakes, pasta blends, pizza crust) that are also free of corn, soy, potato, dairy and nuts.
- Available in retail stores.
- Order direct by phone, fax, mail or internet; shipping charges based on amount purchased; ships via FedEx Ground.

Nana's Cookie Company, 4901 Morena Blvd., Suite 401, San Diego, CA, USA   92130

✦ Phone: 800-836-7534/858-273-5775   FAX: 858-273-3432
Email: nanas@nanascookiecompany.com   www.nanascookiecompany.com

- Produce cookies and cookie bars that are egg and dairy-free and sweetened with fruit juice. The gluten-free cookies are produced in a shared facility on separate baking days and equipment is thoroughly cleaned. Use dedicated baking pans for gluten-free products. Products certified by Gluten-Free Certification Organization (GFCO).
- Available in retail stores.
- Order direct by phone, email or internet; shipping charges based on weight; ships via UPS.

Native Seeds/SEARCH, 3061 N. Campbell Ave., Tuscon, AZ, USA 85719
✦ Phone: 866-622-5561/520-622-5561   FAX: 520-622-5591
  Email: info@nativeseeds.org   www.nativeseeds.org
- Non-profit seed conservation organization.
- Sell products that are native to southwestern USA and northwestern Mexico (beans, seeds, chili powder, whole chilies, salsas, sauces, baking mixes, jelly, syrup, herbal teas, amaranth, cornmeal and mesquite meal). Many products are gluten-free.
- Shop in person or order direct by phone, fax, mail or internet; shipping charges based on amount purchased; ships via UPS or USPS.

Nature's Own Bakery, 481 Wellham Road, Unit 7, Barrie, ON, Canada L4N 8Z6
✦ Phone: 800-353-3178/705-721-0919   FAX: 705-721-3345
  Email: info@naturesownbakery.ca   www.naturesownbakery.ca
- Specialty commercial bakery.
- Produce breads, buns, cookies, pizza crusts, bread crumbs, granola and baking mixes. A variety of products are gluten-free.
- Gluten-free products manufactured on dedicated equipment in a segregated area of the shared facility. Products are tested using an ELISA test for gluten.
- Available in retail stores.
- Order direct by phone, shipping charges based on amount purchased; ships via UPS.

Nature's Hilights Inc., P.O. Box 3526, Chico, CA, USA 95927
✦ Phone: 800-313-6454/530-342-6154   FAX: 530-342-3130
  Email: cynthia64@msn.com
- Gluten-free specialty company; dedicated GF facility.
- Produces "Nature's Hilights" gluten-free pizza crust and soy cheese pizza.
- Available in retail stores.
- Order direct by phone, fax or mail; shipping charges based on amount purchased; ships via FedEx Ground.

Nature's Path Foods Inc., 9100 Van Horne Way, Richmond, BC, Canada V6X 1W3
✦ Phone: 888-808-9505/604-248-8777   FAX: 604-248-8760
  Email: consumer_services@naturespath.com   www.naturespath.com
- Produce a variety of organic products generally made from whole grains (breads, cereals, waffles, snack bars, cookies and baking mixes). Products sold under the name of Nature's Path Foods, EnviroKidz and Optimum.
- Many products are gluten-free. Specific manufacturing processes are utilized to prevent cross-contamination. All gluten-free products are regularly tested for gluten. Cereals and snack bars are certified by Gluten-Free Certification Organization (GFCO).
- Available in retail stores.
- Order direct by phone or internet; shipping charges based on amount purchased; ships via UPS, FedEx or USPS.

Nelson David of Canada, 7 - 845 Lagimodiere Blvd., Winnipeg, MB, Canada R2J 3M2
✦ Phone: 866-989-0379/204-989-0379   FAX: 204-989-0384
  Email: crennnie244@aol.com
- Gluten-free specialty company; dedicated GF facility.
- Produce "Celimix" gluten-free mixes (breads, biscuits, buns, cakes, cookies, muffins, pancakes, pastry, pizza crusts, Yorkshire pudding), egg replacer and pasta.
- Available in retail stores.
- Order direct by phone or fax; shipping charges based on weight; ships via Canada Post.

New Morning, Attune Foods, 535 Pacific Ave., 3rd Floor, San Francisco, CA, USA 94133
   Phone: 800-641-4508/415-486-2101

www.attunefoods.com

- Produce a variety of cereals and cookies. One cereal is gluten-free.
- Equipment is thoroughly cleaned and strict allergen quality control procedures are used prior to production of gluten-free cereals. Products tested for gluten.
- Available in retail stores.

No Nuts, Mountain Meadows Food Processing Ltd., Site 13, Box 45, RR #1,
      Legal, AB, Canada T0G 1L0
   Phone: 800-961-2470/780-961-2470   FAX: 780-961-3995
   Email: info@peabutter.ca   www.peabutter.ca

- Nut-free alternative spread made from golden peas, canola oil and icing (confectioner's) sugar. Product is gluten and dairy-free.
- Made in a dedicated nut and gluten-free facility.
- Available in retail stores.

Nonuttin' Foods, Inc., 1 - 2911 Allenby Road, Duncan, BC, Canada V9L 6W2
✦   Phone: 866-714-5411/250-715-1481   FAX: 250-248-4942
   Email: info@nonuttin.com   www.nonuttin.com

- Produce granola bars and granolas (made with pure, uncontaminated oats), trail mix, fruit snacks and baking ingredients. All products also free of peanuts, tree nuts, sesame, dairy, egg, sulfites, preservatives, color and artificial flavors.
- Products certified by Gluten-Free Certification Organization (GFCO).
- Owner has a child with severe peanut allergy.
- Available in retail stores or order direct by phone, fax or internet; shipping charges based on weight; ships via FedEx Ground or Canada Post.

Northern Quinoa Corporation, Box 519, Kamsack, SK, Canada S0A 1S0
✦   Phone: 866-368-9304/306-542-3949   FAX: 306-542-3951
   Email: quinoa@quinoa.com   www.quinoa.com

- Process a variety of gluten-free products (quinoa, amaranth, buckwheat, flax, legumes, millet, spices and wild rice) in a dedicated GF facility.
- Quinoa is available as whole grain, flakes, flour and pasta.
- Company has developed a process to remove the bitter-tasting saponin coating from quinoa, making it ready to use and fast cooking.
- Available in some retail stores.
- Order direct by phone or internet; shipping charges based on weight; ships via Canada Post or UPS Ground.

Nu-World Amaranth, Nu-World Foods, P.O. Box 2202, Naperville, IL, USA 60567
✦   Phone: 877-692-8899/630-369-6819   FAX: 630-369-6851
   Email: customerservice@nuworldfamily.com www.nuworldfoods.com

- Gluten-free specialty company; dedicated facility free of gluten, dairy, egg, soy and nuts.
- Products tested for gluten in house and samples also tested by an independent lab. Products certified by Gluten-Free Certification Organization (GFCO).
- Produce a variety of amaranth and amaranth-based products (bread crumbs, cereals, flat breads, flour, pre-gel powder, side dishes, toasted bran flour).
- Also mill other gluten-free flours (millet, quinoa, sorghum, teff).
- Available in retail stores.
- Order direct by phone, fax, mail or internet; shipping charges based on amount purchased; ships via FedEx Ground.

O'Doughs, 3727 Chesswood Drive, North York, ON, Canada M3J 2P6
✦   Phone: 416-342-5700   FAX: 416-636-9985
    Email: eatwell@odoughs.com   www.odoughs.com

- Gluten-free specialty company; dedicated GF facility; products certified by Gluten-Free Certification Organization (GFCO).
- Produce a variety of breads, buns, cakes and pizza crusts..
- Available in retail stores.
- Order direct by phone, fax, mail or internet; shipping charges based on weight; ships FedEx 2-day in styrofoam containers with dry ice.

Omega Nutrition, 1695 Franklin. St, Vancouver, BC, Canada V5L 1P5
                            6515 Aldrich Rd., Bellingham, WA, USA 98226
✦   Phone: 800-661-3529   FAX: 604-253-4228 (Canada)
        604-253-4677 (Canada)   FAX: 360-384-0700 (USA)
        360-384-1238 (USA)
    Email: info@omeganutrition.com   www.omeganutrition.com

- Over 400 natural health products such as specialty oils (flax, borage, sesame, sunflower, hazelnut, olive, pistachio, pumpkin, safflower), flavorings, nutritional supplements, flax seed meal and seed butters.
- Available in retail stores.
- Order direct by phone, fax, mail or internet; shipping charges based on weight; ships a variety of ways.

Omega Smart Inc., 9 Delta Drive, Londonderry, NH, USA 03053
✦   Phone: 603-425-6800   FAX: 603-425-6822
    Email: info@omegasmartbar.com   www.omegasmartbar.com

- Produce gluten-free, dairy-free whole food meal replacement bars made from organic dried fruits, nuts, ground flax seed, soy flour, soynuts and agave syrup. Dedicated gluten-free facility.
- Available in retail stores.
- Order direct by phone, fax, mail or internet; shipping charges based on weight; ships via FedEx Ground.

Only Oats™ (see Avena - formerly FarmPure Foods)

The Organic Bistro, Food Collective, Inc., 1882 Mcgaw Ave., Suite A, Irvine, CA, USA 92614
✦   Phone: 866-328-8638/949-797-0014   FAX: 949-797-0041
    Email: info@theorganicbistro.com   www.theorganicbistro.com

- Produce gluten-free frozen organic entrées with whole grains (brown rice or quinoa), vegetables and poultry or salmon. Microwave or oven bake.
- Made in a facility with dedicated gluten-free production periods. Equipment thoroughly cleaned.
- Available in retail stores.
- Order direct by internet; shipping charges based on weight; ships in insulated, reusable coolers; ships FedEx Ground.

Orgran, Roma Food Products, 47-53 Aster Ave., Carrum Downs, Vic 3201, Australia

✦ Phone: 03 9776 9044 (Australia)   FAX: 03 9776 9055 (Australia)

       877-380-3422/845-278-8164 (USA)   FAX: 845-278-6277 (USA)

     Email: info@orgran.com   www.orgran.com

       healthflavors@gmail.com (USA)

- Roma Food Products is Australia's major manufacturer of alternative grain, pasta and health foods.
- Produce "Orgran" wheat-free, gluten-free products (cereals, cookies, crisp breads, crumbs, fruit bars, licorice mixes, pasta and soups) in a dedicated GF facility. Products are tested for gluten using the ELISA test.
- All Orgran products are also dairy, yeast, egg and GMO-free and vegan. Most of the products are also soy, tree nut and peanut-free.
- Available in retail stores.
- Order direct via internet from several distributors.

Pacific Foods, 19480 SW 97th Ave., Tualatin, OR, USA 97062

     Phone: 503-692-9666   FAX: 503-692-9610

     Email: info@pacificfoods.com   www.pacificfoods.com

- Produce a variety of non-dairy beverages (almond, grain, hazelnut, hemp, rice and soy), ice teas, broths, soups, entrées and side dishes. Many of their products are gluten-free.
- Strict food allergy safety procedures utilized to prevent cross-contamination. Products tested for gluten on every batch.
- Available in retail stores.

Pamela's Products, 200 Clara Ave., Ukiah, CA, USA 95482

     Phone: 707-462-6605   FAX: 707-462-6642

     Email: info@pamelasproducts.com   www.pamelasproducts.com

- A variety of "Pamela's" cookies, biscotti, baking mixes (bread, chocolate brownie and baking/pancake), cakes, cheesecakes and frostings. All products are gluten-free.
- Gluten-free products made on 100% dedicated gluten-free machinery.
- Available in retail stores and from select online specialty companies.

PaneRiso/Kingsmill, Canbrands Specialty Foods, P.O. Box 117,

       Gormley, ON, Canada L0H 1G0

✦ Phone: 905-888-5008   FAX: 905-888-5009

     Email: info@canbrands.ca   www.canbrands.ca

- Gluten-Free specialty company; dedicated GF facility.
- Produce PaneRiso/Kingsmill brands of gluten-free breads, croûtons, bread crumbs, cookies, pizza crusts and baking mixes. Most products are free from dairy, egg and trans fat.
- Available in retail stores.
- Order direct by phone, fax, mail or internet; shipping charges based on weight; ships via courier (Canpar).

Pastamaiza (see Pastariso)

Pastariso, Maplegrove Gluten-Free Foods, 13112 Santa Anna Ave., Unit A2-A3,
Fontana, CA, USA 92337

✦ Phone: 909-823-8230 FAX: 909-823-2708
Email: info@maplegrovefoods.com www.maplegrovefoods.com

- Gluten-free specialty company; dedicated GF facility.
- MapleGrove Gluten-Free Foods produce a large variety of pastas sold under the name "Pastariso" (white and brown rice pasta, rice pasta and cheese dinners), "Pastamaiza" (corn pasta) and "Pastato" (potato and rice pasta and cheese dinners). Pasta products certified by Gluten-Free Certification Organization (GFCO).
- Also produce "CelifibR" soup base and bouillon cubes.
- Available in retail stores.
- Order direct by internet.

Pastato (see Pastariso)

PatsyPie Gluten-Free Bakery, 3060 rue Brabant-Marineau, Ville St. Laurent, QC,
Canada H4S 1K7

✦ Phone: 877-287-9743/514-333-7253 FAX: 514-333-1916
Email: info@patsypie.com www.patsypie.com

- Gluten-free specialty company; dedicated GF facility.
- Produce "PatsyPie" cookies, biscotti, brownies and muffins. Contains no preservatives.
- Available in retail stores.
- Order direct by phone, fax or internet; shipping charges based on weight; ships via UPS.

Perfect 10 Natural Energy, Leed Products Inc., #2 - 68 Schooner St.,
Coquitlam, BC, Canada V3K 7B1

✦ Phone: 888-239-3282/604-540-1000 FAX: 604-540-1030
Email: info@perfect10bars.com www.perfect10bars.com

- Dedicated gluten-free facility.
- Produce snack bars made from dried fruits, nuts and seeds that are also dairy-free.
- Available in retail stores.
- Order direct by phone or internet; shipping charges based on weight; ships via USPS, DHL Ground or Canada Post.

Perky's (see Enjoy Life)

Philly Swirl, 1102 N. 28th St., Tampa, FL, USA 33605

Phone: 877-379-4757/813-353-8645 FAX: 813-241-2591
Email: alex@phillyswirl.com www.phillyswirl.com

- Produce a variety of frozen dessert novelties (including dairy-free [sorbet cups, Popperz, Stix] and dairy-containing [cupcakes, Fudge Stix, Fruit & CreamStix]) in a dedicated peanut and tree nut-free facility.
- All products are gluten-free except cupcakes. Cupcakes are made in a separate facility.
- Available in retail stores.

Plum-M-Good, Van Rice Products, #8 -1350 Valmont Way, Richmond, BC,
Canada V6V 1Y4

Phone: 604-273-8038 FAX: 604-273-7324

- Variety of organic and regular rice cakes that are gluten-free. Products are tested for gluten.
- Available in retail stores.

Premier Japan, Edward & Son's Trading Co., Inc., P.O. Box 1326, Carpinteria, CA, USA 93014

✦ Phone: 805-684-8500　　　　　　　　FAX: 805-684-8220
　Email: edwardsons@aol.com　　　　　www.edwardandsons.com
　　　or info@edwardandsons.com

- Produce organic oriental sauces including "wheat-free" teriyaki and hoisin that are gluten-free. Made in a shared facility; products tested for gluten by an independent lab.
- Available in retail stores.
- Order direct by phone, fax, mail or internet; shipping charges based on weight; ships via FedEx Ground or USPS.

PureFit Nutrition, Inc., 216 Technology, Suite F, Irvine, CA, USA　92618

✦ Phone: 866-787-3348/949-679-7997　　　FAX: 949-679-7998
　Email: info@purefit.com　　　　　　　www.purefit.com

- Variety of nutrition energy bars made from soy protein, soy flour, soy nuts and other ingredients. Bars are gluten and dairy-free and high in protein (18 grams).
- Available in retail stores.
- Order direct by internet; shipping charges based on weight; ships via UPS or FedEx Ground.

PurFoods, LLC, 718 S.E. Shurfine Drive, Ankeny, IA, USA　50021

✦ Phone: 866-942-7873/515-963-0641
　Email: julie.hanes@purefoods.com　　　www.purefoodsfreshstart.com

- Produce ready to heat (microwave or oven) and eat prepared fresh meals that are fresh made and do not add preservatives for packaging. Special packaging permits refrigerated shelf-life of 2 weeks from delivery.
- A variety of entrées (beef, pork, poultry and fish), casseroles, salads, vegetables, desserts, snacks and breakfast items are gluten-free sold as "PureFoods Fresh Start Gluten-Free Meals".
- Gluten-free products made in a shared facility. Strict allergen control program to prevent cross-contamination; products tested for gluten using ELISA test.
- Order direct by phone or internet; shipping charges based on amount purchased; ships via FedEx (2 day) in styrofoam containers with a gel pack (can re-use the packs).

Quaker, Pepsi-QTG Canada, 14 Hunter Street East, Quaker Park, Peterborough, ON, Canada　K9J 7B2

Phone: 800-267-6287　　　　　　　　www.quakeroats.ca

- Manufacture a large variety of products (cereals, juices, snacks and bars, rice and pasta side dishes, syrups and mixes).
- Most of the large rice cakes and "Crispy Mini Rice Chips" are gluten-free. Made in a dedicated GF facility.
- Available in retail stores.

Quaker Oats, A Unit of PepsiCo Beverages and Foods, P.O. Box 049003, Chicago, IL, USA　60604

Phone: 800-856-5781/312-821-1000　　　www.quakeroats.com
　　　　　　　　　　　　　　　　www.quakerricesnacks.com

- Manufacture a large variety of products (cereals, juices, snacks and bars, rice and pasta side dishes, syrups and mixes).
- Many of the large rice cakes and "Quakes" (mini rice cakes) are gluten-free. Some products contain barley gluten or barley malt flour and are NOT gluten-free. Products made in a shared facility; strict quality control procedures to prevent cross-contamination.
- Available in retail stores.

Real Foods, Pty Ltd., 47 Campbell Road, St. Peters NSW 2044, Australia
    Phone: 61 2 8595 6600   FAX: 61 2 8595 6601
                                    www.cornthins.com

- Produce crispbreads (Rice Thins and Corn Thins) in a variety of flavors. All products are gluten-free except the Rye & Caraway Corn Thins (only available in Australia).
- Strict allergen management program and quality control procedures to prevent cross-contamination.
- Available in retail stores and some internet grocery stores.

The Really Great Food Company, P.O. Box 2239, St. James, NY, USA 11780
✦   Phone: 800-593-5377/631-361-3553   FAX: 631-361-6920
    Email: support@reallygreatfood.com   www.reallygreatfood.com

- Gluten-free specialty company; dedicated GF facility.
- Produce "Really Great Food Company" gluten-free mixes (biscuits, breads, cakes, cookies, muffins, pancake, pie, pizza).
- Also carry other companies' products (cookies, flours, sauces, snacks, soups, vitamins and baking accessories).
- Available in some retail stores.
- Order direct by phone, fax, mail or internet; shipping charges based on amount purchased; ships via UPS Ground.

Redbridge, Anheuser-Busch, Inc., One Busch Place, St. Louis, MO, USA 63118
    Phone: 800-342-5283   www.anheuser-busch.com
                                    www.redbridgebeer.com

- Produce a variety of ales, beers and lagers including a gluten-free beer (Redbridge) made from sorghum in a 12 oz. (340 mL) bottle.
- Available in some liquor stores, grocery and health food stores.

Rice Expressions, P.O. Box 1430, Pacific Palisades, CA, USA 90272
    Phone: 310-820-4808   FAX: 310-820-2559
    Email: info@riceexpressions.com   www.riceexpressions.com

- Produce frozen pre-cooked, organic rice (brown, white, pilaf and tex-mex varieties) in plastic pouches that are heated in the microwave for 3 minutes.
- All products are gluten-free.
- Available in retail stores.

Rice Works, Shearer Foods, Canada, Inc., #1900 – 1030 West Georgia Street, Vancouver, BC, Canada V6E 2Y3
    Phone: 866-581-4431   FAX: 604-654-8448
    Email: info@riceworkssnacks.com   www.riceworkssnacks.com
        info@glutenfreesnacksforme.com   www.glutenfreesnacksforme.com

- Whole grain brown rice snack crisps in a variety of flavors.
- Produced on dedicated GF equipment; products tested by an independent lab for gluten.
- Available in retail stores.

Rizopia Food Products Inc., 330 Middlefield Road, Toronto, ON, Canada   M1S 5B1

✦   Phone: 416-609-8820   FAX: 416-609-8825
    Email: info@rizopia.com   www.rizopia.com

- Gluten-free specialty company; dedicated GF facility; products tested for gluten.
- A large variety of rice pastas (white, brown, organic brown and organic wild). Also available in bulk sizes.
- Available in retail stores.
- Order direct by internet from online stores.

Road's End Organics, Edward & Son's Trading Co., Inc., Box 1326, Carpinteria, CA, USA   93014

✦   Phone: 805-684-8500   FAX: 805-684-8220
    Email: edwardson@aol.com   www.edwardandsons.com
        info@edwardandsons.com

- Produce organic pastas, mixes and dips that are free of dairy, egg and nuts.
- A variety of products including some "Mac & Chreese" pasta, "Chreese" cheese mixes, dips and gravy mixes are gluten-free.
- Gluten-free products made in a dedicated GF facility and are tested for gluten by an independent lab.
- Available in retail stores.
- Order direct by phone, fax, mail or internet; shipping charges based on weight; ships via FedEx Ground or USPS.

The Ruby Range LLC, 1231 Willow Lane, Estes Park, CO, USA   80517

✦   Phone: 970-577-0888   FAX: 303-279-5366
    Email: ldcleene@msn.com   www.therubyrange.com

- Gluten-free specialty company; dedicated GF facility; products tested for gluten, certified by the Gluten-Free Certification Organization (GFCO).
- A variety of "Ruby Range" mixes (all purpose, cakes, cookies, cupcakes, pancakes), as well as flours and baking ingredients. Mixes contain mesquite, teff and other gluten-free flours.
- Order direct by phone, fax, mail or internet; shipping charges based on amount purchased; ships via USPS.

Rustic Crust, 31 Barnstead Road, Pittsfield, NH, USA   03263

✦   Phone: 603-435-5119   FAX: 603-435-5141
    Email: info@rusticcrust.com   www.rusticcrust.com

- Produce shelf-stable organic pizza crusts, frozen flatbread pizzas, pizza sauce and pizza kits. One pizza crust is gluten-free that is produced in a gluten-free facility and certified by the Gluten-Free Certification Organization (GFCO).
- Available in retail stores.
- Order direct by internet; shipping charges based on weight; ships via FedEx Ground.

St. Claire's Organics, 2275 West Midway Blvd., Suite A, Broomfield, CO, USA 80020

✦ Phone: 303-357-5682 FAX: 303-558-4111
Email: sales@stclaires.com www.stclaires.com

- A variety of organic candies (licorice, mints, tarts and aromatherapy pastilles) and hot cocoa mixes. All products are free of gluten, dairy, corn, soy and nuts. Contain no artificial colors, flavors or preservatives.
- Available in retail stores.
- Order direct by phone, fax,mail or internet; shipping charges based on weight; ships via FedEx or USPS.

San-J International, 2880 Sprouse Dr., Richmond, VA, USA 23231

✦ Phone: 800-446-5500/804-226-8333 FAX: 804-226-8383
Email: sales@san-j.com www.san-j.com

- Produces tamari soy sauces (liquid, powder, low salt/lite), sauces (Asian, barbecue), instant miso soups and rice crackers.
- Wheat-free tamari soy sauces and rice crackers are gluten-free. Wheat-free soy sauces are certified by the Gluten-Free Certification Organization (GFCO). Rice crackers produced in Japan in a shared facility and are not tested for gluten.
- Available in retail stores.

Savory Choice, Savory Creations International, 2121 S. El Camino Real, Suite C-210, San Mateo, CA, USA 94403

Phone: 866-472-8679/650-638-1024 FAX: 650-638-1178
Email: info@savory-creations.com www.savory-creations.com
www.savorychoice.com

- Major provider of "clean label" broth concentrates (regular and low sodium) and demi-glace for foodservice and food manufacturers, as well as broth concentrates for consumers.
- Produced by thermal processing of stock and natural flavors to obtain a concentrate with an intense flavor and aroma. Do not contain gluten, MSG, hydrolyzed vegetable proteins or preservatives.
- Available in shelf-stable Bag-in-Box and Stock Pot in Pouch (foodservice) and stick pouches (retail).
- Consumer products available in some retail stores.
- Foodservice products available from Sysco, US Foodservice, Shalit Foods and other distributors.

Schär, Dr. Schar GmbH, Winkelau 9, I-39014 Postal (BZ) Italy

✦ Phone: 39 0473 293300 FAX: 39 0473 293399
Email: info@schar.com www.schar.com

Schär USA Inc., 1050 Wall Street West, Suite 370, Lyndhurst, NJ USA 07071
Phone: 201-355-8470 FAX: 201-355-8624

- Gluten-free specialty company; dedicated GF facility.
- Extensive line of "Schar" gluten-free mixes (all-purpose, bread, cake), baked products (breads, baguettes, cakes, cookies, crackers, pizza crusts, rolls) and pasta.
- Products available in retail stores in North America.
- Order direct by internet; shipping charges based on weight; ships via FedEx (Ground, 2-day, next day).

Shiloh Farms (see GardenSpot Distributors)

Silk, White Wave Foods Company Consumer Affairs, 12002 Airport Way,
Bloomfield, CO, USA 80021
Phone: 888-820-9283/303-635-4000   www.silksoymilk.com
                                          www.silksoybeverage.ca

- Produce an extensive line of soy products (milk, yogurt and creamers). All products are gluten-free.
- Available in retail stores.

Simply Asia Foods Inc., 2342 Shattuck Ave., PMB 322, Berkley, CA, USA 94704
✦ Phone: 800-967-8424/410-527-8670
   Phone: 800-209-8707 (Canada)
   Email: information@simplyasia.net   www.simplyasia.com

- A variety of Asian flavored noodles (rice or wheat) with sauces.
- Some rice noodle soup products are gluten-free. Rice noodles made in a dedicated facility. Sauces made in a shared facility.
- Available in retail stores.
- Order direct by phone or internet in the US; shipping charges based on amount purchased; ships via UPS.

Soya World Inc., P.O. Box 3018, Vancouver, BC, Canada V6B 3X5
   Phone: 888-401-0019/604-291-0910   FAX: 604-291-0981
   Email: consumer@soyaworld.com   www.soyaworld.com

- One of North America's largest producers of fresh and shelf-stable soy beverages ("So Good Fortified Soy", "So Nice Soyganic", "Sunrise Soy"), soy yogurt ("So Nice") and non-dairy frozen desserts and cones ("So Good").
- Beverages, frozen desserts (in tubs) and yogurts are gluten-free.
- Available in retail stores.

Sunrise Soya Foods, 729 Powell Street, Vancouver, BC, Canada V6A 1H5
   Phone: 800-661-2326/604-253-2326   FAX: 604-251-1083
   Email: consumer-info@sunrise-soya.com   www.sunrise-soya.com

- Variety of tofu products and soy beverages. Many are gluten-free.
- Available in retail stores.

Sunstart Bakery, 30 Woodside Road, Industrial Estate, Ballymena, Ireland, BT42 4QJ
✦ Phone: 08 70 95 02510   FAX: 08 70 95 02520
                                             www.sunstartbakery.com

Sunstart USA, 1005 N. Commons Drive, Aurora, IL, USA 60504
   Phone: 630-851-2111   FAX: 630-851-7744
   Email: beckytt@sbcglobal.net   www.sunstartusa.com

Sunstart (in Canada) – Canbrands Specialty Foods, P.O. Box 117, Gormley, ON,
                                          Canada L0H 1G0
   Phone: 905-888-5008   FAX: 905-888-5009
   Email: info@canbrands.ca   www.canbrands.ca

- Gluten-free specialty company; dedicated GF facility.
- Produce cookies and bars that are also free of eggs, nuts and trans fats.
- Available in retail stores.
- Order direct by phone, fax or internet; shipping charges based on weight; ships via UPS.

Sylvan Border Farm, 7425 Clard Road, Unit A, Paradise, CA, USA 95969

✦ Phone: 530-327-7716 FAX: 530-327-7709
Email: sylvanborderfarm@saber.net www.sylvanborderfarm.com

- Gluten-Free specialty company; dedicated GF facility; ELISA-test products for gluten.
- Produce "Sylvan Border Farm" gluten-free baking mixes packed in oxygen-free pouches with a shelf-life of 2 years. Mixes made with healthy gluten flours such as brown rice, quinoa, amaranth and garbanzo bean.
- Available in retail stores.
- Order direct by phone, fax or internet; shipping charges based on product weight; ships via UPS Ground.

Taste Adventure, Will-Pak Foods Inc., Suite 200, 3350 Shelby St.,
Ontario, CA, USA 91764

✦ Phone: 800-874-0883/909-945-4554 FAX: 909-899-7822
Email: taste_adv@earthlink.net www.tasteadventure.com

- Low-fat soups, beans, quick cuisine entrées and chilies. Many products are gluten-free.
- Available in retail stores.
- Order direct by phone, fax, mail, internet; shipping charges based on weight; ships via UPS Ground.

The Teff Company, P.O. Box A, Caldwell, ID, USA 83606

✦ Phone: 888-822-2221/208-455-0375
Email: teffworld@gmail.com www.teffco.com

- Grow and mill only teff grain (brown and ivory varieties); dedicated GF facility.
- Grain and flour available in various sizes.
- Available in retail stores.
- Order direct by internet; shipping charges included in product price; ships via UPS Ground.

Terra, Hain-Celestial Group, Consumer Relations Department,
4600 Sleepytime Drive, Boulder, CO, USA 80301

✦ Phone: 800-434-4246 FAX: 303-581-1520
Email: consumerrelations@hain-celestial.com www.terrachips.com

- Variety of chips made from exotic root vegetables (taro, sweet potato, yucca [cassava], batata and parsnip). Several products are gluten-free.
- Available in retail stores.
- Order direct by internet, shipping charges based on weight; ships via FedEx.

Thai Kitchen, Simply Asia Foods Inc., P.O. Box 13242, Berkley, CA, USA 94712

✦ Phone: 800-967-8424/410-527-8670
Phone: 800-209-8707 (Canada)
Email: info@thaikitchen.com www.thaikitchen.com

- Asian products include a variety of plain and flavored rice noodles, rice side dishes, sauces, soups and coconut milk. Many products are gluten-free. Rice noodles made in a dedicated facility.
- Available in retail stores.
- Order direct by mail, or internet in the US; shipping charges are a flat rate; ships via UPS or DHL.

Think Products!, Prime Health Dietary Supplements Inc., 1650 Palma Drive, Suite 201,
Ventura, CA, USA 93003

✦ Phone: 866-988-4465/805-644-4848 FAX: 805-644-3511
Email: customerservice@thinkproducts.com www.thinkproducts.com

- Produce a variety of nutrition snack bars sold under the names thinkThin, thinkThin Desserts and thinkThin Bites. Bars made with soy and/or whey protein and sweetened with maltitol.
- Available in retail stores.
- Order direct by phone, fax, mail or internet; shipping charges based on weight; ships via FedEx.

Tinkyada, Food Directions Inc., 120 Melford Drive, Unit 8,
Scarborough, ON, Canada M1B 2X5

Phone: 416-609-0016 FAX: 416-609-1316
Email: jojo@tinkyada.com www.tinkyada.com
www.ricepasta.com

- Gluten-free specialty company; dedicated GF facility.
- Brown rice (with rice bran), organic brown rice and white rice pastas in a variety of shapes. Products also available in bulk.
- Available in retail stores.

Tom Sawyer Gluten-Free Products, 2155 W. Highway 89A, Suite 106,
Sedona, AZ, USA 86336

✦ Phone: 877-372-8800/928-282-6629 FAX: 928-282-5937
Email: tomsawyer@esedona.net www.glutenfreeflour.com

- Gluten-free specialty company; dedicated GF facility; products tested for gluten by an independent lab.
- Produce gluten-free all purpose flour mix from white rice, sweet rice and tapioca flours, xanthan gum and gelatin.
- Available in some retail stores.
- Order direct by phone, fax, email or internet; shipping charges included in product price; ships via UPS.

Twin Valley Mills LLC., RR #1, Box 45, Ruskin, NE, USA 68974

✦ Phone: 402-279-3965
Email: sorghumflour@hotmail.com www.twinvalleymills.com

- Grow and mill only sorghum grain in a dedicated GF facility; randomly tests for gluten.
- Sorghum flour available in 2.5 lbs. and 25 lb. containers; whole sorghum available in 30 lb. container.
- Order direct by phone, mail and email; shipping charges based on weight; ships via UPS Ground.

Udi's Gluten-Free Foods, 7010 Broadway, Suite 430, Denver, CO, USA 80221

✦ Phone: 303-657-6366 FAX: 303-657-5373
Email: glutenfree@udisfood.com www.udisglutenfree.com

- Gluten-free specialty company; dedicated gluten-free facility; products certified by Gluten-Free Certification Organization (GFCO).
- Produce bagels, breads, cinnamon rolls, granola (made with certified gluten-free oats), muffins and pizza crusts.
- Products available in retail stores.
- Order direct by internet; shipping charges based on weight; ships via UPS 2 day air.

Vance's Foods, P.O. Box 627, Gilmer, TX, USA 75644

✦ Phone: 800-497-4834 FAX: 800-497-4329
Email: info@vancesfoods.com www.vancesfoods.com

- Produce dairy substitutes ("SNO*E Tofu", "Darifree"), as well as hot chocolate mixes (made with whey) and a sugar substitute.
- "Darifree" is a potato-based non-dairy substitute which is gluten and casein-free. Available as dry powder beverage mixes.
- Order direct by phone, mail or internet; shipping charges based on weight; ships via UPS Ground.

Van's International Foods, 3285 East Vernon Ave., Vernon, CA, USA 90058

Phone: 323-585-5581 FAX: 323-585-4084
Email: customerservice@vansintl.com www.vansintl.com

- Produce frozen waffles (Belgian, organic, mini, regular and wheat-free), pancakes and French Toast.
- Wheat-Free waffles (large and mini), Wheat-Free French Toast sticks and Wheat-Free Pancakes are gluten-free.
- Strict quality control procedures to prevent cross-contamination. Every batch is tested for gluten.
- Available in retail stores.

Wellness Foods Inc., 337 Grace St., Toronto, ON, Canada M6G 3A8

✦ Phone: 800-547-5790/416-836-9926
Email: info@wellnessfoods.ca www.wellnessfoods.ca

- Produce high protein, low-fat snack bars that are gluten and dairy-free, vegan and kosher. Made with non GMO soy crisps and sweetened with agave nectar.
- Dedicated gluten-free facility.
- Available in retail stores.
- Order direct by internet; flat rate shipping charge; ships via Canada Post and CanPar.

The Wizard's, Edward & Son's Trading Co., Inc., P.O. Box 1326, Carpinteria, CA, USA 93014

✦ Phone: 805-684-8500 FAX: 805-684-8220
Email: info@edwardandsons.com www.edwardandsons.com
or edwardson@aol.com

- Produce organic sauces including wheat-free "vegetarian worcestershire" and "hot stuff piquante" sauces that are gluten-free. Made in a shared facility; products tested for gluten by an independent lab.
- Available in retail stores.
- Order direct by phone, fax, mail or internet; shipping charges based on weight; ships via FedEx Ground or USPS.

GLUTEN-FREE BAKERIES

NOTE: The majority of gluten-free bakeries listed below produce only gluten-free items in dedicated gluten-free facilities. However, there are several bakeries listed in this section that produce gluten-free products in a shared facility (some in segregated areas) on dedicated equipment or equipment that has been thoroughly cleaned and sanitized to prevent cross-contamination.

Azna Gluten Free, 2647 Cameron Park Drive, Cameron Park, CA, USA 95682
Phone: 530-677-5810   FAX: 530-677-1010
Email: orders@aznaglutenfree.com   www.aznaglutenfree.com

- Gluten-free specialty bakery; dedicated GF facility.
- Produce breads, brownies, cakes, pizza crust, rolls, scones and waffles.
- Available in some retail stores.
- Shop in person or order direct by phone or internet; shipping charges based on weight; ships via UPS.

Bittersweet Bakery, 2105 Cliff Road, Eagan, MN, USA 55122
Phone: 651-686-0112   FAX: 651-686-0550
Email: info@bittersweetgf.com   www.bittersweetgf.com

- Gluten-free specialty bakery; dedicated GF facility.
- Produce bars, breads, cakes, cookies, cupcakes, muffins, pies, pizza crust, rolls and baking mixes.
- Available in some retail stores.
- Shop in person or order direct by phone; shipping charges based on weight; ships via UPS Ground.

Choices Best Rice Bakery, 2595 West 16th Ave., Vancouver, BC, Canada V6K 3B9
Phone: 604-736-0301   FAX: 604-736-0331
Email: rice-bakery@choicesmarket.com   www.choicesmarket.com

- Gluten-free specialty bakery; dedicated GF facility.
- Extensive line of fresh baked goods (e.g., breads, brownies, cakes, cookies, muffins, pies, rolls, scones, tarts), frozen products (bread, pie & tart shells, cookie dough and waffles), granola and museli cereals and mixes.
- Bakery is part of Choices Market, western Canada's largest retailer of natural and organic foods.
- Available in the bakery and Choices Market's Stores.
- Order direct by phone.

Crave Bakery, 325 Montcalm Street, San Francisco, CA, USA 94110
    Phone: 415-826-7187
    Email: info@cravebakery.com   www.cravebakery.com

- Gluten-Free specialty wholesale bakery; produced in a shared facility; gluten-free products made on dedicated equipment with GF ingredients that are isolated from other ingredients; strict quality control and cleaning procedures utilized to prevent cross-contamination; ingredients and final products tested for gluten by an independent lab.
- Produce brownies, cookies, cakes, cupcakes and tarts; all products are also casein-free.
- Owner of bakery has gluten intolerance.
- Available in retail stores on west coast (USA).
- Order direct by internet; shipping charges based on weight; ships via UPS.

Wheatless in Seattle (formerly Da Vinci Bakery and Cafe), 10003 Greenwood Ave. N.,
                                              Seattle, WA, USA 98133
    Phone: 206-782-5735
    Email: wheatlessinseattle@yahoo.com   www.wheatlessinseattle.net

- Gluten-free specialty bakery; dedicated GF facility.
- Produce breads, brownies, cakes, cookies, pies, rolls, squares, tarts and breakfast items.
- Owner and family members have gluten intolerance.
- Some products sold to pizza restaurants and retail stores.
- Shop in person.

Deby's Gluten-Free, Inc., 2369 S. Trenton Way, Suite M, Denver, CO, USA 80231
    Phone: 866-473-2155/303-283-4060   FAX: 303-337-0544
    Email: info@debysglutenfree.net   www.debysglutenfree.com

- Gluten-free specialty company, bakery and cafe; dedicated gluten, peanut and shellfish-free facility; ingredients tested for gluten.
- Large variety of baked products (breads, cakes, cookies, crackers, muffins, pies, pie crusts, pizza crusts, rolls, tarts, tortillas), baking mixes and entrées. Many products are also dairy-free. Also sell other companies' products.
- Owner of company and family members have celiac disease.
- Some of Deby's products are individually packaged and sold to foodservice distributors for sale to health care institutions and restaurants.
- Available in retail stores sold under the name "8 Free Foods".
- Cafe open for breakfast, lunch and dinner.
- Shop in person or order direct by mail, phone, fax, email, internet; shipping charges based on weight; ships via USPS Priority or DHL. Entrées shipped in a freezer shipping box with dry ice.

Earth's Oven Gluten-Free Bakery, #316 - 2066 - 18th Ave. NE,
Calgary, AB, Canada   T2E 8N5

Phone: 403-686-4810 (retail)   FAX: 403-217-2603
403-620-6930 (wholesale)
Email: earthsoven@gmail.com   www.earthsoven.com

- Gluten-free specialty bakery; dedicated GF facility.
- Produce breads, cakes, cookies, muffins, pies, squares and frozen entrées (beef & chicken burgers, Mexican foods).
- Available in some local stores.
- Shop in person or order direct by phone or email; shipping charges based on weight; ships via UPS or local courier.

Farmer's Kitchen Cafe, 624 - 4th Street, Davis, CA, USA   95616

Phone: 530-756-1862   FAX: 530-756-7210
Email: roseanne@naturalfoodworks.com   www.farmerskitchencafe.com

- Gluten-free specialty bakery and cafe; dedicated GF facility.
- Produce an extensive variety of baked products (bagels, breads, cakes, cookies, muffins, pies, rolls), pasta, soups and frozen entrées.
- Cafe serves gluten-free items prepared in the dedicated GF bakery. Also will serve a bread (made offsite containing gluten) prepared on a separate cutting board and with a separate knife.
- Shop in person or order direct by phone or internet for pickup. Some items can be shipped. Contact store for details.

Flying Apron Bakery, 3510 Fremont Ave. North, Seattle, WA, USA   98103

Phone: 206-442-1115
Email: flyingapron@msn.com   www.flyingapron.net

- Gluten-free specialty bakery and cafe; dedicated GF facility.
- Produce bars, breads, cakes, cookies, muffins, scones as well as entrées.
- Use certified gluten-free oats in some products.
- Open for lunch and dinner.
- Shop in person or order direct by phone or internet; shipping charges based on weight; ships via UPS.

French Meadow Bakery™, 1000 Apollo Road, Eagan, MN, USA   55121

Phone: 877-669-3278/651-286-7861   FAX: 651-454-3327
Email: glutenfree@frenchmeadow.com   www.frenchmeadow.com

- Certified organic bakery (bagels, breads, brownies, cookies, pizza crusts, rolls, tortillas).
- Wide variety of product lines, including gluten-free, vegan, yeast-free and kosher parve.
- Produce gluten-free breads, brownies, cakes, cookies, cookie dough, cupcakes, muffins, pizza crust, rolls and tortillas. All are casein-free, lactose-free and peanut-free.
- Gluten-free products manufactured on dedicated equipment in a dedicated gluten and nut-free facility. Tested by an independent lab and also certified by the Gluten-Free Certification Organization (GFCO).
- Available in retail stores.
- Order direct by phone or internet; shipping charges based on amount purchased; ships via UPS.

Gluten-Free Creations Bakery, 2940 E. Thomas, Phoenix, AZ, USA 85016
    Phone: 602-522-0659   FAX: 602-954-8047
    Email: glutenfreeenews@cox.net   www.glutenfreecreations.com
- Gluten-free specialty company; dedicated GF facility; certified by the Gluten-Free Certification Organization (GFCO).
- Produce a variety of baked products (bagels, breads, cakes, cookies, donuts, muffins, pizza crusts), bread crumbs and graham cracker crumbs, as well as mixes.
- Owner has celiac disease.
- Available in some retail stores and restaurants.
- Shop in person in the bakery.
- Order direct by phone, fax, mail or internet; shipping charges based on weight; ships via UPS Ground.

Gluuteny Bakery, 1923 Murray Ave., Pittsburgh, PA, USA 15217
    Phone: 412-521-4890
    Email: orders@gluuteny.com   www.gluuteny.com
- Gluten and casein-free bakery; dedicated gluten and casein-free facility.
- Produce breads, cakes, cookies, mixes, muffins, pizza crust and tarts.
- Shop in person or order direct by phone or internet; shipping charges based on weight; ships via UPS.

The Grainless Baker, 360 J & J Road, Moscow, PA, USA 18444
    Phone: 570-689-9694   FAX: 570-503-0092
    Email: info@thegrainlessbaker.com   www.thegrainlessbaker.com
- Gluten-free retail and wholesale bakery; dedicated GF facility.
- Produce bagels, breads, cakes, cookies, muffins, pies, pizza and rolls.
- Owner has family members with celiac disease.
- Available in retail stores.
- Shop in person or order direct by phone; shipping charges based on amount purchased; ships via UPS Ground.

Greyston Bakery (formerly Good Juju Bakery), 104 Alexander Street,
                                      Yonkers, NY, USA 10701
    Phone: 800-289-2253/914-375-7534   FAX: 914-375-1514
    Email: judithm@greystonbakery.com   www.greystonbakery.com
- Gluten-free specialty bakery; dedicated GF facility; purchase dedicated GF ingredients.
- Produce breads, muffins and cookies.
- Bakery representative has celiac disease and is a registered nurse.
- Shop in person or order direct by mail, phone, fax, email or internet; shipping charges based on weight; ships via FedEx Ground or 2 day.

Haley's Corner Bakery, 10216 SE 256th Street, Suite 111, Kent, WA, USA 98030
    Phone: 253-852-4486
    Email: info@haleyscorner.com   www.haleyscorner.com
- Gluten-free specialty bakery; dedicated GF facility.
- Produce breads, cakes, cookies, muffins, pies, pizza, rolls and scones.
- Owner has family members with celiac disease.
- Shop in person.

Heaven Mills Bakery, 5614 New Utrecht Ave., Brooklyn, NY, USA 11219
    Phone: 347-770-8065   FAX: 347-770-8067
    Email: info@heavenmills.com   www.heavenmillsglutenfree.com

- Gluten-free specialty bakery; dedicated GF facility and certified kosher by the Tartikov Kashrus Agency.
- Produce breads, cakes, cookies, matzah (made with pure, uncontaminated gluten-free oats), muffins, pizza as well as mixes.
- Available in some retail stores.
- Order direct by internet only.

Island Gluten-Free Bakery, 1880 Stickney Point Road, Sarasota, FL, USA 34231
    Phone: 941-923-0002
    Email: islandgfbakery@mindspring.com   www.islandgfbakery.com

- Gluten-free specialty bakery; dedicated GF facility.
- Produce breads, cakes, muffins, scones, mixes and entrées (lasagna, pizza, quiche). Many products are also casein-free.
- Shop in person or order direct by phone or internet; shipping charges based on weight; ships via UPS.

Jake Bakes, P.O Box 643, Boonton, NJ, USA 07005
    Phone: 973-588-3513   FAX: 973-299-9327
    Email: info@jakebakes.com   www.jakebakes.com

- Gluten-free bakery; dedicated GF facility.
- Produce bars, cookies, granola and other items. Use certified gluten-free oats in cookies and granola.
- Order direct by phone or email; shipping charges based on weight; ships via UPS or USPS.

Joan's GF Great Bakes, Inc., 1905A Bellmore Ave., Bellmore, NY, USA 11710
    Phone: 516-804-5600   FAX: 516-804-5602
    Email: info@gfgreatbakes.com   www.gfgreatbakes.com

- Gluten-free specialty bakery; dedicated gluten and peanut-free facility.
- Produce bagels, cookies, muffins, pizza and rolls.
- Available in retail stores.
- Shop in person or order direct by mail, email or internet; shipping charges based on weight; ships via UPS. Frozen items packed with insulated foam, gel packs and/or dry ice.

Jubilee Kafe, 299 South Street, London, ON, Canada N6B 1B6
    Phone: 519-432-1683   www.jubileekafe.com

- Gluten-free specialty bakeshop; dedicated GF facility.
- Produce breads, buns, cakes, cookies, granola, muffins, pies, squares, as well as soups and entrées (e.g., lasagna, perogies, quiche).
- Also sell gluten-free products from other companies.
- Family members have celiac disease.
- Shop in person.

Kathy's Creations, LLC., 2010 Crestview, Alliance, OH, USA 44601
    Phone: 866-821-8183/330-821-8183
    Email: info@kathyscreationsbakery.com   www.kathyscreationsbakery.com
- Gluten-free specialty bakery; dedicated GF facility.
- Produce breads, brownies, cakes, cookies, muffins, pies, pizza crusts and rolls.
- Also available in some retail stores.
- Shop in person.

Les Glutineries, 2416 rue Dessaulles, Saint-Hyacinthe, QC, Canada J2S 2V1
    Phone: 450-252-4588

Les Glutineries, 7800 boul. Taschereau, Brossard, QC, Canada J4X 1V7
    Phone: 450-672-2919   www.lesglutineries.com
- Gluten-free specialty store and bakery; dedicated GF facility.
- Over 1200 items (frozen, refrigerated and shelf-stable). Also produce over 350 items including entrées, pizza, quiche, soups and desserts.
- Shop in person or phone orders for pick up at either location.

The Little Aussie Bakery, 3610 Avenue B., San Antonio, TX, USA 78209
    Phone: 210-826-7877   FAX: 210-826-8830
    Email: rita@thelittleaussiebakery.com   www.thelittleaussiebakery.com
- Gluten-free specialty bakery and cafe; dedicated GF facility.
- Baked products such as breads, buns, cakes, cookies, pies, pizzas, as well as flours and mixes.
- Cafe open for Sunday brunch, lunch and dinner throughout the week except Monday.
- Shop in person or order direct by phone; shipping charges based on weight; ships via FedEx.

Molly's Gluten-Free Bakery, N 47-W-28270 Lynndale Road, Pewaukee, WI, USA 53072

Phone: 262-369-1404   FAX: 262-369-1404

Email: mollysgfbakery@yahoo.com   www.mollysglutenfreebakery.com

- Gluten-free bakery; dedicated gluten and nut-free facility.
- Produce breads, buns, cakes, cookies, cupcakes, pies, pie crust, rolls and squares.
- Many products also dairy and egg-free.
- Owner has a child with celiac disease.
- Shop in person.

Mountain Top Café and Bakery, #103 – 1124 Lonsdale Ave.,
Vancouver, BC, Canada V7M 2H1

Phone: 604-960-9605   FAX: 604-960-9605

Email: info@emountaintop.com   www.emountaintop.com

- Gluten-Free bakery and cafe; dedicated GF facility.
- Produce breads, cakes, cookies, muffins, pies, as well as mixes.
- Cafe open for breakfast and lunch.
- Available in some retail stores.
- Order in person or direct by phone or internet; shipping charges based on weight; ships via Greyhound or courier.

Organic Bliss Bakery, 3723 N. King Road, Toledo, OH, USA 43617

Phone: 419-517-7799   FAX: 419-517-7796

Email: info@organicblissmarket.com   www.organicblissmarket.com

- Gluten-free specialty bakery; dedicated GF facility.
- Produce breads, buns, cakes, cookies, cupcakes, pies, pizza crusts and scones.
- Also serve breakfast and lunch items.
- Shop in person or order direct by phone or email; shipping charges based on weight; ships via FedEx Ground.

Outside The Breadbox, Inc., 2027 W. Colorado Ave., Colorado Springs, CO, USA 80904

Phone: 719-633-3434   FAX: 719-633-0068

Email: info@outsidethebreadbox.com   www.outsidethebreadbox.com

- Gluten-Free specialty bakery; dedicated GF facility; products tested for gluten using ELISA test.
- Produce baked products (bagels, breads, cakes, cookies, crackers, muffins, pies, pizza crusts, rolls).
- Also carry other companies' products (e.g., gluten-free oats, pasta).
- Owned by a family whose child has celiac disease.
- Available in some retail stores.
- Shop in person or order direct by phone, fax, email or mail; shipping charges based on weight; ships via UPS Ground.

Panne Rizo, 1939 Cornwall Ave., Vancouver, BC, Canada V6J 1C8
✦   Phone: 604-736-0885   FAX: 866-340-3722/604-736-0825
      Email: info@pannerizo.com   www.pannerizo.com
- Gluten-Free specialty bakery, deli and cafe; dedicated GF facility.
- Produce gluten-free breads, bread crumbs, buns, special occasion cakes, cookies, crackers, mixes, muffins, pies, pastries, pizza crusts, pizza, ready-to-eat entrées and soups.
- Also carry other companies' products (cereals, cookies, crackers, pasta, soup cubes).
- Available in the Panne Rizo store or in some retail stores in western Canada.
- Order direct by phone, fax, email, mail or internet; shipping charges based on weight; ships via FedEx.

Quejos Bakery & Cafe, 4129 Main Street, Vancouver, BC, Canada V5V 3P6
      Phone: 604-420-0832
      Email: info@quejos.com   www.quejos.com
- Gluten-free specialty bakery; dedicated GF facility.
- Produce "quejos" a Brazilian bread made from cassava (manioc), cookies, muffins, pizza wraps and squares.
- Also sell products from other companies (e.g., cereals, mixes, pasta).
- Quejos products sold in other retail stores.
- Shop in person or order direct by internet; shipping charges based on amount purchased (Canadian orders) or weight (USA orders); ships via UPS or other couriers.

Rose's Wheat-Free Bakery & Café, 2901 Central Street, Evanston, IL, USA 60201
      Phone: 847-859-2723   FAX: 847-859-2726
      Email: rosesbakery@gmail.com   www.rosesbakery.com
- Gluten-free bakery; dedicated GF facility.
- Produce breads, cakes, cookies, pies, pie crust, pizza, pizza crusts, rolls and squares.
- Owner has family members with gluten intolerance.
- Cafe open for lunch and dinner on select days.
- Shop in person or order direct by internet; shipping charges based on weight; ships via UPS Ground.

Schroedter's Farm Market Café & Bakery, 1492 Highway 62 South, RR #1,
Bloomfield, ON, Canada   K0K 1G0

Phone: 613-393-2823

- Specialty bakery & cafe; gluten-free products made in separate kitchen on dedicated equipment.
- Produce breads, cookies, doughnuts, muffins, pies, tarts, turkey pies, sausages.
- Also sell other companies' gluten-free products.
- Owners have wheat sensitivity.
- Cafe open for lunch. Separate food preparation area for gluten-free items.
- Shop in person.

The Sensitive Baker, 108361/2 Washington Blvd., Culver City, CA, USA   90232

Phone: 310-815-1800   FAX: 310-815-0113

Email: gf-bakers@thesensitivebaker.com   www.thesensitivebaker.com

- Specialty bakery whose products are gluten and casein-free; certified kosher by the RCC; dedicated gluten and casein-free facility.
- Produce bagels, breads, brownies, cakes, cookies, muffins, pizza crusts and rolls.
- Also available from gfmeals.com
- Shop in person or order direct by mail, phone, fax, email or internet; shipping charges based on amount purchased; ships via UPS Ground in southern California or 2nd day air for other locations; items shipped in special styrofoam containers with dry ice.

The Silly Yak Bakery & Bread Barn, 7866 Mineral Point Road,
Madison, WI, USA   53717

Phone: 608-833-5965   FAX: 608-833-5611

Email: sillyyakbakery@gmail.com   www.sillyyakbakery.com

- Specialty bakery that produces gluten-free products 3 days/week in a dedicated GF facility. Products routinely tested for gluten and are certified by the Gluten-Free Certification Organization (GFCO).
- Produce breads, cakes, cookies, muffins, mixes, pies, pizza crusts and scones.
- Also carry other gluten-free companies' products.
- Shop in person or order direct by mail, phone, fax, email or internet; shipping charges based on weight; ships via USPS Priority Mail.

Silly Yak Bakery in Village Bulk Foods, 172 Second Ave. West,
Qualicum Beach, BC, Canada   V9K 1S7
Phone: 250-752-2857   FAX: 250-752-2857

- Gluten-free specialty bakery; dedicated GF facility located within Village Bulk Foods.
- Produce breads, cookies, muffins, pie crusts, perogies, rolls, tarts, tart shells and bread mixes.
- Owner has food allergies.
- Shop in person.

Sinfully Gluten-Free, 79 South Main Street, Miamisburg, OH, USA 45342
Phone: 937-866-3000
Email: contact@sinfullygf.com   www.sinfullygf.com

- Gluten-free specialty bakery and cafe; dedicated GF facility.
- Produce breads, brownies, cakes, cookies and gift baskets.
- Also sell other companies' products.
- Cafe open for lunch and dinner.
- Shop in person or order direct by phone or internet; shipping charges based on weight; ships via UPS or USPS.

Sterk's Bakery, 137 Queen Street, Dunnville, ON, Canada   N1A 1H6
Phone: 905-701-1905   FAX: 905-701-0278
Email: sterksbakery@gmail.com   www.sterksbakery.net

- Gluten-free specialty company; dedicated GF facility.
- Owners have celiac disease.
- Produce a variety of bagels, breads, buns, cakes, cookies, mixes, muffins and pizza crusts.
- Also carry other companies' gluten-free products (cereals, crackers, flours, pasta, soup bases).
- Available in some retail stores and gluten-free specialty shops.
- Shop in person in the bakery.
- Order direct by phone, fax, email or internet; shipping charges based on amount purchased; ships via UPS Ground.

Sunny Valley Wheat Free, 7032 South 188th Street, Kent, WA, USA 98032
Phone: 425-251-0909   FAX: 425-251-6655
Email: deann@sunnyvalleywheatfree.com   www.sunnyvalleywheatfree.com

- Gluten-free specialty company; dedicated GF facility.
- Produce a variety of baked products (e.g., breads, desserts and rolls) and frozen convenience meals (e.g., lasagna, pizza and quiche).
- Available in retail stores.

Sweet Christine's Gluten-Free Confections, 132 West State Street, Kennett Square, PA, USA 19348

    Phone: 610-444-5542   FAX: 610-444-3963

    Email: cruggio@sweetchristinesglutenfree.com   www.sweetchristinesglutenfree.com

- Gluten-free specialty bakery; dedicated GF facility.
- Produce brownies, cookies and mixes.
- Owner has celiac disease.
- Also available in some retail stores.
- Shop in person or order direct by internet; shipping charges based on weight; ships via USPS Priority Mail or UPS Ground.

Sweet Escape Pastries, LLC., 600 S. Sunset Street, Suite D, Longmont, CO, USA 80501

    Phone: 720-204-2062

    Email: melissa@sweetescpastries.com   www.sweetescpastries.com

- Gluten-free specialty bakery; dedicated gluten and nut-free facility.
- Produce breads, buns, cakes, English muffins and pizza crusts.
- Owner and family members have celiac disease.
- Shop in person or order direct by phone or email for pick up orders.

Sweet Sin Bakery, 123 West 27th Street, Baltimore, MD, USA 21218

    Phone: 410-366-5777/410-464-7211   FAX: 410-366-5788

    Email: renne@glutenfreedesserts.com   www.glutenfreedesserts.com

- Specialty gluten-free bakery; dedicated GF facility.
- Produce breads, cakes, cookies, muffins, mini desserts, tarts.
- Available in retail stores and some local cafes.
- Order direct by phone or email, shipping charges based on weight; ships via FedEX. Cakes shipped frozen in a container with dry ice.

The Twisted Bakery, 1470 East Villard Street, Dickinson, ND, USA 58601

    Phone: 701-483-4726   FAX: 701-483-4725

    Email: thetwistedbakery@hotmailcom   www.qualityglutenfree.com

- Gluten-free specialty bakery; dedicated GF facility.
- Produce breads, brownies, cakes, cookies, kuchen, mixes, muffins and rolls.
- Available in retail stores.
- Shop in person or order direct by mail, phone or internet; shipping charges based on weight; ships via UPS.

Whole Foods Market Gluten-Free Bakehouse, 2800 Perimeter Park Drive, Suite C, Morrisville, NC, USA 27560

    Email: glutenfree.bakehouse@wholefoods.com   www.wholefoodsmarket.com

- Gluten-free specialty bakery; dedicated GF facility; ingredients and finished products tested for gluten in their on-site testing lab.
- Produce a variety of items (breads, buns, cakes, cookies, granola, muffins, pies, pie crusts, pizza crust, scones).
- Products are frozen on the day they are baked and shipped to Whole Foods Market Stores in the USA and Canada.
- Whole Foods Market is the largest retailer of natural and organic foods with over 270 stores in the USA, Canada and U.K.

Gluten-Free Stores & Distributors

Against The Grain, 2292 West 5400 South, Taylorsville, UT, USA 84118
  Phone: 801-955-4418   FAX: 801-955-4323
  Email: iamglutenfree@againstthegrainslc.com   www.againstthegrainslc.com
- Gluten-free specialty retail store.
- Sell over 1000 items (frozen, refrigerated, fresh and shelf-stable) and books from a variety of companies.
- Shop in person or order direct by mail, phone, fax or email; shipping charges based on weight; ships via USPS.

The Allergy Free Shop, 8803 SW 132 Street, Miami, FL, USA 33176
  Phone: 877-212-2828/305-254-2828   FAX: 305-254-2851
  Email: info@allergyfreeshop.com   www.allergyfreeshop.com
- Retail store specializing in allergen-free and gluten-free foods and related products (e.g., cleaning products, equipment and books).
- Over 700 gluten-free products (frozen, refrigerated and shelf-stable).
- Owner has children with food allergies.
- Shop in person or order direct by mail, phone, fax, email or internet. Free shipping on orders over $150.00. Flat rate $9.88 on orders under $150.00. Ships via UPS.

AllergyGrocer, LLC, 7135 Minstrel Way, Suite 101, Columbia, MD, USA 21045
  Phone: 888-476-3350/410-309-9343   FAX: 410-290-5689
  Email: info@allergygrocer.com   www.allergygrocer.com
- Gluten-free online retail store that sells over 900 products.
- Carry "Miss Roben's" mixes and other companies' products such as baked products, beverages, cereals, cookies, condiments, crackers, desserts, entrées and side dishes, ingredients, pasta, snacks and soups.
- Order direct by phone, fax or internet; shipping charges based on amount purchased; free shipping on orders over $100.00; ships UPS Ground or USPS.

Alternative Eating, 116 South Main Ave., Scranton, PA, USA 18504
  Phone: 570-344-6568   FAX: 570-344-6537
  Email: gluten-free@alternativeeating.net   www.alternativeeating.net
- Gluten-free specialty retail store.
- Over 500 items (frozen, refrigerated, fresh and shelf-stable), books, gift baskets and body products.
- Owner is both a registered dietitian and registered nurse. Offers nutrition counselling by appointment.
- Shop in person or order direct by mail, phone, fax or email; shipping charges based on weight; ships via FedEx, UPS or USPS.

DeLiteful Foods and Cafe DeLite, Glendale Plaza, 4040 Quakerbridge Road,
Lawrenceville, NJ, USA 08619

Phone: 609-586-7122 FAX: 609-586-2078
Email: info@delitefulfood.com www.delitefulfood.com

- Specialty food retail store with an extensive selection of gluten-free and allergen-free products (frozen, fresh and shelf-stable).
- Cafe serves light breakfast and lunches. Gluten-free products made on dedicated equipment.
- Shop in person or order direct by mail, phone, fax or email; shipping charges based on weight; ships via USPS.

GardenSpot Distributors, 191 Commerce Drive, New Holland, PA, USA 17557

Phone: 800-829-5100/717-354-4936 FAX: 877-829-5100/717-354-4934
Email: info@gardenspotdist.com www.gardenspotdist.com

- Full service wholesale distributor of organic, natural and specialty foods over 1000 products (e.g., breads, baked products, cereals, dried fruits, flours, grains, frozen foods, meats, nuts, seafood, snack foods).
- Over 400 gluten-free products from a variety of companies.
- Order direct by phone, fax or internet; shipping charges based on weight; ships via FedEx or UPS Ground.

G.F. Joe's Market, 5739 Littlerock Road SW, Suite 103, Tumwater, WA, USA 98512

Phone: 360-628-8010 FAX: 360-628-8011
Email: gfjoe@gfjoes.com www.gfjoes.com

- Gluten-free specialty retail store.
- Sell over 1600 gluten-free and allergen-free products (frozen, refrigerated and shelf-stable) and books.
- Owner has celiac disease.
- Shop in person or order direct by internet; shipping charges based on weight; ships via FedEx.

GlutenFree.com USA, P.O. Box 840, Glastonbury, CT, USA 06033
Canada (Head Office), 2055 Dagenais West, Laval, QC H7L 5V1

Phone Orders: 800-291-8386 Fax Orders: 450-963-0137
Email: pantry@glutenfree.com www.glutenfree.com

- Gluten-free online retail store that sell over 650 items from 100 companies.
- Carry "Gluten-Free Pantry" mixes and "Glutino" products, as well as other companies' products such as baked items, baking ingredients, beverages, cereals, cookies, condiments, crackers, entrées and side dishes, pasta, snacks, soups, vitamins, toaster bags, books and other publications.
- Order direct by phone, fax or internet; shipping charges based on weight; ships via UPS.

Gluten-Free Specialty Market, 2612 J Street, Suite 1, Sacramento, CA, USA 95816
    Phone: 916-442-5241   FAX: 916-441-5199
    Email: info@glutenfreespecialty.com   www.gfspecialty.com

- Gluten-free specialty retail store.
- Sell over 2400 items (frozen, refrigerated, fresh and shelf-stable) and books.
- Owner has celiac disease.
- Shop in person or order direct by mail, phone, fax, email or internet; shipping charges based on weight; ships via FedEx, UPS, or USPS.

Gluten Free Store, 807 Waukegan Road, Northbrook, IL, USA 60062
    Phone: 888-212-0169/847-513-6515   FAX: 847-513-6514
    Email: Kathy@glutenfreestoreusa.com   www.glutenfreestoreusa.com

- Gluten-free specialty retail store.
- Over 750 items (frozen and shelf-stable) from a variety of companies.
- Shop in person or order direct by mail, phone, fax, email or internet; shipping charges based on weight; ships via UPS Ground.

Gluten-Free Cupboard, 1833 - 3rd Ave. S.E., Rochester, MN, USA 55904
    Phone: 507-529-1132   FAX: 507-529-8003
    Email: info@glutenfreecupboard.com   www.glutenfreecupboard.com

- Gluten-free specialty retail store.
- Sells over 900 items (frozen and shelf-stable).
- Owners have celiac disease.
- Shop in person or order direct by mail, phone, fax or email; shipping charges based on weight and handling fee; ships via courier or USPS.

Gluten-Free Grocery, 1922 Mannheim Road, Westchester, IL, USA 60154
    Phone: 708-483-8785   FAX: 708-483-8786
    Email:gfgrocery@gmail.com   www.gfgrocery.com

- Gluten-free specialty retail store.
- Over 800 products (frozen and shelf-stable).
- Owner has celiac disease.
- Shop in person. Order direct by phone or internet; ships via UPS.

Gluten-Free Mall, Inc., 4927 Sonoma Highway, Suite C1, Santa Rosa, CA, USA 95409
    Phone: 866-575-3720/707-509-4528   FAX: 707-324-6060
    Email: info@glutenfreemall.com   www.glutenfreemall.com

- Gluten-free internet shopping mall carrying hundreds of gluten-free products from dozens of companies from around the world, as well as gluten-free books and cookbooks, celiac awareness t-shirts, supplements and other items.
- Ships all products from a central warehouse with one shipping charge based on weight; ships via UPS.
- Ships dry goods and frozen products separately. Frozen products shipped in special freezer pack containers.

Gluten-Free Supermarket, 1850 West 169th Street, Suite B, Gardena, CA, USA 90247
    Phone: 800-806-4737/310-366-7612   FAX: 310-366-6938
    Email: sales@authenticfoods.com   www.glutenfree-supermarket.com

- Gluten-free online retail store.
- Carry a variety of gluten-free products (cereals, pasta, snacks), "Authentic Foods" mixes, flours and other baking supplies, as well as books.
- Order direct by phone, fax, mail or internet; shipping charges based on weight; ships via UPS Ground or USPS.

Gluten-Free Trading Company, 3116 South Chase Ave., Milwaukee, WI, USA 53207
    Phone: 888-993-9933/414-747-8700   FAX: 414-747-8747
    Email: info@food4celiacs.com   www.food4celiacs.com

    Delafield/Pewaukee Location:
    N47W2870 Lynndale Road (CTH JK), Pewaukee, WI, USA 53027
    Phone: 262-369-8700

- Gluten-free specialty retail store.
- Sell over 1000 gluten-free items from over 120 companies from around the world.
- Shop in person or order by phone, mail, fax or internet; shipping charges based on weight; ships via FedEx Ground or USPS.

Goodday Gluten-Free, 514B North Western Ave. Lake Forest, IL, USA 60045
    Phone: 877-395-2527/847-615-1207   FAX: 847-615-1209
    Email: shop@gooddayglutenfree.com   www.gooddayglutenfree.com

- Gluten-free specialty store and internet shopping mall that carry over 500 gluten-free items.
- Shop in person in the retail store or order direct by phone, fax, mail or internet; shipping charges based on amount purchased; ships via UPS Ground or USPS.

Granny's Gluten-Free Zone, 3419 W. Eisenhower Blvd., Loveland, CO, USA 80537
    Phone: 970-669-9986   FAX: 970-669-9946
    Email: orders@grannysglutenfree.com   www.grannysglutenfree.com

- Gluten-free specialty retail store.
- Sell a variety of items (frozen, fresh and shelf-stable) and books.
- Owner has celiac disease.
- Shop in person or order direct by phone, fax, mail, email or internet; shipping charges based on weight; ships via UPS Ground.

Healthy Haven, 80 Main Road, Tiverton, RI, USA 02878
    Phone: 401-816-5844
    Email: info@healthyhaven.necoxmail.com   www.healthyhavenri.com

- Retail store specializing in gluten-free and allergen-free products.
- Sell over 800 gluten-free products (frozen and shelf-stable), books and gift baskets.
- Owner has celiac disease.
- Shop in person.

Herbalicious ... Everything Nutritious, 612 West Main Street,
Mount Pleasant, PA, USA 15666

Phone: 724-542-9745 FAX: 724-542-9746
Email: herbal@winbeam.com www.everythingnutritious.com

- Gluten-free specialty retail store operated by a registered dietitian.
- Carry a wide variety of gluten-free products (frozen and shelf-stable baked products, cereals, cookies, crackers, mixes, pastas, soups).
- Also sells other food products, supplements, toiletries, gift baskets and books.
- Shop in person or order direct by phone, fax or internet; shipping charges based on weight; ships via UPS Ground.

Jakes Gluten-Free Store, 12646 West Fairview Ave., Boise, ID, USA 83713

Phone: 208-322-5935 FAX: 208-322-6421
Email: info@jakesglutenfreestore.com www.jakesglutenfreestore.com

- Gluten-free specialty store.
- Sell over 1000 items (frozen, refrigerated and shelf-stable), as well as supplements and books.
- Owner and family members have celiac disease.
- Shop in person or order direct by mail, phone, fax, email or internet; shipping charges based on weight; ships via UPS Ground.

Karma Foods, 634 Kinderkamack Road, River Edge, NJ, USA 07661

Phone: 201-986-1225 FAX: 201-986-0540
Email: karmafood@aol.com www.karmafoodsdist.com

- Gluten-free specialty distributor that carries a large selection of products from various gluten-free companies. Over 200 items such as bagels, breads, cakes, cookies, crackers, muffins, pasta, rolls and frozen entrées.
- Sell products to health food and grocery stores, restaurants and health care facilities.
- Can order direct if there is no retail outlet in the area.

Lil's Dietary Shop, 2738 W. 111th Street, Chicago, IL, USA 60655

Phone: 773-239-0355 FAX: 773-239-0357
Email: lilsdietaryshop@sbcglobal.net www.lilsdietary.com

- Specialty food retail store with an extensive selection of gluten-free, allergen and sugar-free, as well as low protein products (frozen, refrigerated and shelf-stable). Also carry books.
- Shop in person or order direct by mail, phone, fax, email or internet; shipping charges based on weight or amount purchased; ships via UPS Ground. Frozen foods shipped in styrofoam containers with ice packs.

Lingonberries Market, 6300 NE 117 Ave., Vancouver, WA, USA 98662
    Phone: 360-260-4411   FAX: 360-260-7459
    Email: christina@lingonberriesmarket.com   www.lingonberriesmarket.com

- Gluten-free specialty retail store.
- Sell over 2000 items (frozen, refrigerated, fresh and shelf-stable) and books.
- Owner has celiac disease.
- Shop in person or order by phone, mail, fax or email; shipping charges based on weight; ships via UPS Ground.

Livefreeda Inc., P.O. Box 11204, Yakima, WA, USA 98909
    Phone: 425-891-4998   FAX: 360-378-3673
    Email: info@livefreeda.com   www.livefreeda.com

- Gluten-free meal program that provides 28 days of breakfast, lunch, dinner, snack and dessert items. Includes shelf stable and frozen products that are shipped directly to customer. All products are gluten-free and are taste tested. Also includes 28 day menu developed and approved by registered dietitians.
- Order direct by internet and phone.
- Free shipping. Dry and frozen products shipped in different containers but entire shipment sent at the same time. Frozen products are shipped in dry ice.

Lorenzo's Specialty Foods Ltd., 1060 St. Mary's Road,
                        Winnipeg, MB, Canada R2M 3S9
    Phone: 866-639-1711/204-253-1300   FAX: 204-253-4049
    Email: hello@lorenzosfoods.ca   www.lorenzosfoods.ca

- Gluten-free specialty retail store and bakery; dedicated GF facility operated by a family with celiac disease.
- Carry a variety of gluten-free products (frozen, fresh and shelf-stable) from many companies, as well as books.
- Also produce fresh baked goods (breads, cakes, cookies, pies and squares).
- Shop in person.

Med-Diet Laboratories Inc., 3600 Holly Lane N., Suite 80, Plymouth, MN,
                        USA 55447
    Phone: 800-633-3438/763-550-2020   FAX: 763-550-2022
    Email: meddiet@med-diet.com   www.med-diet.com

- Distributor of a variety of products for special dietary needs (gluten-free, cardiac, critical care, diabetes, dysphagia, low protein).
- Gluten-free baking mixes, breads, cookies, crackers and pastas from Allergaroo, Domata, Dr. Lucy's, Ener-G Foods, General Mills, Gillian's Foods, Gluten-Free Sensations, Glutino, PaneRiso/Kingsmill, Orgran and Schär.
- Order direct by phone, fax, or internet; shipping charges based on weight; ships via FedEx.

Paramed Inc., 995 Wellington, Suite 220, Montreal, QC, Canada H3C 1V3
    Phone: 888-606-6676/514-395-2458   FAX: 514-395-2396
    Email: info@paramedinc.com   www.paramedinc.com

- Gluten-free specialty food distributor. Carry products from Ener-G Foods, Canbrands, Cheecha, Hot Kids and other companies.
- Order direct by phone or fax; ships via Purolator.

Quattrobimbi Imports Inc., 48 Lawridge Drive, Rye Brook, NY, USA 10573
    Phone: 866-618-7759/914-819-0494   FAX: 914-937-3437
    Email: info@quattrobimbi.com   www.quattrobimbi.com

- Importer and distributor of Italian gluten-free products from Bi-Aglut, Galbusera (crackers and cookies), Molino di Ferro (Le Veneziane Cookies & corn pasta), Pedon's (Easyglut baking mixes). All products made in dedicated GF facilities.
- Products sold to various retail stores.
- Order direct by internet; shipping charges based on weight; ships via FedEx or UPS.

Shalit Foods Inc., 601 Magnetic Drive, Unit 24, Toronto, ON, Canada M3J 3J2
    Phone: 800-969-6991/416-663-2727   FAX: 416-650-5643
    Email: info@shalitfoods.com   www.shalitfoods.com

- Foodservice supplier of a large variety of products for health care facilities, college/ university dining services, airlines, hotels and restaurants in Canada and the U.S.
- Also offer a selection of complete meals and bulk entrées for health care facilities, including products that are suitable for gluten-free, lactose-free and renal diets. Complete meals are packed in three compartment trays which includes a protein, starch and vegetables.
- Contact company for ordering information.

Simply Gluten-Free, 1321 E. Thousand Oaks Blvd., #A108, Thousand Oaks, CA, USA 91362
    Phone: 805-777-4877   FAX: 805-777-0064
    Email: simplyglutenfree@gmail.com   www.simplyglutenfree.org
    www.simply-glutenfree.com

- Gluten-free specialty retail store.
- Sell over 1200 products (fresh, frozen, refrigerated and shelf-stable), as well as gift baskets, gift items and books.
- Owner has celiac disease.
- Shop in person or order direct by mail, phone, fax, email or internet; shipping charges based on weight; ships via UPS. Also offer local delivery service.

Specialty Food Shop, 555 University Ave., Toronto, ON, Canada M5G 1X8
    Phone: 800-737-7976/416-813-5294   FAX: 416-977-8394
    Email: sfs.admin@sickkids.ca   www.specialtyfoodshop.com

- Specialty food retail store located in the Hospital for Sick Children.
- Carries over 600 specialty products (gluten-free, low-protein, dysphagia, food allergies and intolerances, nutritional supplements, enteral feeding equipment, specialized infant feeding products/equipment and books).
- Large variety of gluten-free products from North American and European companies.
- Dietitians on staff for inquiries.
- Shop in person or order direct by phone or internet; shipping charges based on weight; ships via Purolator.

Sydney's Health Market, 810 - 30th Avenue S., Moorhead, MN, USA 56560
    Phone: 218-233-3310   FAX: 218-233-3378
    Email: info@sydneyshealthmarket.com   www.sydneyshealthmarket.com

- Retail store specializing in gluten-free, allergen-free and organic products.
- Sell over 4000 items (frozen and shelf-stable) and books.
- Owner has a child with celiac disease.
- Shop in person or order direct by mail, phone, fax, email or internet; shipping charges based on weight; ships via UPS Ground.

APPENDIX A

Enriched Gluten-Free Products		
Company	**Products**	**Nutrients Added**
De Boles	Multi Grain pasta (penne, spaghetti), Rice Plus golden flax pasta (angel hair, spirals)	Thiamin, riboflavin, niacin, iron and folic acid
Duinkerken Foods	Mixes (breads, biscuit, cookie, muffin, pizza, waffle)	Thiamin, riboflavin, niacin, folic acid and iron
Ener-G Foods	All breads (except yeast-free), buns, rolls, pizza shells, brown English muffins, crackers, melba toast, bread crumbs, croûtons, brownies, doughnut holes, plain doughnuts, pound cake	Thiamin, riboflavin, niacin, iron and folic acid
Enjoy Life	Bagels	Thiamin, riboflavin, niacin, folate, calcium, magnesium, Vitamin B_6
	Granola Cereals	Thiamin, niacin, pantothenic acid, iron, zinc, magnesium, folate, Vitamin B_6
	Snack Bars	Thiamin, riboflavin, niacin, folate, Vitamin B_6
Food-Tek	All mixes except icings	Thiamin, riboflavin, niacin, folic acid
Gluten-Free Creations Bakery	All breads, bagels, pizza crusts, cakes, cookies, brownies, donuts, muffins, bread crumbs, graham cracker crumbs and mixes (except "Baking Mix")	Thiamin, riboflavin, niacin, iron, folic acid and calcium
Glutino	Original corn breads, Premium (corn breads, bagels, pizza crusts)	Thiamin, riboflavin, niacin, Vitamin B_6, iron and calcium
Kinnikinnick	All breads (including yeast-free), bagels, buns, English muffins, pizza crusts, bread crumbs and tapioca rice bread mix	Thiamin, riboflavin, niacin, iron and folic acid
Pastato	Fortified potato pasta (elbows, spaghetti and penne)	Thiamin, riboflavin, niacin, folic acid, Vitamin B_6, pantothenic acid, iron and magnesium
Schär	Hearty White Bread	Thiamin, riboflavin, niacin and iron
	Multigrain Bread	Calcium and folic acid

Appendix B

Gluten-Free Products Designed/Suitable For Foodservice	
Company/ Distributor Name	**Products**
Apetito	Frozen, fully cooked complete meals in individual trays (single serve) and bulk (in foil trays). Heat in microwave or oven. Seven products are gluten-free and also suitable for lactose-free and renal diets.
Celinal Foods	Single-serve microwave bread and cake mixes, soup bases, pasta, instant gravy mix and soy sauce. All are gluten-free.
Ener-G Foods	Shelf-stable gluten-free breads available in 2 slice vacuum-sealed packages.
French Meadow Bakery	Frozen pizza crusts on foil pans ready-to-bake (24/package), Chocolate Chip Cookie and Fudge Brownie (single-serve, individually wrapped), small iced cakes.
Glutenfreeda Foods	Frozen, single serve burritos. Heat in microwave.
	Gluten-free oatmeal and granola in single-serve packages.
Kari-Out	"Panda Brand" gluten-free soy sauce in single-serve packets.
Kettle Cuisine	Single-serve, gluten-free frozen soups that are microwavable.
Marsan Foods	"Balanced Cuisine" frozen soups (in bulk pouches) and frozen entrées (in single-serve trays and bulk pouches). Heat in microwave or oven. Many products are gluten-free.
My Own Meals	Single-serve, shelf-stable, fully cooked meals in individual trays that are in vacuum sealed packages. Heat in microwave. Five products are gluten-free.
Nature's Path Foods	Single-serve cereal in small bag and cup.
Organic Bistro	Single-serve, gluten-free frozen organic entrées. Heat in microwave or oven.
Savory Creations	"Savory Choice" soup broth concentrates (regular, reduced sodium and low sodium) and demi-glace in shelf-stable bag-in-box and stock pot in-a-pouch. All are gluten-free.
Swiss Chalet	"Cuisine Sante" shelf-stable soup and soup bases, roux and sauces. All are free of gluten, major allergens and MSG.

* In addition to the above, there are many other companies and their products included in this guide that can be purchased by health care facilities, college/university dining services and restaurants.

APPENDIX C

Companies and Products with Gluten-Free Oats	
AllergyFree Foods	Oatmeal Raisin Bites
Andrea's Fine Foods	Oatmeal Cookies, Oatmeal Cookie Dough
Avena (formerly FarmPure Foods) [Only Oats™]	Breakfast Blends Hot Cereal (various flavors), Oat Flakes (Regular, Quick), Mixes (Cookie, Muffin, Pancake), Steel Cut Oat Pearls, Oat Flour, Oat Bran
Bittersweet Bakery	Monster Cookies
Bob's Red Mill	Gluten-Free Whole Grain Rolled Oats, Gluten-Free Steel Cut Oats
Cream Hill Estates (Lara's)	Oat Flour, Oat Groats, Rolled Oats
Deby's Gluten-Free	Oatmeal Cookie Dough
Flying Apron Bakery	Berry Oat Wondies, Carrot Muffins, Flying Aprons
Gifts of Nature	Gluten-Free Rolled Oats, Gluten-Free Whole Groats
Gluten-Free Creations Bakery	Honey Oat Bread, Honey Oat Bread Mix, Oatmeal Raisin Cookies
Glutenfreeda Foods	GF Granola (various flavors), Instant Oatmeal (various flavors)
Gluten-Free Oats®	Old Fashion Rolled Oats, Oat Groats
Greyston Bakery (formerly Good Juju Bakery)	Oatmeal Raisin Cookies
Heaven Mills Bakery	Gluten-Free Matzah
Holly's Oatmeal	Gluten-Free Oatmeal Porridge (Plain and Cranberry)
Jake Bakes	Cookies and Granola
Mountain Top Café and Bakery	Dad's Cookies, Date Squares, Dream Bars, Granola, Granola Crunch Cereal, Rice Honey Oats Bread
Nonuttin' Foods	Granola Bars, Granola Clusters
Outside The Breadbox	Egg-Free Oat Bread, Oatmeal Cookies, Oatmeal Cookies with Cranberries, Pizza Crust, Vegan Quinoa Muffins
PaneRiso/Kingsmill	Apple Crisp Mix
PureFit Nutrition	Granola Crunch Bar
Rose's Wheat Free Bakery & Café	Oatmeal Cookies (Plain, Cranberry Chocolate Chip and Sugar-Free Raisin)
Sweet Christine's Gluten-Free Confections	Oatmeal Raisin Cookies
The Grainless Baker	Oatmeal Cookies
The Sensitive Baker	GF Oat Mini Loaf, GF Oat Loaf Mix
The Silly Yak Bakery	Oatmeal Cookies, Oatmeal Cookie Dough
The Twisted Bakery	Oatmeal Raisin Cookies, Oatmeal Raisin Cookie Mix
Udi's Gluten-Free Foods	Granola (various flavors)
Whole Foods Gluten-Free Bakehouse	Fruit and Nut Granola, Honey Oat Bread

Appendix D

Gluten-Free Certification Organization (GFCO)

- Program of the Gluten Intolerance Group of North America (GIG). It is modeled after high standard kosher and organic certification programs.

- GFCO's mission is to "provide an independent service to supervise gluten-free food production according to a consistent, defined, science-based standard that is confirmed by field inspections, in order to achieve consumer confidence and safety".

- Certification requires regular audits, onsite product testing and random independent gluten testing by the GFCO.

- Third party auditors (with years of experience in food manufacturing audits) conduct the gluten-free inspections.

- Products meeting the GFCO certification standards can use the "GF Logo" on the package label.

- Website includes information about certification procedures and a listing of retail products, manufacturing facilities and commercial ingredients that are GFCO certified.

Phone: 253-218-2957   FAX: 253-833-6675   www.gfco.org

GLUTEN-FREE RESOURCES
Canadian Celiac Organizations

Canadian Celiac Association (CCA)
5025 Orbitor Drive, Bldg. 1, Suite 400
Mississauga, ON, Canada L4W 4Y5
Phone: 800-363-7296/905-507-6208
FAX: 905-507-4673
www. celiac.ca
Email: info@celiac.ca

Fondation Québécoise de la Maladie Coeliaque (Quebec Celiac Foundation)
4837 rue Boyer, Bureau 230
Montreal, QC, Canada H2J 3E6
Phone: 514-529-8806
FAX: 514-529-2046
www.fqmc.org
Email: info@fqmc.org

American Celiac Organizations

American Celiac Disease Alliance (ACDA)
2504 Duxbury Place
Alexandria, VA, USA 22308
Phone: 703-622-3331
www.americanceliac.org
Email: info@americanceliac.org

Celiac Disease Foundation (CDF)
13251 Ventura Blvd., Suite #1
Studio City, CA, USA 91604-1838
Phone: 818-990-2354
FAX: 818-990-2379
www.celiac.org
Email: cdf@celiac.org

Celiac Sprue Association/USA, Inc. (CSA)
P.O. Box 31700
Omaha, NE, USA 68131-0700
Phone: 877-272-4272/402-558-0600
FAX: 402-558-1347
www.csaceliacs.org
Email: celiacs@csaceliacs.org

Gluten Intolerance Group of North America (GIG)
31214 - 124th Ave. S.E.
Auburn, WA, USA 98092-3667
Phone: 253-833-6655
FAX: 253-833-6675
www.gluten.net
Email: info@gluten.net

National Foundation for Celiac Awareness (NFCA)
P.O. Box 544
224 South Maple Street
Ambler, PA, USA 19002-0544
Phone: 215-325-1306
FAX: 215-643-1707
www.celiaccentral.org
Email: info@celiaccentral.org

International Celiac Organizations

ARGENTINA: www.celiaco.org.ar
AUSTRALIA: www.coeliacsociety.com.au
AUSTRIA: www.zoeliakie.or.at
BELGIUM: www.coeliakie.be
          http://vcv.coeliakie.be
BRAZIL: www.acelbra.org.br
CHILE: www.coacel.cl
CZECH REPUBLIC: www.coeliac.cz
CROATIA: www.celiajakija.hr
DENMARK: www.coeliaki.dk
FINLAND: www.keliakialiitto.fi
FRANCE: www.afdiag.org

GERMANY: www.dzg-online.de
GREECE: www.koiliokaki.com
HUNGARY: www.coeliac.hu
IRELAND: www.coeliac.ie
ISRAEL: www.celiac.org.il
ITALY: www.celiachia.it
LUXEMBURG: www.alig.lu
NETHERLANDS: www.coeliakievereniging.nl
NEW ZEALAND: www.coeliac.co.nz
NORWAY: www.ncf.no
PAKISTAN: www.celiac.com.pk
POLAND: www.celiakia.org.pl

International Celiac Organizations Cont'd

PORTUGAL: www.celiacos.org.pt
RUSSIA: www.celiac.spb.ru
SLOVAKIA: www.celiakia.sk
SLOVENIA: www.drustvo-celiakija.si
SPAIN: www.celiacos.org;
　　　　www.celiacscatalunya.org

SWEDEN: www.celiaki.se
SWITZERLAND: www.zoeliakie.ch
　　　　www.coeliakie.ch
　　　　www.celiachia.ch
UNITED KINGDOM: www.coeliac.co.uk
URUGUAY: www.acelu.org

Celiac Education, Research & Treatment Centers

Celiac Center at Beth Israel Deaconess Medical Center, Harvard Medical School
Boston, MA
Phone: 617-667-1272　　　　　　　　　　　www.bidmc.harvard.edu/celiaccenter

Celiac Disease Center at Columbia University
New York, NY
Phone: 212-342-4529　　　　　　　　　www.celiacdiseasecenter.columbia.edu

Celiac Disease Clinic at Mayo Clinic
Rochester, MN
Phone: 507-284-5255 (Patients)　　　　　　www.mayoclinic.org/celiac-disease
　　　　507-284-2631 (Clinicians)

Celiac Disease Clinic, Department of Internal Medicine, Gastroenterology, University of Iowa Hospitals and Clinics
Iowa City, IA
Phone: 319-356-4060　　　　　　　　　　　　　www.uihealthcare.com

Celiac Disease Program at Boston Children's Hospital, Gastroenterology and Nutrition Division
Boston, MA
Phone: 617-355-6058 (appointments)　　　www.childrenshospital.org/celiac
　　　　617-355-2127 (Celiac Support Group)

Celiac Group at University of Virginia Health System, Digestive Health Center of Excellence
Charlottesville, VA
Phone: 434-243-9309　　www.healthsystem.virginia.edu/internet/digestive-health/patientcare.cfm

Stanford Celiac Sprue Management Clinic, Stanford University Medical Center
Stanford, CA
Phone: 650-723-6961
　　　　www.stanfordhospital.com/clinicsmedservices/clinics/gastroenterology/celiacsprue.html

University of Chicago Celiac Disease Program
Chicago, IL
Phone: 773-702-7593　　　　　　　　　　　www.celiacdisease.net

University of Maryland Center for Celiac Research
Baltimore, MD
Phone: 800-492-5538 (Appointments)　　　　www.celiaccenter.org
　　　　410-328-6749

William K. Warren Medical Research Center for Celiac Disease and the **Clinical Center for Celiac Disease at the University of California**
San Diego, CA
Phone: 858-822-1022　　　　　　　　　　http://celiaccenter.ucsd.edu

Resources for Health Professionals and/or Consumers

National Institutes of Health (NIH) Celiac Disease Awareness Campaign
www.celiac.nih.gov

NIH Consensus Development Conference on Celiac Disease
http://consensus.nih.gov/2004/2004CeliacDisease118html.htm

National Digestive Diseases Information Clearinghouse (NDDIC)
http://digestive.niddk.nih.gov/   (Click on "A-Z" list and then "C" and "Celiac Disease")

Children's Digestive Health and Nutrition Foundation (CDHNF): Celiac Disease Resources
www.cdhnf.org
www.celiachealth.org

Canadian Celiac Association Website for Health Professionals/Consumers
www.celiacguide.org

**American Dietetic Association Nutrition Evidence Analysis Project
"Gluten Intolerance/Celiac Disease" section**
http://www.adaevidencelibrary.com/topic.cfm?cat = 1403

Dietitians of Canada Practice-Based Evidence in Nutrition (PEN): "Celiac Disease" section
http://www.dieteticsatwork.com/pen/ViewPublicCurrentTopics.asp

Health Canada Celiac Disease Links
http://www.hc-sc.gc.ca/fn-an/securit/allerg/cel-coe/index-eng.php
http://www.hc-sc.gc.ca/fn-an/pubs/securit/gluten_conn-lien_gluten-eng.php
http://www.hc-sc.gc.ca/fn-an/securit/allerg/cel-coe/oats_cd-avoine-eng.php

American College of Gastroenterology: Digestive Health SmartBrief
Free email newsletter: http://www.smartbrief.com/dhsb/?campaign = acg

Shelley Case's Website (Free Handouts and Resources for Health Professionals & Consumers)
www.glutenfreediet.ca

Celiac Disease & Gluten-Free Diet Resources

Real Life with Celiac Disease: Troubleshooting and Thriving Gluten-Free
✦   369-page book written by Melinda Dennis (dietitian), Dr. Daniel Leffler (Director of Clinical Research,
    Celiac Center at Beth Israel Deaconess Medical Centre in Boston) and more than 50 international
    celiac experts. Includes 53 chapters on a wide variety of topics on celiac disease and gluten-related
    disorders. Each chapter features a patient case study with a specific problem and/or questions
    followed by a discussion about treatment recommendations, lifestyle changes and outcomes.
✦   Cost: $18.95 (U.S.); ISBN 978-1-60356-008-5
    American Gastroenterology Association Press   www.reallifewithceliacdisease.com

Celiac Disease: A Hidden Epidemic (Revised and Updated Edition)
✦   352-page book by Dr. Peter H. R. Green, director of the Celiac Disease Center at Columbia University
    in New York, and science writer Rory Jones, who has celiac disease. Comprehensive information
    about celiac disease including symptoms, diagnostic tests, related conditions and complications,
    treatment, lifestyle issues and resources.
✦   Cost: $22.95 (U.S.); ISBN 978-0-06-17281-6-7
    Harper Collins   www.harpercollins.com

Celiac Disease for Dummies

✦ 384-page book by Dr. Ian Blumer (internal medicine) and Dr. Sheila Crowe (gastroenterologist). Very comprehensive and practical information about celiac disease including symptoms, diagnostic tests, associated conditions, complications, treatment, nutritional considerations, alternate and complimentary therapies, follow-up, frequently asked questions and resources.

✦ Cost: $19.99 (U.S.); $23.99 (CDN); ISBN 978-0-470-16036-7
Dummies   www.dummies.com

Celiac Disease: The Road to Diagnosis

✦ 75-page booklet written by Dr. Mohsin Rashid, pediatric gastroenterologist and member of the Canadian Celiac Association Professional Advisory Board. Features a collection of short stories of individuals with celiac disease describing their long and often difficult road to diagnosis. After each story, Dr. Rashid highlights key medical points called "Clinical Pearls".

✦ Free online version available for health professionals and consumers.
http://celiacstories.ca   E-mail: info@celiacstories.ca

American Dietetic Association's Easy Gluten-Free: Expert Nutrition Advice with More than 100 Recipes

✦ 288-page book by Tricia Thompson (dietitian) and Marlisa Brown (dietitian and chef). Provides an overview on label reading and cross-contamination issues, nutritional tips, gluten-free grains, healthy recipes, meal plans and resources.

✦ Cost: $15.95 (U.S.); $18.95 (CDN); ISBN 978-0-470-47609-3
John Wiley & Sons   www.wiley.com

The Gluten-Free Nutrition Guide

✦ 245-page book by dietitian Tricia Thompson. Includes the basics of the GF diet; ingredient and labeling information; worksheets to assess your dietary intake and tips to improve its nutritional quality; 50 recipes and resources.

✦ Cost: $16.95 (U.S.); ISBN 978-0-07-154541-9
McGraw Hill   www.mhprofessional.com

Complete Gluten-Free Diet and Nutrition Guide: With a 30-day Meal Plan & Over 100 Recipes

✦ 272-page book by dietitian Alexandra Anca and Theresa Santandrea-Cull (culinary expert). Provides information about celiac disease including symptoms, diagnosis and management, as well as foods allowed and to avoid, shopping tips, substitutions, nutritional considerations, healthy meal plans and recipes.

✦ Cost: $24.95 (U.S.); $27.95 (CDN); ISBN 978-0-7788-0252-5
Robert Rose   www.robertrose.ca

The Complete Idiot's Guide to Gluten-Free Eating

✦ 304-page book by Eve Adamson and dietitian Tricia Thompson. Includes an overview of celiac disease and gluten intolerance; foods/ingredients allowed and to avoid; label reading guidelines; menu suggestions; recipes; substitutions; nutrition information; eating out and resources.

✦ Cost: $16.95 (U.S.); ISBN 978-1-59257-683-8   Alpha Books

Living with Celiac Disease: Abundance Beyond Wheat and Gluten (2nd Edition)

✦ 199-page book by Claudine Crangle, who has been living with celiac disease for over 30 years. Provides an overview of celiac disease and practical information on the gluten-free diet including foods and ingredients allowed and to avoid, shopping, food preparation tips, recipes, eating away from home, traveling, healthy lifestyle advice and resources.

✦ Cost: $24.95 (U.S.); $28.95 (CDN); ISBN 978-1-55369404-5
Your Health Press   www.yourhealthpress.com

Celiac Disease: A Guide to Living with Gluten Intolerance

✦ 160-page book by Sylvia Llewelyn Bower (nurse); Mary Kay Sharrett (dietitian) and Steve Plogsted (pharmacist). Includes information on symptoms, diagnosis, dermatitis herpetiformis, complications, healthy gluten-free diet guidelines, GF baking, recipes, medications, resources and the emotional aspects of celiac disease.

✦ Cost: $16.95 (U.S.); ISBN 978-1-932603-25-5
Demos Medical Publishing   www.demosmedpub.com

Canadian Celiac Association *Pocket Dictionary: Acceptability of Foods and Food Ingredients for the Gluten-Free Diet*
- ✦ 60-page pocket-size dictionary of more than 300 foods and food ingredients and over 300 food additives listed in alphabetical order for easy reference. Easy-to-understand description of each item and food ingredients classified by category (allowed, not allowed, or to check). Written by dietitians with expertise in celiac disease who did extensive research into ingredient manufacturing practices and food-labeling regulations in the USA, Canada and Europe.
- ✦ Cost: $6.95 members, $9.95 non-members; ISBN 0-921026-21-8
- ✦ Also available on a CD-Rom for $19.95. The hard copy and CD-Rom available from the Canadian Celiac Association (see below).
- ✦ An online downloadable version is available from Clan Thompson (see page 348).
  Canadian Celiac Association
  Phone: 800-363-7296/905-507-6208   www.celiac.ca

Gluten-Free Living **magazine**
- ✦ Quarterly national publication devoted to the gluten-free lifestyle. Covers diet and ingredient concerns, practical lifestyle coping skills, recipes and medical and research information. Reviewed by a medical and dietetic advisory board.
- ✦ Subscriptions are $34 (1 year) or $54 (2 years). Canada: $40 (1 year) or $66 (2 years) in US funds. Send cheque, money order or Visa/MasterCard/Discover Card number, expiration date, security code to:
  Gluten-Free Living, P.O. Box 375, Maple Shade, NJ, USA 08052; by phone at 800-324-8781; or online at www.glutenfreeliving.com

Living Without **magazine**
- ✦ National magazine published 6 times per year featuring inspirational and educational articles about allergies, food allergies and intolerances, as well as celiac disease. All recipes are gluten-free. Ingredient substitutions are provided for common food allergies. Published by Belvoir Media Group, the magazine is reviewed by an advisory board (MD's, dietitians and directors of American Celiac organizations).
- ✦ Subscriptions are $23 (1 year) or $42 (2 years) in US funds.
- ✦ To subscribe: online at www.livingwithout.com or call 800-474-8614
            Living Without, P.O. Box 420235, Palm Coast, FL, USA 32142-0235.

Celiac.com
- ✦ On-line resource since 1995 providing information and support for celiac disease and the gluten-free diet. Site provides a searchable database of over 2,000 articles on celiac disease, recipes, message board, celiac calendar and a bookstore. Owned and managed by Scott Adams who has celiac disease.
- ✦ Forum of over 31,000 members at www.glutenfreeforum.com
- ✦ Quarterly newsletter *Journal of Gluten Sensitivity* by Celiac.com available by subscription.
- ✦ www.celiac.com   Email: info@celiac.com

New Era Productions Educational Resources
- ✦ **Understanding Celiac Disease and Gluten Intolerance DVD**
  Two-disc DVD set (2 hours) featuring Dr. Michelle Pietzak (aka "Gluten-Free MD"), Dr. Fasano, Dr. Green, Shelley Case, Danna Korn, Andrea Levario and other experts. For patients, physicians and healthcare providers. Cost: $49.95
- ✦ **Celiac Disease & Gluten Intolerance Audio CD**
  Two-disc audio CD (85 minutes) featuring Dr. Michelle Pietzak who explains symptoms, diagnosis and treatment. Cost: $25
- ✦ **New Era Productions**
  P.O. Box 171, Lumberton, NC, USA 28358 Phone: 866-963-9372/910-674-3934
  FAX: 760-406-4201   Email: info@neweraproductions.com
  www.neweraproductions.com   www.glutenfreemd.com

Clan Thompson Celiac Resources

✦ *Celiac SmartList of Foods for Palm OS Handhelds, Pocket PC's, Windows Mobile, Blackberry Smartphones, Windows or Macs*
Includes gluten status of over 19,400 products found in USA supermarkets, health food stores and online. Can search by name of food, category or manufacturer.

✦ *Celiac SmartList of Drugs for Palm OS Handhelds, Pocket PC's, Windows Mobile, Blackberry Smartphones, Windows or Macs*
Includes gluten status of over 3,300 prescription and over-the-counter medications; cosmetics, personal care items, etc., found in the USA. Can search by name of product, category or manufacturer.

✦ *Celiac SmartList of Canadian Foods for Palm OS Handhelds, Blackberry Smartphones, Windows or Macs*
Includes gluten status of over 3,200 products found in Canadian supermarkets. Can search by name of food, category, or manufacturer.

> **Note:** Information in SmartList software is verified directly with each manufacturer and updated regularly. SmartList software programs stand alone and don't require other programs to open them. Available for USA or Canadian products. Software can be searched by product name, category or manufacturer. Fully functional, free demo versions are available to download. Each program costs $24.95.

✦ *Celiac Ingredient Computer Dictionary for Windows, Pocket PC's and Smart Phones*
Software version of the Canadian Celiac Association's *Pocket Dictionary of Food and Food Ingredients for the Gluten-Free Diet*. Information is applicable for USA and Canada. Contains over 700 listings of ingredients and additives with an assessment of their acceptability for the GF diet.
Cost is $20 and can be purchased and downloaded at www.clanthompson.com/dictionary

> All resources available from:
> **Clan Thompson**, 42 Green St., Bridgton, ME, USA 04009
> www.clanthompson.com   Email: celiac@clanthompson.com

Cooking Resources: Cookbooks

The Gluten-Free Gourmet Bakes Bread: More Than 200 Wheat-Free Recipes by Bette Hagman
✦ Cost: $18.00   ISBN 0-8050-6078-2   Owl Books

The Gluten-Free Gourmet Cooks Comfort Foods: Creating Old Favorites with the New Flours by Bette Hagman
✦ Cost: $27.50   ISBN 0-8050-7453-8   Henry Holt and Co.

The Gluten-Free Gourmet Cooks Fast and Healthy: Wheat-Free and Gluten-Free with Less Fuss and Less Fat by Bette Hagman
✦ Cost: $18.00   ISBN 0-8050-6525-3   Owl Books

More From the Gluten-Free Gourmet: Delicious Dining Without Wheat by Bette Hagman
✦ Cost: $18.00   ISBN 0-8050-6524-5   Owl Books

The Gluten-Free Gourmet: Living Well Without Wheat (**Second Edition**) by Bette Hagman
✦ Cost: $18.00   ISBN 0-8050-6484-2   Owl Books

The Gluten-Free Gourmet Makes Dessert: More Than 200 Wheat-Free Recipes for Cakes, Cookies, Pies and Other Sweets by Bette Hagman
✦ Cost: $18.00   ISBN 0-8050-7276-4   Owl Books

100 Best Gluten-Free Recipes by Carol Fenster
✦   Cost: $16.95   ISBN 978-0-470-47583-6   John Wiley & Sons

1,000 Gluten-Free Recipes by Carol Fenster
✦   Cost: $35.00   ISBN 978-0-470-06780-2   John Wiley & Sons

Gluten-Free 101: Easy Basic Dishes Without Wheat by Carol Fenster
✦   Cost: $19.95   ISBN 1-889374-08-3   Savory Palate, Inc.

Cooking Free: 220 Flavorful Recipes for People with Food Allergies and Multiple Food Sensitivities by Carol Fenster
✦   Cost: $18.95   ISBN 1-58333-215-4   Avery

Wheat-Free Recipes & Menus: Delicious, Healthful Eating for People with Food Sensitivities by Carol Fenster
✦   Cost: $16.95   ISBN 1-58333-191-3   Avery

Books can be ordered direct from:
Savory Palate, Inc.
8174 S. Holly, #404, Centennial, CO, USA   80122-4004
Phone: 800-741-5418   www.savorypalate.com

Wheat-Free Gluten-Free Cookbook for Kids and Busy Adults by Connie Sarros
✦   Cost: $16.95   ISBN 978-0-07-162747-4   McGraw Hill

Wheat-Free Gluten-Free Dessert Cookbook by Connie Sarros
✦   Cost: $16.95   ISBN 978-0-07-142372-4   McGraw Hill

Wheat-Free Gluten-Free Reduced Calorie Cookbook by Connie Sarros
✦   Cost: $16.95   ISBN 978-0-07-142375-5   McGraw Hill

Books can be ordered direct from:
Gluten-Free Cookbooks
3800 Rosemont Blvd., #103-D, Fairlawn, OH, USA   44333
Phone: 330-670-1356   www.gfbooks.homestead.com

---

125 Best Gluten-Free Bread Machine Recipes by Donna Washburn and Heather Butt
✦   Cost: $24.95 (U.S.), ($27.95 (CDN)   ISBN 978-0-7788-0238-9   Robert Rose

Complete Gluten-Free Cookbook: 150 Gluten-Free, Lactose-Free Recipes, Many with Egg-Free Variations by Donna Washburn and Heather Butt
✦   Cost: $24.95 (U.S.), $27.95 (CDN)   ISBN 978-0-7788-0158-0   Robert Rose

125 Best Gluten-Free Recipes by Donna Washburn and Heather Butt
✦   Cost: $19.95 (U.S.), $19.95 (CDN)   ISBN 0-7788-0111-X   Robert Rose

The Best Gluten-Free Family Cookbook by Donna Washburn and Heather Butt
✦   Cost: $18.95 (U.S.), $19.95 (CDN)   ISBN 0-7788-0065-2   Robert Rose

250 Gluten-Free Favorites by Donna Washburn and Heather Butt
✦   Cost: $24.95 (U.S.), $27.95 (CDN)   ISBN 978-0-7788-0225-9   Robert Rose

Books can be ordered direct from:
Quality Professional Services, 1655 County Road 2, Mallorytown, ON, Canada   K0E 1R0
Phone: 613-923-2116   www.bestbreadrecipes.com

Gluten-Free Every Day Cookbook: More than 100 Recipes from the Gluten-Free Chef by Robert Landolphi
✦   Cost: $16.99 (U.S.), $20.99 (CDN)   ISBN 978-0-7407-7813-1   Andrews McMeel Publishing

Gluten-Free Baking with the Culinary Institute of America by Chef Richard J. Coppedge Jr., C.M.B.
- ✦   Cost: $18.95 (U.S.), $20.99 (CDN)   ISBN 978-1-59869-613-4   Adams Media

Gluten-Free Baking: More Than 125 Recipes for Delectable Sweet and Savory Baked Goods Including Cakes, Pies, Quickbreads, Muffins, Cookies and Other Delights by Rebecca Reilly
- ✦   Cost: $16.00   ISBN 978-1-4165-3599-7   Simon and Schuster

Bake Deliciously! Gluten and Dairy Free Cookbook by Jean Duane, Alternative Cook
- ✦   Cost: $24.95 (U.S.)   ISBN 978-0-9787109-0-3   Alternative Cook, LLC Publisher

Books can be ordered direct from:
> **Alternative Cook, LLC,** 8200 S. Quebec Street, Suite A3-220, Centennial, CO, USA 80112
> Phone: 303-221-0771   www.alternativecook.com

You Won't Believe It's Gluten-Free! 500 Delicious Foolproof Recipes for Healthy Living
by Robyn Ryberg
- ✦   Cost: $21.95   ISBN 978-1-56924-252-0   De Capo Press

Delicious Gluten-Free Wheat-Free Breads by LynnRae Ries and Bruce Gross
- ✦   Cost: $15.95/book $6.99/PDF   ISBN 0-972415-1-6   What No Wheat Publishing

Books can be ordered direct from:
> **What No Wheat Publishing,** 4757 E. Greenway Rd., Suite 107B, #9, Phoenix, AZ, USA 85032-8510
> Phone: 602-485-8751   www.whatnowheat.com

Gluten-Free Cooking For Dummies by Danna Korn and Connie Sarros
- ✦   Cost: $19.99   ISBN 978-0-470-17810-2   For Dummies

Together We're Better for Life: 25 Years & Growing – Gluten-Free Recipes from the Canadian Celiac Association
- ✦   Cost: $10.00   Canadian Celiac Association

Books can be ordered direct from:
> **Canadian Celiac Association,** 5025 Orbitor Drive, Bldg. 1, Suite 400, Mississauga, ON, Canada L4W 4Y5
> Phone: 800-363-7296 or 905-507-6208   www.celiac.ca

Sharing Our Best! A Collection of Recipes by The West End Gluten Intolerance Group
- ✦   Cost: $7.95
Books can be ordered direct from: **TWEGIG**, 10900 Brunson Way, Glen Allen, VA, USA 23060

Incredible Edible Gluten-Free Foods for Kids (see page 355).

Cooking Resources: Miscellaneous

Glutenfreeda.com, Glutenfreeda Foods, Inc.
- ✦   Free on-line gluten-free cooking magazine. Over 5000 gluten-free recipes, as well as articles and seasonal features, gluten-free product testing and menus. Recipe search capability by main ingredient, category or title. On-line cooking classes. *Good For You* column by Shelley Case, R.D.
- ✦   Glutenfreeda, Inc, P.O. Box 487, Burlington, WA, USA 98233
  Phone: 306-755-1300

Gluten-Free Baking and More
- ✦   Free monthly print newsletter dedicated to gluten-free baking and cooking. Founded by Elizabeth Barbone, graduate of the Culinary Institute of America.
- ✦   Members-only resource features hundreds of tested recipes, product reviews, advice and opinions from GF experts, menu ideas and suggestions, substitutions, cooking and baking video, podcasts and other information. By Subscription only for $34.95 per year ($29.99 renewal) or $8.95 per month. Payment in U.S. funds.
- ✦   Gluten-Free Baking and More, P.O. Box 94, Cropseyville, NY, USA 12052
  Phone: 518-279-3884   www.glutenfreebaking.com

Carol Fenster's Downloadable PDF Booklets
✦ *Gluten-free Baking Tips and Techniques from My Kitchen to Yours*
✦ *Dairy-Free & Delicious: Tips for Using Non-Dairy Alternatives in Cooking*
✦ *Egg-Free and Excellent: Cracking the Case for Successful Baking Without Eggs*
   Note: Each booklet is $6.95 and available from **Savory Palate, Inc.** (see page 355).

GFreeCuisine.com
✦ Online gluten-free menu planning service.
✦ Choose dinners and side dishes with minimal preparation time from a list of new gluten-free recipes once a week. Includes a categorized grocery list identifying gluten-free brand names and recipes developed by GF culinary expert Carol Fenster.
✦ Cost: $30 for 3 months; discounts for longer subscriptions.
   Phone: 877-606-6264/303-679-3048   Email: info@gfreecuisine.com

Gluten-Free Customized Menus and Recipes (Downloadable Format)
✦ Ten days of menus with 75-80 recipes for various special diets such as GF diabetics, GF low fat/low carb and others developed by Connie Sarros.
✦ Cost: $10.95; available from **Gluten-Free Cookbooks** (see page 349).

Alternative Cook™ Instructional Cooking DVD's
✦ Gluten-free, dairy-free, low cholesterol cooking instructions featuring six meals, how to use alternative ingredients, cooking tips and recipe booklet included.
✦ Four different DVD's: Italian (75 min.), Mexican (75 min.), Kids' Meals (75 min.) and Chocolate (45 min.) Features culinary expert, Jean Duane who has celiac disease and other food sensitivities.
✦ Cost: $24.95 per video available from **Alternative Cook, LLC** (see page 350).

All You Wanted to Know About Gluten-Free Cooking
✦ DVD (72 minutes) featuring Connie Sarros, gluten-free cookbook author, that discusses all aspects of cooking gluten-free, including conversions about wheat recipes, recipe tips and trouble-shooting and healthy-eating guidelines.
✦ Cost: $18.95 plus shipping, available from **Gluten-Free Cookbooks** (see page 349).

Cooking Gluten-Free! A Food Lover's Collection of Chef and Family Recipes Without Gluten or Wheat (CD-Rom)
✦ Digital cookbook on CD-Rom by Karen Robertson features a wide variety of recipes (many from celebrity chefs).
✦ Cost: $14.99 (U.S.); $16.99 (CDN)
✦ Available from: Celiac Publishing, P.O. Box 99605, Seattle, WA, USA 98139
   www.cookingglutenfree.com

GF Culinary Productions, Inc.
✦ Company that specializes in presenting gluten-free culinary educational events for the public including *The Gluten-Free Culinary Summit*™, *The Art & Science of Gluten-free Gastronomy Lecture Series*™ and *The GF Baking Invitational*™. Events feature culinary institute chef-instructors, restaurant chefs, cookbook authors and industry experts.
✦ Suzanne Bowland, President/Producer, 3065 South Xenia Street, Denver, CO, USA 80231
   Phone: 303-368-9990   www.theglutenfreelifestyle.com   Email: info@prchefs.com

Shopping, Travel and Eating-Out Resources

BeFreeForMe.com

✦ Free web site for consumers with gluten intolerance or food allergies that offers coupons, savings and samples. Also includes product reviews, articles, extensive database of recipes and the "AskBeFreeForMe" column by Shelley Case, RD.

Triumph Dining Resources

Offer a variety of resources that focus on safe gluten-free shopping, travel and dining. Also have a free on-line newsletter.

✦ *The Essential Gluten-Free Grocery Guide* (4th Edition)
30,000 gluten-free products listed, including over 1,000 name brands and store brands. Full color and portable (6 x 9 inches).
Cost: $24.95 (U.S.); ISBN 978-0-9776111-8-8

✦ *The Essential Gluten-Free Restaurant Guide* (5th Edition)
460-page book featuring over 6,500 restaurant locations across the 50 American States recommended by individuals with celiac disease, more than 120 gluten-free lists from chain restaurants and strategies for safely eating out.
Cost: $24.95 (U.S.); ISBN 978-09776111-6-4

✦ *Dining Cards*
Laminated, foldable wallet-sized cards for ten different cuisines (American, Chinese, French, Greek, Indian, Italian, Japanese, Mexican, Thai and Vietnamese). Each cuisine includes three statements: 1) "I cannot eat", 2) "Please check" and 3) "I can eat". One side of card is in English and the other side in the foreign language.
Cost: $2.50/card or $20.95 for ten cards.

Triumph Dining, 124 E. Broad St., 2nd floor, Falls Church, VA, USA 22046
Phone: 800-558-2906   www.triumphdining.com

Gluten-Free Passport Resources

Offer a variety of resources that focus on safe gluten-free dining and travel. Also have an informative website at www.glutenfreepassport.com

✦ *Let's Eat Out with Celiac/Coeliac and Food Allergies! (Enhanced Edition)*
325-page full-color book by Kim Koeller and Robert LaFrance. Details hundreds of menu item choices from 7 international restaurant cuisines for those with gluten/wheat intolerances and allergies to dairy, eggs, fish, shellfish, peanuts, tree nuts, soy and corn. Showcases ingredients, food preparation, cross-contamination, airlines and travel checklists for safe eating everywhere.
Available in print and electronic formats such as ebooks for PCs and smartphones.
Cost: $26.95 (U.S.); ISBN 978-0-9764845-5-4

✦ *Multi-Lingual Food Allergen Phrase Passport:* **Part of the** *Let's Eat Out!* **Series**
Pocket-size guide provides over 1200 phrase translations from English to French, German, Italian and Spanish. Detailing gluten and other food concerns, all phrases translated by professional language services and quality tested by native speakers. Available in print and electronic formats such as ebooks for PCs and smartphones.
Cost: $9.95 (U.S.); ISBN 978-0-9764845-4-7

✦ *Gluten-Free Cuisine Passports:* **Part of the** *Let's Eat Out!* **Series**
Restaurant menu choices from the *Let's Eat Out!* book packaged into 3 pocket-sized guides for easy reference: 1) American Steak & Mexican; 2) Chinese, Indian & Thai; 3) French & Italian Cuisine Passport. Available in print and electronic formats such as ebooks for PCs and smartphones.
Cost for each guide: $6.95 (U.S.) ISBNs 0-9764845-1-X; 0-9764845-3-6; 0-9764845-2-8

✦ ***iPhone/iPad/iPod Touch Applications: iEatOut and iCanEat OnTheGo Gluten & Allergen Free***
Two innovative apps dynamically customize safe meal choices based on gluten, wheat and other food allergens. Reflecting over 300 pages from the *Let's Eat Out!* book, *iEatOut*™ empowers users with knowledge about international cuisines, dishes and ingredients for safe restaurant dining. *iCanEat OnTheGo*™ offers thousands of US fast food menu options and pinpoints what is safe to eat by hiding specific allergen containing items.
Cost through Apple App Store: *iEatOut* - $4.99 (U.S.) and *iCanEat* - $2.99 (U.S.)

✦ ***Gluten-Free Dining by International Restaurant Cuisines*: Part of the *Let's Eat Out!* Series**
1. Sample restaurant menu items, descriptions and questions to ask restaurant staff from the Let's Eat Out! series packaged into individual eBooks for easy reference: 1) Steak & Seafood 2) French 3) Indian 4) Italian 5) Mexican 6) Thai Restaurant Cuisine. Available in electronic format for any smartphone, eReader, tablet and PC
2. Cost for each restaurant cuisine : $2.99 (U.S.) eISBNs: 978-0-9829599-4-7, 978-0-9830577-0-3, 978-0-9829599-3-0, 978-0-9829599-7-8 and 978-0-9829599-5-4
GlutenFree Passport, 27 North Wacker Drive, Suite 258, Chicago, IL, USA 60606
Phone: 312-952-4900   www.glutenfreepassport.com

Bob & Ruth's Gluten-Free Dining & Travel Club
✦ A company specializing in assisting individuals on a gluten-free diet and/or their families with dining out and traveling.
✦ Quarterly newsletter featuring dining out and traveling tips, review of North American restaurant chain menus, recipes, member dining-out and travel experiences and upcoming travel opportunities.
✦ Going Out to Eat & Traveling Gluten-Free workshops
✦ Escorted "Gluten-Free Getaways" – mini (2-3 nights), destination resorts, cruises and tours of exotic places all over the world.
✦ Annual membership fee $40 (U.S.).
Bob & Ruth's, 205 Donerial Court, Havre de Grace, MD, USA 21078
Phone: 410-939-3218   www.bobandruths.com

TheCeliacScene.com
✦ Canada's only comprehensive listing of celiac-endorsed restaurants. Owned, operated and maintained by individuals with celiac disease in cooperation with Chapters of the Canadian Celiac Association. All recommendations are reviewed and must meet specific standards to be listed. Free maps plus links to celiac-friendly fast-food chains across North America.   www.theceliacscene.com

Gluten-Free Restaurant Awareness Program™ (GFRAP)
✦ Program of the Gluten Intolerance Group of North America (GIG) that facilitates a relationship between restaurants and individuals with celiac disease and gluten intolerance.
✦ GFRAP representatives meet with the restaurant to present the program, explain gluten-free diet preparation and provide educational and training materials. Dietitians with expertise in the GF diet review the menus, recipes and ingredients for the restaurant. The restaurant can choose one of three levels of participation: Basic, Advanced or Specialized. All three levels receive educational and training materials. The Basic level receives a review of the GF menu and assistance from a Resource Member and Dietitian; Advanced and Specialized levels receive intensive assistance in menu review by qualified nutrition experts. Specific guidelines must be met in order to be listed on the website and use the GFRAP logo.
✦ Consumers can search participating restaurants in North America by restaurant name or city and/or type of cuisine.   www.glutenfreerestaurants.org

Glutenfreeonthego.com
✦ Free on-line global directory of over 6,000 gluten-free listings of restaurants, bakeries, hotels, resorts, spas, cruises and more. Recommendations submitted by individuals (with celiac disease and others following a gluten-free diet) and gluten-free eating establishments.

Chicken Paradise Bed & Breakfast, 606 Jackson Keller Road, San Antonio, TX, USA 78216
Phone: 210-340-0648   FAX: 210-366-3920
Email: annebarfield@satx.rr.com   www.chickenparadise.com
✦ Suite with all amenities including a small kitchen and outdoor pool. Breakfast prepared in a totally gluten-free kitchen; also can accommodate other food allergies and intolerances.
✦ Owner has celiac disease.

Children's Resources

Raising Your Celiac Child: Guidelines for a Gluten-Free Life DVD
✦ 2 hour DVD by Children's Hospital Boston designed to help both families and clinicians learn more about managing celiac disease. Includes 12 different interactive modules with practical advice on celiac disease, lifestyle management and emotional support.
✦ Cost: $29.95   www.childrenshospital.org/celiac
Phone: 617-355-2127   Email: celiacsupportgroup@childrens.harvard.edu

Kids with Celiac Disease: A Family Guide to Raising Happy, Healthy, Gluten-Free Children
✦ 256-page book by Danna Korn. Provides parents with advice and specific strategies on how to deal with the diagnosis, cope with emotional challenges, and help their child develop a positive attitude. Practical information on menu planning, shopping, food preparation, recipes and eating outside the home (e.g., birthdays, restaurants, camps, vacations).
✦ Cost: $17.95 (U.S.); ISBN 1-89062-72-16
Woodbine House, 6510 Bells Mill Rd., Bethesda, MD, USA 20817
Phone: 800-843-7323   www.woodbinehouse.com   www.glutenfreedom.net

Gluten-Free Friends: An Activity Book for Kids
✦ 57-page illustrated book by registered dietitian Nancy Patin Falini. Designed for children age 4-11. The book features two friendly kids who explain what gluten is, describe how gluten makes them sick and which foods to avoid, and how to make healthy food choices. Easy-to-follow instructions for parents and caregivers to help them guide children through learning activities and explore their thoughts and feelings about living gluten-free.
✦ Cost: $18.95 (U.S.); ISBN 1-889374-09-1
Savory Palate Inc., 8174 S. Holly – PMB #404, Littleton, CO, USA 80122-4004
Phone: 800-741-5418   www.savorypalate.com

No More Cupcakes & Tummy Aches: A Story for Parents and Their Celiac Children to Share
✦ Illustrated book for children ages 3-8 by Jax Peters Lowell. A story of a little girl who learns about living gluten-free and being loved and feeling truly special.
✦ Cost: $22.99 (hard cover); ISBN 1-4134-6255-3
$16.99 (soft cover); ISBN 1-4134-6254-5
Xlibris Publisher   Phone: 888-795-4274/610-915-5214   www2.xlibris.com

How I Eat Without Wheat
✦ 28-page illustrated picture book for toddlers and young children who must follow a diet eliminating gluten and wheat. A story about "a boy who takes a positive approach to his change in diet and restores his health".
✦ Written by Karen Fine, mother of a child with celiac disease.
✦ Cost: $14.95 (U.S.); ISBN 978-1-4259-7570-8
AuthorHouse   Phone: 888-519-5121   www.authorhouse.com

Eating Gluten-Free with Emily: A Story for Children with Celiac Disease
- ✦ Illustrated book for young children by Bonnie J. Kruszka. A story about a 5-year old girl who develops celiac disease and how she makes positive lifestyle changes to manage her disease.
- ✦ Cost: $13.99; ISBN 978-1-4392-1226-4

Incredible Edible Gluten-Free Foods for Kids
- ✦ Cookbook for Kids written by Sheri L. Sanderson. Includes 150 family-tested recipes, general food preparation tips, baking substitutes, as well as an overview of celiac disease and the gluten-free diet, tips for dealing with daycares and schools, and resources.
- ✦ Cost: $19.95 (U.S.); ISBN 978-1-890627-28-7
  Woodbine House, 6510 Bells Mill Rd., Bethesda, MD, USA 20817.
  Phone: 800-843-7323   www.woodbinehouse.com

R.O.C.K. (Raising Our Celiac Kids)
- ✦ Free support group for parents, families and friends of children on a gluten-free diet. Over 100 chapters in the USA and several in Canada. Founded by Danna Korn, mother of a child with celiac disease.
- ✦ www.celiackids.com   Email: rock@celiackids.com

U.S. National School Lunch Program and Celiac Disease
- ✦ Background information and practical guidelines for families navigating the school setting including model and sample 504 Plans, Physician Statements for Students with Special Dietary Needs, State information and sample GF school menu. See www.americanceliac.org

Allergy Resources

Food Allergy Survival Guide: Surviving and Thriving with Food Allergies and Sensitivities
- ✦ 384-page book by registered dietitians Vesanto Melina, Jo Stepaniak and Dina Aronson. Comprehensive resource on food sensitivities and other conditions (e.g., arthritis, asthma, ADHD, Candida, depression, dermatitis, digestive disorders including celiac disease, fatigue, headaches), diagnostic testing, nutritional concerns for various allergies, label reading and substitutions, meal planning, cooking tips, over 100 recipes (free of gluten, dairy, eggs, fish, shellfish, peanuts, tree nuts, soy, yeast and kiwi) with nutritional analysis and resources.
- ✦ Cost: $19.95 (U.S.), $29.95 (CDN); ISBN 1-57067-163-X
  Healthy Living Publications, Box 99, Summertown, TN, USA 38483
  Phone 888-260-8458   www.foodallergysurvivalguide.com

Allergic Living magazine
- ✦ Quarterly magazine for people with food and environmental allergies and intolerances, as well as celiac disease. Includes articles, recipes, product information and "Ask The Expert" columns (Allergist, Celiac, Dermatologist, Dietitian). Magazine editor has food allergies.
- ✦ Website includes a wide variety of information and a special section on celiac disease, the gluten-free diet and gluten-free recipes. The "Ask The Celiac Expert" column is written by Shelley Case, RD.
- ✦ Subscription rates: Canada $17.69 plus GST (1 year); $26.54 plus GST (2 years)
                  USA $19.99 (U.S. funds) for 1 year, $29.99 (U.S. funds) for 2 years
                  (includes postage)
  Allergic Living, 2100 Bloor St. West, Suite 6-168, Toronto, ON, Canada M6S 5A5
  Phone: 888-771-7747/416-604-0110   www.allergicliving.com

Living Without magazine (see page 347)

Let's Eat Out! with Celiac/Coeliac and Food Allergies! (Enhanced Edition) (see page 352)

Diabetes and Celiac Disease Resources

Managing Diabetes and Celiac Disease … Together
+ 50-page booklet that includes an overview of diabetes and celiac disease, meal planning, carbohydrate content of gluten-free flours and recipes with nutritional analysis.
+ Published by the Canadian Celiac Association (CCA) and Canadian Diabetes Association (CDA).
+ Cost: $11.95 (CDN) members; $13.95 (CDN) non-members
  Canadian Celiac Association, 5170 Dixie Road, Suite 204, Mississauga, ON, Canada L4W 1E3
  Phone: 800-363-7296 or 905-507-6208   www.celiac.ca

Diabetes, Celiac Disease and Me! An Introduction to Living with Both Diseases
+ 37-page booklet that includes an overview of diabetes and celiac disease, sample menus, carbohydrate content of selected gluten-free foods and ingredients, and resources.
+ Published by the Gluten Intolerance Group (GIG) and Houston Celiac Disease Support Group.
+ Available in a free "pdf" that can be downloaded from www.gluten.net or www.houstonceliacs.org. Hard copy available for $10 from GIG (see page 349).

Counting Gluten-Free Carbohydrates: A Dietitian Resource for Counseling Individuals with Diabetes and Celiac Disease
+ 142 page online resource written by dietitians Tricia Thompson and Suzanne Simpson. Includes the American Dietetic Association's evidence-based practice guidelines for celiac disease and Type 1 diabetes, as well as an extensive alphabetical list of gluten-free manufacturers and products. The grams of carbohydrate, sugar, fiber, protein and fat are provided for each product. Lists gluten-free cookbooks that provide nutrition information for recipes.
+ Free downloadable PDF available from: www.glutenfreedietitian.com/registration.php?id = cgfc

Pharmaceutical Resources

Clan Thompson Celiac SmartList of Drugs for Palm OS Handhelds, Pocket PC's, Windows Mobile, Blackberry Smartphones, Windows or Macs (see page 348)

Glutenfreedrugs.com
+ On-line resource containing information about over-the-counter and prescription medications listed by therapeutic category or alphabetical product name.
+ Site developed and managed by Dr. Steve Plogsted, PharmD, Nutrition Support Services, Children's Hospital, Columbus, Ohio

Gluten-Free/Celiac Disease Novelty Items

The Silly Yak Shirt Company   181 Lorraine Gate, East Meadow, NY, USA 11554
                                        www.silly-yak.com
+ T-shirts, hats and tote bags with various slogans about celiac disease and gluten-free to raise awareness of celiac disease.
+ Portion of sales goes to the Celiac Disease Center at Columbia University.

Gluten-Free Mall   www.glutenfreemall.com
+ "Gluten-Busters" celiac disease awareness T-shirts.

INDEX

ORDER FORM

GLUTEN-FREE DIET *A Comprehensive Resource Guide*

Number of copies _____ x $26.95 U.S. = $ _____

Number of copies _____ x $26.95 CDN = $ _____

Shipping and handling (see below) = $ _____

Subtotal = $ _____

In Canada add GST (5%) = $ _____
GST# 867639122

Total enclosed = $ _____

Shipping and Handling

	USA	CANADA
1 Book	$5.00	$6.00
2-3 Books	$4.00 per book	$5.00 per book
4 or more Books	contact Case Nutrition Consulting, Inc.	

✦ Please allow 1-3 weeks for delivery. Books shipped by USPS or Canada Post.
✦ Payment Methods: Check (payable to Case Nutrition Consulting, Inc.)
   Credit Card (Visa or MasterCard)
✦ U.S. orders payable in U.S. funds.

NAME: _____

ORGANIZATION: _____

STREET: _____

CITY: _____ STATE/PROV.: _____

COUNTRY: _____ ZIP/POSTALCODE: _____

PHONE: _____ FAX: _____

Email: _____
We do not rent, lease or share our mailing list.

Credit Card Orders: ___Visa ___MasterCard   Expiry: _____/_____

Card Number: _____

Name on Card: _____

Signature: _____

Mail to: **CASE NUTRITION CONSULTING, INC.**,
   1940 Angley Court,   Online Ordering: www.glutenfreediet.ca
   Regina, Saskatchewan,   Email: info@glutenfreediet.ca
   Canada S4V 2V2   Phone/FAX: 306-751-1000